Aspects of cardiovascular nursing

BJN Monograph

edited by
*Jeremy Pope Cruickshank, Martyn Bradbury
and Steve Ashurst*

Quay
Books

Mark Allen
Publishing Ltd

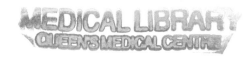

Quay Books Division, Mark Allen Publishing Limited, Jesses Farm, Snow Hill, Dinton, Nr Salisbury, Wiltshire SP3 5HN

© Mark Allen Publishing Group 2000   1003395810

A British Library Cataloguing-in-Publication Data
A catalogue record for this book is available from the British Library

ISBN 1 85642 172 4

Printed in the UK by The Cromwell Press Ltd, Trowbridge, Wiltshire, UK

1
Contents

About the editors

Jeremy Pope Cruickshank

A direct descendent of Florence Nightingale and with over 20 years experience in nursing, Jeremy Pope Cruickshank MSc (Notts), BN (Hons), RGN, PGCE (FE), CMS, Dip PE is currently a Nurse Teacher at the University of Nottingham, where he teaches on the Diploma in Nursing course and participates in the delivery of a variety of post-registration courses. A graduate of the Universities of Wales and Nottingham, he specialises in the acute areas of adult branch nursing. He has travelled to China, Australia and the United States to witness first-hand the cultural differences in healthcare provision. His clinical background is in areas of high dependency/critical care and emergency nursing. Among his professional interests, he is a member of the editorial board of the *British Journal of Nursing* and a member of the commissioning board of Quay Books.

Martyn Bradbury RGN, BSc, MSc, Cert Ed

Following qualification in 1980 he completed an intensive care and cardiac care course at the Royal Sussex County Hospital, Brighton. Later, he was Charge Nurse in acute medicine and then Clinical Supervisor for ITU/CCU and medicine at East Surrey Hospital, Redhill. He was awarded a BSc in Nursing Studies at Brighton Polytechnic in 1987 and a MSc in Health Care from Exeter University in 1995. He is currently employed as a Senior Lecturer within the Institute of Health Studies, Plymouth University, where his responsibilities include teaching 'Applied nursing skills'. He retains a clinical interest in cardiac medicine and engages in practice within the cardiac unit at Torbay Hospital, Torquay.

Steve Ashurst

Having been educated at Wigan Grammar School he graduated with a first class honours degree in Biochemistry from the University of Salford (1977). He was awarded a PhD in Biochemical Pharmacology at the University of Surrey in 1980. Following postdoctoral research at the University of Tennessee and the Wistar Institute in Philadelphia, USA, he commenced nurse training at the Nightingale School, St Thomas's Hospital, London and qualified in 1984. He moved to the Intensive Care Unit in Wrexham in 1985. He is presently nursing 35 hours a week on the Critical Care Unit, incorporating ITU, coronary care, surgical high dependency care and medical high dependency care. He also teaches pharmacology, microbiology, pathology and physiology to several groups of pre- and post-registration nurses and is involved with teaching on several post-registration courses, including respiratory care, diabetes, infection control, critical and intensive care. He is a member of the Nursing Practice Group in Wrexham and a member of the commissioning board of Quay Books.

List of contributors

Renee Adomat is Lecturer in Nursing at the School of Health Sciences, The Medical School, University of Birmingham.

John W Albarran is Senior Lecturer in Critical Care at the Faculty of Health and Social Care, University of the West of England, Bristol.

Ricky Autar is Senior Lecturer in Biological Sciences and Nursing at De Montfort University, Leicester.

Maria Barrell is Head of Midwifery and Neonatal Care at the University of Northumbria, Newcastle upon Tyne.

Charlie Bloe is Senior Nurse for Coronary Care and Medical High Dependency at Falkirk and District Royal Infirmary NHS Trust, Scotland and a freelance lecturer for CB Nursing Updates, Bonnybridge, Scotland.

Martyn Bradbury is Senior Lecturer in Nursing at the University of Plymouth.

Neal F Cook is a Staff Nurse in Neurosurgery, at the Royal Victoria Hospital, Belfast, Northern Ireland.

Jeremy Pope Cruickshank is a Nurse Teacher in the undergraduate division of the Nursing School at the University of Nottingham, Lincolnshire.

Samantha Donohue is Team Leader in the Vascular Unit at the John Radcliffe Hospital, Oxford.

Denise Flisher is Cardiac Services Manager at Bedford Hospital NHS Trust, Bedford.

Janice Gabriel is Oncology Nurse Specialist/Manager at Portsmouth Oncology Centre, Portsmouth NHS Trust, Portsmouth.

Dorothy Gourlay is Senior Staff Nurse at the Western General Hospital NHS Trust, Edinburgh, Scotland.

Chris Higgins is a freelance medical writer from Milborne St Andrew, Dorset.

David Jenkins is Continuing Education Officer at the Head of Nursing Education Office, School of Nursing Studies, Keogh Barracks, Aldershot, Hampshire.

Heather Kapeluch is Business Manager at North Bristol NHS Trust, Frenchay Hospital, Bristol.

Vidar Melby is Lecturer in Nursing at the University of Ulster, Coleraine, Northern Ireland.

Sara Nelson is Cardiac Clinical Case Manager at Bromley Hospital NHS Trust, Bromley, Kent.

Mike Nolan is Director of Research and Professor of Gerontological Nursing at the School of Nursing and Midwifery, University of Sheffield.

Jane Nolan is a Lecturer in the School of Nursing and Midwifery, University of Sheffield.

Karen Noy is Sister in the Cardiac Suite at Kettering General Hospital NHS Trust, Kettering.

David O'Brien is Head of Adult Nursing at the University of Northumbria, Newcastle upon Tyne.

Sue Palmer is District Nurse, Highworth, Wiltshire.

Helen Rogers is Nursing Officer in the Intensive Care Unit, Cambridge Military Hospital, Aldershot.

Terry Shipperley is Clinical Nurse Specialist for physical health at South Downs Health NHS Trust, Brighton.

Carol Wasling is Cardiology/Chief Dietitian in the Department of Nutrition and Dietetics at Bishop Auckland General Hospital, County Durham.

Lynne Marie Whitaker is a Staff Nurse in the Medical Ward at Bassetlaw District General Hospital NHS Trust, Nottinghamshire.

Clare Williams is Nursing Officer in tissue viability, Wrexham Maelor Hospital NHS Trust, Wrexham, Wales.

Philip Woodrow is Senior Lecturer at Whittington Education Centre, Middlesex University, London.

Acknowledgements

I would like to thank my family, Simon, Sue, Oliver and Annabel, but most especially my parents to whom this book is dedicated for all their love, patience and support over the many years. Making you proud of me was my deepest desire. A special dedication to Mr Harry Seymour RGN, RNT in memoriam, a true mentor and friend. I miss your wisdom and guidance. Finally, to thank my fellow editors, Steve and in particular Martyn who over the years of our writing partnership has continued to give me tremendous support, confidence and friendship.

Jeremy P Cruickshank
February 2000

Introduction

Disease of the heart and circulatory system are the most significant cause of morbidity and mortality in western society and represent one of the greatest challenges facing today's healthcare services. While it is increasingly recognised that genetic aspects play an important part in the development of these diseases, many of the contributing factors remain lifestyle dependent and amenable to change through the effective use of education and health promotion (DOH, 1999).

Modern day clinical practice has witnessed a dramatic improvement in the pharmacological and surgical treatments available to manage cardiovascular conditions in recent years. In addition, media attention, especially relating to cardiac drug trials and risk factors, such as diet and smoking, has heightened public awareness and increased the level of knowledge, expectation and informed choice among many patient groups. The modern healthcare team has also had to adapt and change in response to these developments. In particular, nurses have a major and increasingly challenging role to play within the community and hospital setting in addressing all aspects of the prevention, treatment, management and rehabilitation of patients suffering from cardiovascular disease.

This monograph, which considers aspects of cardiovascular nursing, is a selection of peer reviewed articles which have been previously published in the *British Journal of Nursing* (BJN). Its focus, as the title implies, is the management and care required by patients considered to be at risk of, or suffering from, cardiovascular disease. Where appropriate, articles have been amended and updated to incorporate developments in clinical practice that have occurred since the original article was published.

For convenience the monograph has been divided into four sections that reflect the following spheres of practice:

- assessment and prevention in cardiovascular nursing
- nursing management of clients suffering from cardiovascular disorders
- essential psychological and rehabilitation elements in cardiovascular nursing
- developing nursing skills and effective practice in cardiovascular nursing.

This monograph does not set itself the task of presenting a definitive text on cardiovascular nursing. Instead, it seeks to illustrate some of the varied and exciting aspects of cardiovascular care. In so doing, it is hoped that this monograph will prove to be a valuable reference for all nurses and other healthcare personnel, who care for, or have an interest in caring for, patients with cardiovascular disease.

Jeremy Pope Cruickshank
Martyn Bradbury
Steve Ashurst
January, 2000

Reference

Department of Health (1999) *Saving Lives: Our Healthier Nation.* DOH The Stationary Office, London

Section one: Assessment and prevention in cardiovascular nursing

1

Haematology blood testing for anaemia

Chris Higgins

In recognition of the contribution that the clinical laboratory makes to the diagnosis and monitoring of disease, this chapter considers the clinical significance of some common tests performed in the haematology laboratory to investigate anaemia.

Haematology is the study of blood, specifically the cells that circulate in blood, ie. red blood cells (RBCs or erythrocytes), white blood cells (WBCs or leucocytes) and platelets (thrombocytes). There are five types of WBCs in peripheral blood: neutrophils, eosinophils, basophils, monocytes and lymphocytes. RBCs, WBCs and platelets all develop and mature from one cell (the stem cell) in the bone marrow. All blood cells have a limited life span and are constantly being replaced from developing cells in the bone marrow. The function and relationships of these cells are described in *Figure 1.1*.

Apart from the cells in blood, haematology is also concerned with the concentration in blood plasma of many specialised proteins which, in conjunction with platelets, are necessary for the coagulation of blood and therefore prevention of excessive bleeding.

Anaemia is one of many conditions in which haematological blood tests are required for diagnosis; investigation is centred chiefly on the RBC.

Anaemia

The principal function of the RBC is to carry oxygen from the lungs to the tissues and carbon dioxide from the tissues back to the lungs. This is achieved by the protein haemoglobin (Hb) contained in the RBC; each RBC contains around 640 million molecules of Hb. Anaemia is defined as a reduced concentration of Hb in blood (see *Table 1.1*).

The symptoms of anaemia, which are not normally evident until the Hb has dropped below 9–10g/dl, result from an inability to oxygenate tissues effectively and include tiredness, breathlessness on exertion, dizziness and palpitations. The mucous membranes, particularly of the eye, appear pale. The laboratory measurement of Hb confirms the diagnosis of anaemia but reveals nothing about its cause. Further laboratory testing is required.

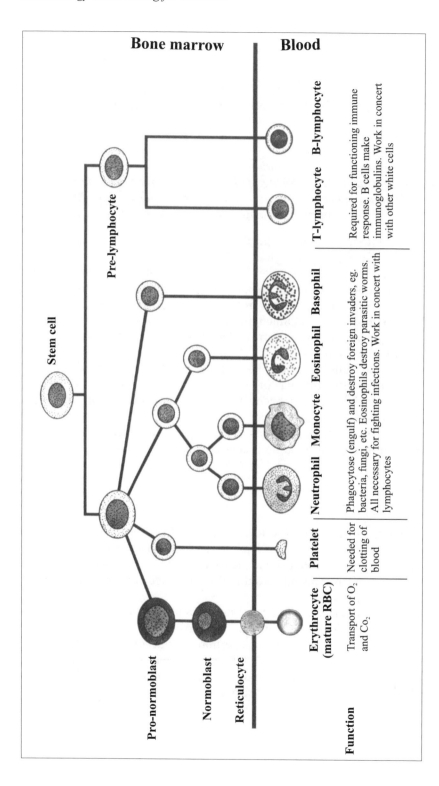

Figure 1.1: Development, relationship and function of blood-borne cells. O_2 = oxygen; CO_2 = carbon dioxide; RBC = red blood cells

Laboratory tests used in the differential diagnosis of anaemia

Table 1.1 lists the first-line laboratory tests used in the differential diagnosis of anaemia.

Until the early 1960s, all haematology tests were performed using manual techniques requiring considerable skill; the principal tool of the haematologist was the microscope, which was used for all blood cell counts. Technological developments over the past 30 years have revolutionised the performance of haematology blood tests. Typically, the modern haematology analyser can produce Hb, RBC and WBC count (including a differential WBC count), platelet count and RBC indices at the rate of 100 samples/hour. The process can be entirely automated, requiring only that samples be loaded onto the analyser. The volume of sample required is usually around 2 ml of venous blood which has been collected into a plastic tube containing anticoagulant to prevent clotting of the specimen. The anticoagulant normally used is potassium-ethylenediamine-tetracetic acid (KEDTA).

While Hb concentration, RBC count and RBC indices provide useful information for investigation of anaemia, further blood tests which are not performed on the routine haematology analyser are useful.

Microscopic examination of RBCs: This involves smearing a drop of blood onto a glass slide, and fixing and staining the specimen so that RBCs can be visualised microscopically. *Table 1.2* lists some of the terms used to describe the shape and staining characteristics of RBCs when viewed under the microscope.

Reticulocyte count: Reticulocytes are immature RBCs (*Figure 1.1*) and normally constitute only 0.5–2% of the RBC population in blood. A high reticulocyte count is a favourable sign since it indicates that the bone marrow is responding to the low Hb by increasing RBC production. The stimulus for RBC production comes from erythropoietin, a hormone which is made predominantly in the kidneys. Erythropoietin production increases as the oxygen content of kidney tissues falls. Anaemia is associated with low levels of oxygen in blood which in turn results in a low oxygen tension in kidney tissues. As the oxygen content of kidney tissues falls, the production of erythropoietin is increased and the hormone is released into the blood. A high blood concentration of erythropoietin stimulates the bone marrow to increase RBC production. This physiological response is described in *Figure 1.2*. (The central role of the kidney in RBC production accounts for the anaemia that usually accompanies chronic renal failure.)

A normal or low reticulocyte count in the blood of an anaemic patient indicates that the bone marrow cannot respond for one reason or another. Reticulocytes are counted from a specially stained blood smear under the microscope and the result expressed as a percentage of total RBC population.

Table 1.1: Laboratory tests used in the differential diagnosis of anaemia	
Hb concentration	Confirms a diagnosis of anaemia and indicates its severity (Hb less than around 6g/dl indicates severe anaemia)
RBC count	The number of RBCs per litre. Since all Hb is contained in RBCs, a low RBC count results in a low Hb and therefore anaemia
RBCs indices	A group of tests which reveal information about the size and Hb content of RBCs: • mean cell volume (MCV), ie. average size of cell • mean (red) cell haemoglobin content (MCH) • mean (red) cell haemoglobin concentration (MCHC)
Hb = haemoglobin; RBCs = red blood cells	

Table 1.2: Some of the more common terms used to describe the appearance of RBCs in a stained blood film	
Normocytic	Average size of cells appears normal
Microcytic	Average size of cells appears smaller than normal
Macrocytic	Average size of cells appears larger than normal
Anisocytic	Cells vary in size
Poikilocytic	Cells vary in shape
Normochromic	Cells stain normally (RBCs appear pink due to the presence of haemoglobin)
Hypochromic	Cells stain less deeply than normal (indicating low concentration of haemoglobin)
RBCs = red blood cells	

Measurement of constituents in serum/plasma: These are substances present in serum/plasma which are necessary for normal RBC or Hb production. Low levels are often associated with anaemia.

Plasma/serum concentration of iron: Iron is required for Hb production.

Plasma/serum concentration of ferritin: Ferritin is a protein in which iron is stored. Serum levels reflect iron stores.

Plasma/serum concentration of vitamin B_{12} and folate: These constituents are required for normal RBC production.

Serum iron concentration is measured by chemical methods, usually on an automated analyser. Ferritin, vitamin B_{12} and folate are, however, measured by a very sensitive and labour-intensive technique which involves the use of radioisotopes and is known as radioimmunoassay.

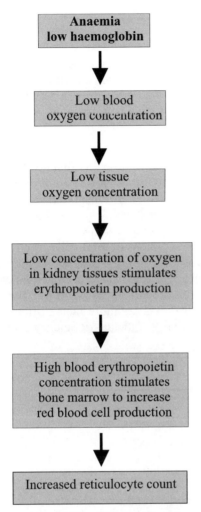

Figure 1.2: Physiological response to anaemia

Haemoglobin electrophoresis: As might be expected, abnormalities in the structure of Hb are often associated with anaemia. The haemo-globinopathies are a relatively rare group of diseases which have in common a congenital abnormality in the globin part of the Hb molecule. The most common of these are thalassaemia and sickle-cell anaemia. Hb electrophoresis is a technique which allows the separation of Hb molecules according to their electrical charge. Abnormal Hb can be separated and identified using this technique.

Bone marrow examination: Since RBCs (along with WBCs and platelets) are made and mature in the bone marrow, the search for a cause of anaemia may require examination of the bone marrow. This involves insertion of a special wide-bore needle into the sternum or iliac crest and aspiration of a small sample of bone marrow. This is then smeared onto a glass slide(s), stained and examined under the microscope. An alternative technique is trephine-biopsy in which a small core of bone is removed and processed histologically before microscopic examination.

Causes of anaemia

Apart from the anaemia associated with acute blood loss, anaemia is also caused by an inability to make sufficient normal Hb or normal numbers of normal RBCs. Occasionally, increased RBC destruction is the cause. Two of the most common causes of anaemia will now be considered, with a detailed description of how the laboratory tests described above are used to make a diagnosis.

Iron deficiency: a hypochromic microcytic anaemia

Iron deficiency is the commonest cause of anaemia worldwide. Hb, which is made in the developing RBCs, consists of four protein chains, each with its own haem group. A the centre of each haem group is an atom of iron; a deficiency of iron therefore results in an inability to make sufficient haemoglobin.

Iron metabolism

The distribution of iron in the body is described in *Figure 1.3*. Seventy-five per cent of the body's iron is held in RBCs. The RBC has a life span of around 120 days, after which it breaks down, releasing iron which is transported back to the iron stores. Normally only about 1 mg of iron per day is lost from the body in desquamating epithelial cells and around 16 mg/month (1.5 mg/day) is lost in menstrual blood loss. This represents less than 0.01% of total body iron. It has been calculated that, if maintained on an iron-free diet, it would take eight years for an adult male and three years for a menstruating female to become clinically iron deficient. In fact, the normal diet contains around 10–15 mg of iron per day and only 5–10% of this is normally absorbed. This is more than sufficient to replace daily physiological losses. For these reasons, dietary deficiency is rarely the sole cause of iron deficiency.

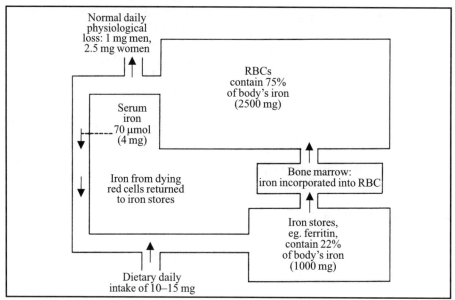

Figure 1.3: Distribution of body iron. RBC = red blood cell

The most common cause of iron deficiency is chronic blood loss, ie. the continuous loss of small amounts of blood over a prolonged period; 500 ml of blood contains 250 mg of iron and unrecognised gastrointestinal bleeding or heavy menstrual blood loss can soon deplete iron strores. Pregnancy is associated with increased blood production and therefore increased demand for iron; this, along with blood loss at delivery, leaves pregnant women particularly vulnerable to iron deficiency.

Laboratory findings (*Table 1.3*)

Iron deficiency results in an inability to produce normal amounts of Hb. Each RBC contains less Hb than normal and is therefore much smaller; these changes are reflected in the RBC indices; MCV, MCH and MCHC are all reduced. Microscopic examination of RBCs reveal hypochromic, microcytic cells.

The reticulocyte count is normal, indicating that the marrow is not responding to the anaemia (it cannot make more red cells in the absence of iron). The concentration of ferritin in plasma is always very low (frequently below the detection limits of current methods), indicating that iron stores are depleted and the plasma concentration of iron is reduced. Although examination of bone marrow is rarely necessary in uncomplicated iron deficiency, microscopic examination of marrow stained with chemicals which react only with iron reveal an absence of iron stores. Finally, investigation of iron deficiency anaemia is not complete until the cause of blood loss has been established.

The laboratory can help if gastrointestinal bleeding is suspected. Very small amounts of blood can be detected in the faeces by the occult blood test which is usually performed in the clinical chemistry laboratory. A positive occult blood implies blood loss from any point in the gastrointestinal tract. Some methods are sensitive enough to detect the blood derived from ingested meat; if these methods are being used it is wise to re-check a positive result from the patient on a meat-restricted diet.

Vitamin B$_{12}$ and folate deficiency: a megaloblastic anaemia

Function of vitamin B$_{12}$ and folate

Vitamin B$_{12}$ and folate are both necessary for the production of DNA, the genetic material held in the nucleus of cells. Although the mature RBCs present in blood do not contain a nucleus, they are derived from immature RBCs in the bone marrow which are nucleated and contain DNA (*Figure 1.1*). The process of maturation of RBCs is characterised by an overall decrease in size of the cell and decreasing amounts of nucleic material. A deficiency of vitamin B$_{12}$ and folate results in abnormal early development of RBCs; the total number of RBCs is reduced and there is a high proportion of immature large RBCs, called megaloblasts, in the bone marrow. The average size of RBCs in peripheral blood is also greater than normal.

Table 1.3: Haematology test results in two different causes of anaemia			
Blood test	**Normal range***	**Anaemia due to iron deficiency**	**Anaemia due to vitamin B$_{12}$/ folate deficiency**
Hb concentration	Male 13.5–17.5 g/dl Female 11.5–15.5 g/dl	Always low, actual concentration reflects severity of anaemia	Always low, actual concentration reflects severity of anaemia
RBC count	Male 4.5–6.5 x 10^{12}/litre Female 3.9–5.6 x 10^{12}/litre	Usually slightly low	Marked reduction, may be as low as 2.0 x 10^{12}/litre
RBC indices: MCV MCHO MCH	80–95 fl 20–35 g/dl 27–34 pg	Reduced Reduced Reduced	Increased Normal Normal
Reticulocyte count	0.5–2.0%	Normal or low	Normal or low
Appearance of RBCs in blood film	Normochromic Normocytic	Microcytic Hypochromic	Macrocytic Normochromic
Serum iron concentration	20–23 µmol/litre	Reduced, often <5µmol/litre	Normal
Serum ferritin concentration	Male 40–340 µg/litre Female 14–150 µtre	Reduced, often <5µg/litre	Normal
Serum vitamin B$_{12}$ concentration Red cell folate concentration	160–925 ng/litre 160–640 ug/litre	Normal Normal	Reduced in vitamin B$_{12}$ deficiency Reduced in folate deficiency
*Normal ranges approximate; consult local laboratory for local normal range. Hb = haemoglobin; MCH = mean cell haemoglobin (weight)			
MCHC = mean cell haemoglobin concentration; MCV = mean cell volume; RBC = red blood cell			

Causes of vitamin B$_{12}$ and folate deficiencies

A deficiency of vitamin B$_{12}$ may result from dietary deficiency or from an inability to absorb the vitamin. We obtain most of our dietary vitamin B$_{12}$ from meat, so that a dietary deficiency is rare except in strict vegetarians, most notably vegans (most Hindu Indians are vegans). Inability to absorb vitamin B$_{12}$ is much more common than a dietary deficiency.

The absorption of vitamin B$_{12}$ takes place in the small intestine and is dependent on the presence of a substance called intrinsic factor which is made in particular cells in the gastric glands deep in the stomach wall. Pernicious anaemia is a condition in which autoimmune damage to these cells results in a deficiency of intrinsic factor and therefore reduced vitamin B$_{12}$ absorption. Lack of intrinsic factor is also the cause of vitamin B$_{12}$ deficiency which can occur after surgical resection of the stomach.

Dietary folate is largely derived from liver and green vegetables and can be easily destroyed in cooking. Folate deficiency occurring alone is usually a result of insufficient folate in the diet.

Laboratory findings (*Table 1.3*)

Whatever the cause, vitamin B_{12} or folate deficiency is associated with normal Hb production (in contrast to iron deficiency anaemia) but with abnormal RBC production. The total RBC count is reduced, so that although each cell contains normal amounts of Hb reflected in a normal MCHC and MCH, the total amount of Hb is reduced. The RBCs are much larger than normal, resulting in a raised MCV. Examination of a blood film reveals large RBCs, often oval in shape, which are well haemoglobinised. Bone marrow examination reveals a higher than normal proportion of large immature RBCs (megaloblasts). The reticulocyte count is normal, indicating inadequate marrow response to the anaemia.

To establish that the cause of all these abnormalities is a deficiency of vitamin B_{12} or folate it is necessary to measure their concentration in plasma; low results indicate a deficiency. The concentration of folate in RBCs is considered a better reflection of folate reserves than serum folate concentration. Once a deficiency is established, the cause must be sought. It may be a dietary deficiency or inability to absorb because of either intestinal disease or a lack of intrinsic factor. The Schilling test is used to establish the cause of a proven vitamin B_{12} deficiency.

Principle of the Schilling test: Radioactively labelled vitamin B_{12} is given orally and the amount of radioactivity appearing in the urine is measured. If the vitamin B_{12} is not absorbed it simply passes through the gut and is excreted in the faeces. In a dietary deficiency, vitamin B_{12} is absorbed, resulting in a relatively high radioactive count in the urine. Conversely, poor absorption is associated with a relatively low radioactive count in the urine. Patients who demonstrate poor absorption proceed to stage two of the test in which a second dose of labelled vitamin B_{12} is given orally, but with intrinsic factor being administered at the same time.

Patients with pernicious anaemia (lack of intrinsic factor) can now absorb the radioactively labelled vitamin B_{12} and will have a high level of radioactivity in the urine. Those with poor absorption due to intestinal disease will continue to have low levels of radioactivity in urine.

Other causes of anaemia

Iron deficiency and vitamin B_{12} or folate deficiency are by far the commonest causes of anaemia but there are many others. Haemolytic anaemias are a group of conditions in which anaemia is caused by increased RBC destruction. Incompatible blood transfusion results in immune destruction of RBCs. The abnormal Hb (HbS) is the cause of RBC destruction in those with sickle-cell anaemia.

Finally, anaemia is associated with any condition in which bone marrow activity is depressed. Aplastic anaemia is a serious condition in which bone marrow stem cell (*Figure 1.1*) development is depressed which results in very low production of not only RBCs but also WBCs and platelets. Some leukaemias are also associated with severe anaemia as a result of bone marrow depression. The blood tests performed in the haematology laboratory provide vital information for the diagnosis of all these conditions.

Key points

* A reduction in the concentration of haemoglobin (Hb), the oxygen-carrying pigment found in red blood cells (RBCs), confirms the presence of anaemia.
* Haematology tests are necessary to elucidate the cause of anaemia; these tests are chiefly centred on the RBC but include the measurement of substances present in blood which are necessary for RBC production and development.
* Iron is required for Hb production and iron deficiency is the commonest cause of anaemia. Iron deficient RBCs are typically smaller than normal and appear less well stained when looked at under the microscope. A low mean cell volume (MCV) and mean cell haemoglobin concentration (MCHC) reflect these changes.
* Iron deficiency may be due to lack of iron intake but more commonly it is the result of iron loss from the body.
* Anaemia may be caused by a deficiency of vitamin B_{12} and folate which are necessary for normal RBC production.
* The anaemia of vitamin B_{12} and folate deficiency results in large immature (megaloblastic) RBCs. A raised MCV is a typical finding.
* Iron, vitamin B_{12} and folate deficiencies are the commonest causes of anaemia, but laboratory tests can help in the elucidation of other rarer causes of anaemia.

Further reading

Hoffbrand AV, Pettit JE (1993) *Essential Haematology.* Blackwell Scientific, Oxford
Roit I (1992) *Essential Immunology.* Blackwell Scientific, Oxford
Zilva JF, Pannall PR, Mayne PD (1991) *Clinical Chemistry in Diagnosis and Treatment.* Edward Arnold, London

2

Calculating patients' risk of deep vein thrombosis

Ricky Autar

Deep vein thrombosis (DVT) constitutes a serious threat to patients' general recovery. DVT in postoperative and bedridden patients is usually preventable and a thromboprophylaxis protocol based on risk assessment categories is strongly recommended. The Autar DVT risk assessment scale was developed to separate risk into no risk, low, moderate and high risk categories. Founded on Virchow's triad in the genesis of DVT, the scale is composed of seven categories of risk factors. When the scale was tested on a trauma/orthopaedic unit a cut-off score of 16 yielded 100% sensitivity, 81% specificity and a correlation coefficient of 0.98. The DVT scale is designed to allow application in diverse clinical specialities. It is recommended that nurses using the Autar DVT scale should evaluate for themselves the best cut-off score to achieve maximum predictive accuracy.

Deep vein thrombosis (DVT) can seriously damage the health of patients. It is often a precursor of pulmonary embolism (PE), an acutely fatal complication. PE initiated by DVT is a serious cause of mortality in surgical and non-surgical patients alike as it is still detected in 10% of hospital autopsies (Sandler and Martin, 1989).

DVT is usually preventable and the National Institutes of Health (NIH, 1986) and the European Consensus Statement (1991) recommend a protocol of venous thromboprophylaxis based on low, moderate and high risk categories (*Table 2.1*).

DVT risk assessment

Although the treatment of DVT is the province of physicians, nurses can proactively identify those at risk, make appropriate referral and implement the appropriate and prescribed venous thromboprophylaxis strategy. A blanket and unquantifiable nursing diagnosis of a potential problem of DVT provides only a crude index of risk measurement. A void has existed in this area of assessment and the Autar DVT scale was developed to fill this gap (Autar, 1994). The objective of the DVT scale is to enable:

- calculation of risk in an individual in the context of multifactoral aetiology

- application of preventive practices consistent with the recommended protocol for the risk category
- provision of quantifiable data for evaluation of practice
- contribution of a body of nursing knowledge, rooted in nursing practice.

Table 2.1: Antithrombotic prophylaxis strategy	
Risk category	**Recommended prophylaxis**
Low risk <5% Minor surgery (<30 min with 0–1 risk factor) Major surgery (<40 years old with no risk factors)	Graduated compression stockings
Moderate risk 5–40% Major surgery >40 years old Major surgery or lower limb surgery in patients on contraceptive pill Major medical illness with prolonged immobilisation (cardiac or inflammatory bowel disease)	Graduated compression stockings and Low dose heparin **or** Graduated compression stockings and Low molecular weight heparin
High risk >40% Major orthopaedic surgery Fractured pelvis, hip, leg Major surgery in patients with malignancy Major surgery in patients with previous thromboembolism or >60 years old Lower limb paralysis	Graduated compression stockings and Adjusted dose of heparin **or** Low molecular weight heparin and intermittent pneumatic compression, except for open limb injury

Sources of data: NIH (1986); European Consensus Statement (1991); Kendall Company (1992); Thromboembolic Risk Factors (THRIFT); Consensus Group (1992); Grace (1993)

The Autar DVT risk assessment scale

The Autar DVT scale (*Figure 2.1*) is modelled on Virchow's triad in the pathogenesis of DVT, which includes changes in: blood composition; blood vessel wall due to trauma; and blood flow due to impaired venous return. The DVT scale comprises seven distinct categories of risk factors, derived from clinically proven research studies. These are: age-specific group; build/body mass index (BMI); mobility/immobility; special risk; trauma risk; surgical intervention; and high risk diseases.

Name:				
Unit No:				
Ward:				

Special risk	**Score**	**Trauma risk**		
Oral contraceptive:		Score item(s) *only* *preoperatively*		
20–35 years	1	Head	1	
35+ years	2	Chest	1	
Pregnancy/puerperium	3	Spinal	2	
		Pelvic	3	
		Lower limb	4	
Age-specific group, age group (years)		**Risk assessment protocol**		
10–30	0	No risk	6	
31–40	1	Low risk	7–10	
41–50	2	Moderate risk	11–14	
51–60	3	High risk	15	
61+	4			
Surgical interventions		**Build/body mass index (BMI)** **Wt(kg)/Ht(m)2**		
Score only one appropriate item		**Build**	**BMI**	**Score**
Minor surgery <30 mins	1	Underweight	16–18	0
Major surgery	2	Average	20–25	1
Emergency major surgery	3	Overweight	26–30	2
Thoracic	3	Obese	31–40	3
Abdominal	3	Very obese	41+	4
Urological	3			
Neurosurgical	3			
Orthopaedic	4			
Mobility		**High risk diseases**		
Ambulant	0	Ulcerative colitis	1	
Limited (uses aids self)	1	Anaemia: sickle cell	2	
Very limited (needs help)	2	polycythaemia	2	
Chair bound	3	haemolytic	2	
Complete bedrest	4	Chronic heart disease	3	
		Myocardial infarction	4	
		Malignancy	5	
		Varicose veins	6	
		Previous DVT or CVA	7	

Scoring: identify appropriate items, add, and record score below

Assessor	**Date**	**Score**

Figure 2.1: Autar DVT risk assessment scale (revised by Autar, 1997)
CVA=cerebrovascular accident; DVT=deep vein thrombosis

Age-specific group

Evidence of the linear relationship between advancing age and the increasing incidence of DVT is compelling (Office of Population Censuses and Surveys [OPCS], 1990). With advancing age, the soleal veins become tortuous and the calf muscle mass decreases (Coon, 1976). Both changes reduce the efficiency of the venous pump and contribute to a decrease in the rate of venous return.

Build/body mass index

Obese patients are at greater risk of developing DVT than their lean counterparts (Kakkar *et al*, 1970; Poller, 1993). Mechanically, obesity increases intra-abdominal pressure and this interferes with venous return. Poller (1993) reported a decrease in fibrinolytic activity in obese patients.

Mobility

The calf muscle pump is the powerhouse of venous return, forcing venous blood towards the heart. Reduced movement of the calf muscles causes a reduction in venous return. Immobility causes venous stasis, which is manifested in at least two forms. Initially there is a decrease in the linear velocity of blood, compromising venous return from the lower extremities. This is followed by dilatation of the veins, delaying further venous return (Caprini *et al*, 1988).

Special risk

This category includes oral contraceptives and pregnancy and the puerperium.

Oral contraceptives: These remain the most popular method of family planning but carry a definite risk of DVT. The controlled investigation of Vessey and Doll (1970) is overwhelmingly supportive of the evidence that oestrogen increases the risk of DVT.

Oral contraceptives cause hypercoagulability of blood by increasing the level of fibrinogen and other clotting factors. They also cause vasodilation and this pre-disposes to venous stasis. Vessey and Doll (1970) reported that DVT occurrence in women aged 35–44 years was 2.5 times greater than in those aged 20–35. For this reason, in the DVT scale, women in the 20–35 age-specific group who are taking oral contraceptives have a weighted score of one, while those aged over 35 score two.

Pregnancy/puerperium: The relative risk of DVT and PE in pregnant or puerperal women is 5.5 times that in non-pregnant and non-puerperal women not taking contraceptives (Coon, 1976). In pregnancy, a pendulous abdomen increases intra-abdominal pressure and this interferes with the venous return mechanism.

The puerperium is the period immediately following delivery until the reproductive organs return to their non-pregnant state. It usually lasts six to eight weeks. Although the oestrogen level is considerably reduced during the puerperium, it remains higher than normal. The plasma composition is also reduced and coagulability is therefore enhanced.

Trauma risk

All patients with accidental trauma, irrespective of the site, carry some risk of DVT (Coon, 1976). In a prospective study of 349 patients admitted to a trauma unit, Geerts *et al* (1994) reported an association between specific injuries and the incidence of DVT (*Table 2.2*). Three of the patients died of massive PE before venography could be performed to confirm DVT.

The highest incidence of DVT reported for lower limb injuries is associated with venous stasis, intimal vessel wall damage and hypercoagulability, which comprise the triad predisposing to DVT (Wheeler, 1988). Enforced immobility following lower limb trauma is also a contributory factor in the pathogenesis of DVT.

Table 2.2: Incidence of DVT in trauma patients			
Injury	**No of patients**	**No of DVTs**	**DVT%**
Face, chest, abdomen	129	65	50
Major head	91	49	54
Pelvic	100	61	61
Spinal	66	41	62
Tibial	86	66	77
Femoral fractures	74	59	80
Source of data: Geerts *et al* (1994) DVT = deep vein thrombosis			

Surgical intervention

Venous stasis, hypercoagulability and vessel wall trauma are present in all surgery. Virchow's triad makes surgery the primary risk factor in the genesis of DVT. Some surgical procedures are associated with a comparatively higher incidence of DVT than others (*Table 2.3*). The risk following orthopaedic surgery is greater than that following other procedures, partly because of the trauma to the tissue surrounding the deep vein and partly because of the difficulty in moving the injured limb to maintain venous return. The enormous range in the reported incidence of DVT in abdominal and gynaecological surgery is due to the varying nature, type and duration of the surgical procedures. The positive correlation between the duration of surgery and the frequency of DVT (Borrow and Goldson, 1981) is illustrated in *Table 2.4*.

Table 2.3: Incidence of DVT according to type of surgery		
Type of surgery		**Incidence of DVT (%)**
Orthopaedic	knee replacement	84
	hip replacement	30–65
	open meniscectomy	20–25
Other surgery	abdominal	3–51
	thoracic	26
	gynaecological	7–45
	retropubic prostatectomy	24–51
	transvesical prostatectomy	7–11
	neurosurgery	29–43
Source of data: Madden and Hume (1976); European Consensus Statement (1991); Grace (1993); Autar (1996a). DVT = deep vein thrombosis		

Table 2.4: Correlation between duration of surgery and incidence of DVT	
Duration of surgery	**Incidence of DVT (%)**
<2 hours	20
2–3 hours	47
>3 hours	62
Source: Borrow and Goldson (1981). DVT = deep vein thrombosis	

High risk diseases

Inflammatory bowel disease, particularly ulcerative colitis, blood dyscrasias such as polycythaemia, sickle cell anaemia and haemolytic anaemia, and malignancy are all associated with increased blood viscosity. In postoperative patients, the presence of carcinoma increases the risk of DVT about 1.5-fold when compared with all patients without cancer, regardless of other risk factors (Kakkar *et al*, 1970). Ancillary predisposing risk factors such as old age and immobility may also coexist in patients with malignancy (Sue-Ling *et al*, 1986). The high risk diseases category illustrated in *Table 2.5* includes cardiovascular diseases which, in association with enforced immobility, contribute to venous stasis.

Table 2.5: Incidence of DVT associated with cardiovascular diseases		
Study	**Cardiovascular disease**	**DVT(%)**
Maurer *et al* (1971)	Myocardial infarction	20–40
Coon (1976)	Chronic heart disease	10–20
Warlow (1978)	Cerebrovascular accident	46–53
Kakkar *et al* (1970)	Varicose veins	56
Kakkar *et al* (1970) Nicolaides and Irving (1975)	Previous DVT	68
Source of data: Autar (1996b). DVT = deep vein thrombosis		

Practical application

Each risk factor in a category is assigned a risk score, according to its estimated importance. Factors carrying little or no risk are allocated a score of 0–1, rising to 2–3 for low to moderate risk factors respectively. A score of 4 or more is indicative of a very high risk of DVT. The risk factors are additive and a summation of the cumulative effects of the risk factors provides an algorithm for determining the risk category. In the low risk category one high risk factor may be present; this rises to two to four high risk factors in the moderate risk category. In the high risk category, more than four factors are present (Caprini *et al*, 1988).

Calculating an individual patient's/client's risk category is simple. An individual risk is assessed in a multifactoral aetiology. All the risk factors appropriate to the individual are identified. However, for patients in the trauma risk category, the risk factor is scored only preoperatively. This category ceases to apply if and when patients have undergone appropriate surgery in the surgical intervention category. The appropriate surgery, by its very therapeutic and corrective nature, addresses the trauma and therefore nullifies scoring in the trauma risk category. Concurrent scoring of the trauma risk factor and the surgical intervention category has the adverse effect of inflating the total score and overpredicts the risk.

All the scores derived from the identified risk factors are added up. The overall aggregate score identifies the risk category for that individual (*Table 2.6*). Patients' health status often fluctuates and daily DVT risk scoring for a minimum period of a week following admission not only

Table 2.6: DVT risk assessment protocol	
Risk category	**Score range**
No risk	6
Low risk	7–10
Moderate risk	11–14
High risk	15
DVT = deep vein thrombosis	

enables the risk continuum to be monitored, but also allows patients' general progress to be evaluated.

Consistency/sensitivity/specificity

Consistency is the extent to which replication produces similar results. The consistency of the DVT scale was tested on a limited sample of 30 patients on two trauma wards. On admission, each patient was independently risk assessed with the DVT scale by two registered nurses. This provided comparative data for two reliability studies on the two wards. The data analysed yielded a percentage agreement of 70% and 80% respectively and a Pearson moment correlation coefficient of 0.98 for both studies (Autar, 1994). This acceptably high percentage agreement and strong positive correlation of 0.98 confirm the interrater reliability of the DVT risk assessment scale.

Sensitivity, in this situation, is the percentage of patients/clients who will develop DVT and are so predicted, and specificity is the percentage who do not develop DVT and are so predicted (Lilienfeld and Lilienfeld, 1980). The admission score of each patient was analysed to diagnose the true positives (who will develop DVT) and true negatives (who will not develop DVT). A cut-off score of 16 achieved 100% sensitivity, 81% specificity and gave false positives in 19% of the study population.

Sensitivity and specificity are inversely related (Mausner and Kramer, 1985). A sensitivity of 100% is achieved at the expense of a specificity of 81%; however, alteration in the cut-off score can alter the sensitivity and specificity of an assessment tool. Nurses will have to evaluate for themselves the best cut-off score to enhance the predictive accuracy of this diagnostic tool. It is only by employing an accurate risk assessment tool that appropriate resources and effective interventions can be targeted.

With the current emphasis on objectivity and evidence-based practice, risk assessment tools are becoming increasingly popular. However, such assessment instruments are not tablets of stone. Nurses using the Autar DVT scale should not be complacent in its application and evaluation, but must exercise rigorous clinical judgement to substantiate decision-making in relation to risk assessment.

Key points

* Deep vein thrombosis (DVT) is usually preventable.
* A systematic and objective DVT risk assessment strategy into risk categories facilitates the choice of the most appropriate venous thromboprophylaxis.
* The Autar DVT scale was developed as an objective risk calculator.

* The design of the scale enables its practical application in diverse clinical areas.
* Nurses using the scale in diverse clinical specialities must evaluate for themselves the best cut-off score to achieve maximum predictive accuracy.

References

Autar R (1994) *Nursing assessment of clients at risk of deep vein thrombosis (DVT). The Autar DVT scale*. Unpublished MSc dissertation, University of Central England, Birmingham

Autar R (1996a) *Deep Vein Thrombosis: The Silent Killer*. Quay Books, Mark Allen Publishing, Dinton, Wiltshire

Autar R (1996b) Nursing assessment of clients at risk of deep vein thrombosis (DVT): the Autar DVT scale. *J Adv Nurs* **23**(4): 763–70

Borrow M, Goldson H (1981) Postoperative venous thrombosis: evaluation of five methods of treatment. *Am J Surg* **141**: 245–51

Caprini J, Scurr JH, Hasty JH (1988) Role of compression modalities in a prophylactic program for deep vein thrombosis. *Semin Thromb Hemost* **14**: 77–87

Coon WW (1976) Epidemiology of venous thromboembolism. *Ann Surg* **186**: 149–64

European Consensus Statement (1991) *Prevention of Venous Thromboembolism*. Med-Orion Publishing, London

Geerts W, Code K, Gray R *et al* (1994) A prospective study of venous thromboembolism after major trauma. *N Engl J Med* **331**(24): 1601–6

Grace R (1993) Thromboprophylaxis: a review. *Br J Hosp Med* **49**(10): 720–6

Kakkar VV, Howe C, Nicolaides AN *et al* (1970) Deep vein thrombosis of the legs: is there a high risk group? *Am J Surg* **120**: 527–30

Kendall Company (1992) *The Guide to Protocol Development for the Prevention of Deep Vein Thrombosis and Pulmonary Embolism*. Kendall Healthcare Products, Basingstoke, Hampshire

Lilienfeld AM, Lilienfeld DE (1980) *Foundation of Epidemiology*. 2nd edn. Oxford University Press, Oxford: 150–9

Madden JL, Hume M, ed (1976) *Venous Thromboembolism: Prevention and Treatment*. Appleton-Century-Crofts, New York

Maurer BJ, Wray R, Shillingford JP (1971) Frequency of deep vein thrombosis after myocardial infarction. *Lancet* **ii**: 1385–7

Mausner JS, Kramer S (1985) *Epidemiology: An Introductory Text*. WB Saunders, Philadelphia

NIH (1986) Consensus Development Conference on the prevention of venous thrombosis and pulmonary embolism. *JAMA* **256**: 744–9

Nicolaides AN, Irving D (1975) Clinical factors and the risk of deep vein thrombosis: In: Nicolaides AN, ed. *Thromboembolism Aetiology: Advances in Prevention and Management*. MTP, Lancaster: 193–204

OPCS (1990) *Mortality Statistics. Cause: England and Wales*. A publication of the government statistical services. DH2, No 17. HMSO, London

Poller L, ed (1993) *Recent Advances in Blood Coagulation: 6.* Churchill Livingstone, Edingburgh

Sandler DA, Martin JF (1989) Autopsy proven pulmonary embolism in hospital patients: are we detecting enough deep vein thrombosis? *J R Soc Med* **82**: 203–5

Sue-Ling HM, McMahon MJ, Johnson D *et al* (1986) Pre-operative identification of patients at risk of deep vein thrombosis after elective major abdominal surgery. *Lancet* **i**: 1173–6

Thromboembolic Risk Factors (THRIFT) Consensus Group (1992) Risk of and prophylaxis for venous thromboembolism in hospital patients. *Br Med J* **305**: 567–74

Vessey MP, Doll R (1970) Postoperative thromboembolism and the use of oral contraceptives. *Br Med J* **iii**: 123–6

Warlow C (1978) Venous thromboembolism after stroke. *Am Heart J* **96**: 283–5

Wheeler HB (1988) Venous thromboembolism following trauma. *J Intensive Care Med* **3**: 65–6

3

Pre-admission preparation days for cardiac surgical patients

Sara Nelson

Traditionally, pre-operative information has been provided on admission, the day before surgery. This was thought not to be the ideal time. An exploratory pilot study was undertaken to evaluate a new information service for patients about to undergo cardiac surgery. Questionnaires were administered to 20 patients who had attended a pre-admission education programme and 20 patients who had received information from the ward staff on admission. The aim was to assess whether patients' fears and anxieties were reduced by the provision of pre-operative information before admission for surgery. One hundred per cent of the patients felt that they benefited from attending the pre-admission programme and 76% felt that their anxieties were relieved.

Introduction

In September 1992, following an operational review, the role of cardiothoracic co-ordinator was developed at Royal Brompton Hospital. This developmental role was seen as providing a link between the patients, community and hospital staff, both before admission, and following discharge, with emphasis on patient and staff education. Its specific remit was to hold pre-admission preparation clinics for both cardiac and thoracic surgical patients; the latter had commenced a year before.

With the support of management, time was allocated to explore what was going on at other hospitals. At that time (1992) very little was happening elsewhere. It was mainly orthopaedic centres who were running pre-admission clinics and these were very different from what we could hope to achieve. The emphasis tended to be on pre-clerking which would have been difficult for us because of the different waiting list practices and the nature of the surgery. Our aim was to be more educational. One hospital we visited was running preparation days similar to those we envisaged, and seeing what their staff had implemented gave us the confidence that we could achieve our objectives.

A literature review provided us with valuable information about anxiety and information-giving. Wilson Barnett (1986) found that patients needed to understand what was happening to them before they could interpret events in ways that reduce their stressful and potentially threatening nature. This is exactly the situation that patients find themselves in when admitted to hospital for cardiac or thoracic surgery. According to Lazarus (1966), anxiety and stress are caused by fear; lack of knowledge about a situation, or not knowing how one will cope with it, makes one unable to control events or anticipate occurrences. This is particularly important for the cardiac patient who will require ventilation on an intensive care unit (ICU) after surgery and may have to undergo a number of invasive procedures.

Research has demonstrated that stress and anxiety can have a detrimental effect on recovery after surgery and that effective preoperative information reduces stress, anxiety and pain levels (Hayward, 1975; Boore, 1978).

Preoperative information at Royal Brompton Hospital has traditionally been provided on the day of admission. However, Wilson Barnett (1986) suggested that this may not be the best time as patients were too distracted by other events to receive and retain information. It was felt that some patients received hurried explanations, of varying quality, about their impending surgery at a time of immediate perceived threat; this is not conducive to learning as patients are too anxious about their admission and the other things that are happening to them to take everything in (Lepzcyk *et al*, 1990).

Yet we know that the provision of information helps to reduce stress (Johnson *et al*, 1973; Byshee, 1988) and leads to better postoperative outcomes (Hathaway, 1986). Other studies have shown that patients who attend preoperative classes do better postoperatively (Hartfield and Cason, 1981; Devine and Cook, 1983; Rice and Johnson, 1984).

Information booklets

Dobree (1990) found that providing patients with booklets ten days before admission was useful and enabled the patients to take an active role in their own care. We resolved to take this one step further by offering a new information service to patients and their relatives with the aim of providing high quality information for patients about to undergo cardiac surgery. Patients are given the opportunity to attend the clinic a few weeks before surgery so that they may receive information about their admission, in a relaxed informal group situation. If they are unable to attend, they are offered an information pack which is sent to them by post.

Guidance on best timing for the pre-admission preparation clinic was influenced by Cupples' work in 1991 which suggests that the ideal time for teaching patients is 5–14 days before admission. It was therefore decided to implement pre-admission preparation clinics. The objective was to give patients and their relatives better information before surgery, with the expectation that they would suffer less anxiety and therefore experience less pain and other complications in the immediate postoperative period.

The proposal was supported by the surgeons and so members of the multi-disciplinary team were approached for assistance, all of whom offered their commitment.

The pre-admission preparation programme for patients awaiting cardiac surgery commenced in January 1993. Patients and their relatives were invited to attend a seminar which lasted approximately three hours (*Table 3.1*).

Table 3.1: Pre-admission preparation clinic seminar schedule	
Time	**Activity**
1100	Welcome and coffee
11.15–11.45	Explanation and discussion of preoperative care
11.45–12.00	Physiotherapy: teaching breathing exercises
12.00–12.30	Video: Intensive care, your recovery after surgery
12.30–13.00	Discussion about how the heart works and general questions with a cardiologist
13.00–13.45	Sandwich lunch provided
13.45–14.15	Discussion about postoperative care, discharge and rehabilitation after surgery
14.15–14.30	Video: Life after heart surgery
14.30	Close and optional tour of the ward and intensive care

The purpose of the clinic is to provide quality information in a relaxed atmosphere that is conducive to learning (*Table 3.2*).

Wilson Barnett (1979) found that pain, loss of independence, alteration of body image and unknown diagnostic results were all threatening aspects of hospitalisation. Many other factors can add to the anxiety a patient experiences when faced with admission to hospital (*Table 3.3*).

Elms and Leonard (1966) reported that explanations about hospital routine, facilities and treatments reduced anxiety on admission. Weiler (1968) reinforced this opinion with his study finding that the information considered most useful by one hundred patients comprised:

Table 3.2: Aims of the pre-admission preparation clinic
The aims of the clinic are:
• to provide information, two to four weeks prior to admission
• to reduce patients' anxiety pre-admission
• to encourage family involvement and reduce their anxieties
• to identify those patients requiring extra support, ie. psychological, physical, social, transport and convalescence.

- explanations about oxygen, deep breathing and coughing
- visiting hours
- communications with relatives.

The period immediately before admission is often one of elevated anticipatory anxiety and we wanted to try to alleviate this. Consequently, the preparation programme was structured to take these factors into account.

Table 3.3: Factors which add to the degree of anxiety that patients experience when facing admission for surgery	
Personality	Health status
Social support network	Self-esteem
Lack of knowledge of terminology used	Perception of ward environment
Unfamiliarity of facilities	Lack of recognition of staff
'Being cut'/mutilation	Fear of the unknown and equipment
Not knowing where to go and when	Fear of pain

Pre-admission clinics

The day (*Table 3.1*) begins with a talk from a member of the ward staff about the admission procedure and what will happen to the patient during the first few days of his/her stay in hospital.

Next, a demonstration and discussion of the importance of breathing exercises and early mobilisation after surgery is given by a physiotherapist. The benefits of preoperative teaching about deep breathing, coughing and leg exercises to prevent postoperative complications are well documented (Healy, 1968; Lindeman and Van Aernam, 1971).

A cardiologist then discusses the importance of reducing cardiac risk factors as a message to take home to their families and answers any questions the patients and their families may have. Lunch is followed by a discussion about getting 'back to normal' after surgery. The information is reinforced by showing videos about the intensive care unit and 'returning to normal'.

Aims of study

When the cardiac clinics had been in operation for six months, an audit tool was developed to evaluate progress. This took the form of a questionnaire to find out whether the information offered before admission for cardiac surgery had reduced patients' fears and anxiety postoperatively.

Methodology

A convenience sample of forty was selected from a population of approximately 150 patients attending for cardiac surgery during the two months of data collection.

Study participants

Subjects were selected from English-speaking patients aged between 20 and 90 years who had undergone routine planned cardiac surgery. The modal age group of patients having surgery was 60–69 years for both sets of patients. The range was 40–79 years in the intervention group and 30–89 years in the control group. In both groups, 70% were males. This was fairly representative of usual ward admission patterns for adults with heart disease.

The pre-admission group (PA)

Twenty patients were chosen from a group who attended a preoperative preparation clinic day two to four weeks before admission for cardiac surgery.

The routine admission group (RA)

Twenty patients were randomly selected from inpatients who had **not** attended the preparation clinics. Emergency cases were excluded as these patients are more anxious and have less time to prepare, and would therefore be unsuitable as a control group. The RA group still received information from the ward staff as it would not have been ethical to eliminate this. One confounding variable was the quality or standard of the education given by different ward staff, but this is being researched in another study.

Questionnaires were developed to gather demographic and descriptive data. These were slightly different for the two groups. Answers were specific with closed questions and boxes to tick for 'yes' or 'no' responses. These were used to facilitate analysis, although space was allowed for patients' comments in order to obtain qualitative data as well.

Because both time and finances were limited, there was no separate researcher to administer the questionnaires. Consequently, whoever led the clinics also performed this task which may have lead to bias as the physical presence of a researcher can affect responses. An attempt was made to redress this by having a covering letter signed by someone else. An envelope was provided for patients to return the questionnaire, thereby ensuring privacy and confidentiality.

There is generally a poor response rate from this method of distribution and retrieval. Hence, in our study the questionnaires were distributed by hand to reduce costs and hopefully improve the return rate.

A pilot study to verify the questionnaire was carried out. Two patients from each group were used to test its reliability. The only alteration made was to collect data about the type of operation the patients had undergone.

Data gathering consisted of issuing questionnaires 24–48 hours prior to discharge following cardiac surgery. This allowed patients to have recovered sufficiently from surgery to be able to concentrate on the questionnaire and for the experience to be fresh in their mind.

Manley (1992) noted that recall of past events may be done badly depending on time lapse and perceived importance of events. One patient commented, 'Memory or the horrors fade quickly so it is important to be asked as soon as possible for information on this'.

The fears reported and the numbers reporting fears were calculated. The number of patients feeling anxious, and whether those anxieties were reduced by prior information, was recorded and compared between the groups.

Findings

Eighty five per cent (17) of the PA group completed the questionnaire and 95% (19) of the RA group completed the questionnaire. It is possible that there was a lower response from the PA group as the questionnaire administered to this group contained six more questions.

Fear of surgery

Patients were asked if they had any fears and what these were. The main fears expressed before surgery were of:

- not surviving surgery
- not coming round after anaesthetic
- surgery itself
- successful outcome
- functioning of the leg after the vein had been removed.

There was little difference between the groups in the number of patients expressing fears before surgery. Only 29% (5) of the PA group had fears compared with 37% (7) in the RA group. However, of these, only 71% (5) of those in the RA group who had fears said they were reduced by the information provided by the ward staff, compared with 100% (5) in the PA group.

All of the patients who had attended the pre-admission clinic said that their fears had been relieved by the information provided. Twenty nine per cent who had received information from the ward on admission said that their fears about the surgery had not been relieved. However, both groups felt that they had been adequately prepared for their surgery.

Information giving

Two patients from the RA group felt that the medical staff could improve on their techniques of informing patients. One said, 'The doctors spoke in medical terms, too fast for me to comprehend... An orderly drew me a sketch and it all became clear'.

Two patients (12%) from the PA group wanted more practical information, eg. the length of time they could expect to be in theatre. They also wanted to receive the information package earlier in the day to avoid unnecessary note taking.

All of the patients and relatives who attended the pre-admission clinic were given the opportunity to visit the intensive care unit. Fifty nine per cent (10) of the patients took this offer and all of them found this useful. However, only 42% (8) of the patients educated by the ward staff were offered this opportunity and 37% (3) of these visited the intensive care unit; all who did visit found it beneficial.

Eighty two per cent (14) of the PA group wanted to know everything about their condition, either to understand it or to influence their treatment, compared with only 47% (9) of the RA group.

Pain

Overall, both groups of patients thought that their pain was better or the same as could be expected. Only 11% (2) in each group felt that it was worse.

Additional comments

Thirty one per cent (6) of the patients who did not attend the clinic felt that this service may have been beneficial. One disadvantage was that those who did not attend the course were given no information to help them answer the question as to whether they felt they may have benefited from a pre-admission service. Place of residence was not recorded and those who declined to attend the clinic may have done so because of the travelling distance and expense of attending, or because of work commitments.

However, comments from those who thought they might have benefited included being given 'peace of mind' and 'making me feel better in myself'. One patient who had not attended the clinic expressed feelings of having been overlooked as he had not heard from the hospital for nine months.

Seventy-six per cent (13) of patients attending the pre-admission programme felt their anxieties had been relieved while 12% (2) said that they had stayed the same. One patient reported that his anxieties had been heightened. Despite this, 100% (17) of the patients felt that they had benefited from attending and that it had been worthwhile making the journey.

Conclusion/discussion

The objectives of the programme were met as nearly all of the patients stated that their fears had been relieved, with only one patient saying that his anxieties had been increased. The audit raises questions as to which type of patient chooses to attend the group. A greater number of the PA group wanted information about their condition in order to influence treatment or understand it. This could be their way of coping with stress. According to Johnson *et al* (1978), 'Patients who attend preoperative teaching classes are usually those who have decided they need and want the information offered'.

It is possible that patients who attended the clinic were 'copers' who wanted to meet their problems head on and use the information constructively. Byshee (1988) found that such people tend to respond well to information.

Raleigh *et al* (1990) suggested that significant others were more anxious than the patients before a preparation seminar, therefore they recommended that relatives and/or partners should be included. Our findings were similar in that

88% (15) of patients brought someone with them, and the majority of these felt that it had been beneficial.

The fears that patients reported feeling were comparable to those reported in other studies, which found that pain, body image, losing control, the anaesthetic and not waking up were patients' biggest fears (Carnevelli, 1966; Wilson-Barnett, 1979; Dobree, 1990).

Patients are generally concerned about the level and type of pain they are likely to experience. Seers (1987) found that pain and anxiety post-operatively are closely correlated. The study reported here however, only determined whether patients' anxieties were increased or reduced, and whether their pain was as they had expected. Pain was measured subjectively and was generally lower than expected in both groups of patients. Further studies could obtain more objective results by measuring pain scores and the amount of analgesia required.

The pre-admission preparation programme attempted to reduce patients' stresses by improving the provision of information. The study does have a number of limitations, that need to be acknowledged. The number of patients in the sample was small, and so the results may not be reliable and could be due to chance. The small sample size also means that the sample cannot be considered representative of the population. A much larger, randomised, controlled study is needed before firm conclusions can be drawn. However, with regard to preoperative information-giving, this small exploratory study does provide replication evidence.

Action taken

The purpose of audit is action, and so the report was sent to all cardiologists and surgeons at the Royal Brompton Hospital to raise their awareness of the clinic. The problems encountered in setting up the clinic were highlighted and these were discussed with appropriate staff. Once the benefits of the programme had been identified, recommendations to increase patient throughput in these clinics were made. Information about the length of time that patients can expect to spend in theatre is now provided during the talks, and an information sheet containing key points from the overheads has been developed to prevent unnecessary note taking.

Using the Dynamic Standard Setting System (DySSSy; Royal College of Nursing, 1990) a group of nurses involved in the clinics have gone on to develop a nursing standard about information-giving pre- and post-operatively for cardiac patients, with the aim of improving practice and auditing activity on the ward generally.

Practical problems, identified by the co-ordinator, such as 'lack of help' and 'carrying equipment around' were resolved by recruiting a voluntary worker, installing a cupboard and making better use of portering services.

Recommendations for future research

This exploratory study not only reflected many of the issues concerning patient education found in the literature, but also raised questions that could be addressed in future research. No attempt was made to control for case-mix severity and the closed questions concerning pain and anxiety elicited mainly 'yes' or 'no' answers. Therefore, a randomised controlled clinical trial was designed to evaluate the effect of pre-admission education on patients' anxiety, depression, pain and well-being following cardiac surgery.

We are now in the third year of this trial which is aiming to recruit 275 patients and is expected to be completed by 1999. The outcome measures being studied are:

- hospital anxiety and depression scale (Zigmund and Snaith, 1983)
- well-being questionnaire (Cox and Gotts, 1987)
- health status (SF36)
- measure of pain.

Meanwhile, the results of the initial audit enabled improvements to be made and we demonstrated that the pre-admission clinics offer positive reassurance to both patients and their relatives and provide a quality service.

Key points

* Admission for cardiac surgery can be stressful for both patients and relatives.
* The pre-admission education programme attempted to reduce patients' stresses by better information provision.
* Pre-admission clinics offer positive reassurance to both patients and relatives.

Acknowledgements

I would like to thank Caroline Shuldham, Director of Nursing and Quality, Royal Brompton Hospital for her support and encouragement, and to Smith and Nephew Foundation for a bursary to support my BSc (Hons) in Health Studies, undertaken at Greenwich University, during which this audit was undertaken.

References

Boore J (1978) *Prescription for Recovery*. RCN, London

Brazier JE, Harper R, Jones NMB *et al* (1992) Validating the SF36 health survey questionnaire: new outcome measure for primary health care. *Br Med J* **305**: 160–64

Byshee JE (1988) The effect of giving information to patients before surgery. *Nurs* **3**(30): 36–39

Carnevelli DL (1966) Preoperative anxiety. *Am J Nurs* **7**: 1536–38

Cox T, Gotts G (1987) *General well being questionnaire: General Well Being Manual*. University of Nottingham, UK

Cupples SA (1991) Effects of Timing and Reinforcement of pre-Operative Education on Knowledge and Recovery of Patients Having Coronary Artery Bypass Graft Surgery. *Heart Lung* **20**(6): 654–60

Devine E, Cooke R (1983) A meta-analytical analysis of psychoeducational interventions on length of post surgical stay. *Nurs Res* **32**(5): 267–74

Dobree L (1990) Pre-operative advice for patients. *Nurs Stand* **24**(48): 28–30

Elms R, Leonard R (1966) Effects of nursing approaches during admission. *Nurs Res* **15**(1): 39–48

Hartfield M, Cason C (1981) Effect of information on emotional responses during barium enema. *Nurs Res* **30**:151–55

Hathaway D (1986) Effect of pre-operative instruction on post-operative outcomes: a meta-analysis. *Nurs Res* **35**(5): 269–275

Hayward J (1975) *Information: A prescription against pain*. RCN, London

Healy KM (1968) Does pre-operative instruction make a difference? *Am J Nurs* **68**(1): 62–7

Johnson JE, Morrissey JF, Leventhal H (1973) Psychological preparation for an endoscopic examination. *Gastrointest Endosc* **19**(4): 180–82

Johnson J, Rice V, Fuller S *et al* (1978) Sensory information instruction in a coping strategy and recovery from surgery. *Res Nurs Health* 1: 4–17

Lazarus RS (1966) *Psychological Stress and the Coping Process*. McGraw Hill Book Company, New York

Lepzcyk M, Raleigh EH, Rowley C (1990) Timing of pre-operative patient teaching. *J Adv Nurs* **15**(3): 300–306

Lindeman CA, Van Aernam B (1971) Nursing intervention with the pre-surgical patient. The effects of structured and unstructured pre-operative teaching. *Nurs Res* **20**: 319–332

Manley BFJ (1992) *The design and analysis of research studies*. Cambridge University Press, Cambridge

Raleigh EH, Lepzcyk M, Rowley C (1990) Significant others benefit from pre-operative information. *J Adv Nurs* **15**: 941–45

Rice V, Johnson J (1984) Pre-admission self instruction booklets, post-admission exercise performance and teaching time. *Nurs Res* **33**(3): 147–151

Rice VH, Mullen MH, Jarosz P (1992) Pre-admission self instruction. Effect on post-admission and post-operative indicators in coronary artery bypass graft patients: partial replication and extension. *Nurs Res* **15**: 253–59

Royal College of Nursing (1990) *Quality patient care, the dynamic standard setting system*. Scutari, Harrow

Seers K (1987) *Pain, anxiety and recovery in patients undergoing surgery.* PhD unpublished thesis, University of London

Weiler MC (1968) Post-operative patients evaluate pre-operative instruction. *Am J Nurs* **68**: 1465–7

Wilson-Barnett J (1979) *Stress in hospitalised patients. Psychological reactions to illness and health care.* Churchill Livingstone, Edinburgh

Wilson-Barnett J (1986) The prevention and alleviation of stress in patients. *Nurs* **10**: 432–36

Zigmund AS, Snaith RP (1983) *The Hospital Anxiety and Depression Scale. Acta Psychiatrica Scandinavia* **67**(6): 361–70

4

The importance of assessing patients with leg ulceration

Terry Shipperley

The treatment of leg ulceration consumes a significant portion of NHS resources, in terms of both equipment and manpower. Recent developments in diagnosis and treatment of these wounds has led to improved healing rates. This chapter reviews the literature relating to the assessment of patients with leg ulceration. It stresses the importance of holistic assessment, including medical and social history, and explains the importance of each aspect of the assessment process. The factors involved in clinical assessment of the wound and details of how to undertake the Doppler procedure are also outlined. With this knowledge the nurse can determine the origin of the ulcer and tailor the care and treatment to the patient's individual needs.

Leg ulceration affects around 580000 people in Britain, approximately 1% of the population, and costs the NHS £300–600 million per annum (Department of Health, 1989). Between 65% and 88% of all cases are managed by the primary healthcare team at an estimated cost of £1200 per patient per year (Callum *et al*, 1988).

The most common cause of leg ulceration is venous disease, but a significant proportion of leg ulcers develop as a result of other conditions (*Table 4.1*). Studies have shown that most ulcers do not have a single cause and may arise from a combination of causative factors (Callam *et al*, 1987b; Cherry *et al*, 1991).

If treatment is to be appropriate and effective, it is vital that accurate assessment is carried out before treatment is commenced, to identify the cause of the ulcer and any physical, psychological and/or social factors that may impede the patient's progress. Ertl (1993a) stresses the importance of treating the whole person and not just the offending lesion. The aim of all leg ulcer treatment is to improve the blood supply to the limb; however, the method used to achieve this will depend on the underlying cause. Therefore, aetiology must be ascertained before active treatment can begin.

Table 4.1: Causes of leg ulceration	
Causes	
Venous disease	70%
Arterial disease	8–10%
Mixed venous/arterial disease	10%
Rheumatoid arthritis	5%
Diabetes	5%
Local trauma, infections, burns, neoplasms	1%
Source: Kenrick et al (1993)	

It is now widely accepted that compression bandaging is the most effective treatment for venous insufficiency (Blair *et al*, 1988). However, arterial disease may be present in 50% of patients over 75 years of age (Cornwall *et al*, 1986), and failure to recognise this can result in inappropriate use of compression, leading to pressure necrosis, loss of limb or even death (Callam *et al*, 1987a).

The primary objective of assessment is to build up a profile of the patient and to identify and prioritise any factors that may have an influence on the healing process or wound management plan. It is important for the district nurse to have a knowledge of the factors that predispose to leg ulceration so that she may develop a management and preventive care strategy; however, it is also necessary for the nurse to ascertain and interpret the patient's beliefs about the ulcer, the future and his/her attitude to coping (Ross, 1987).

Thus, assessment consists of much more than looking at the wound and deciding which dressing to use. This chapter discusses the areas that should be explored in a thorough, holistic assessment of a patient with leg ulceration.

Social history

The patient's standard of living and level of intelligence may have a bearing on treatment outcomes. For example, cold damp rooms may encourage the patient to sit too close to the fire and nights spent sitting in a chair with legs dependent (ie. hanging down) rather than retiring to a cold bedroom are a major cause of oedematous legs (Cullum and Roe, 1995a).

Wise (1986) found that people with high isolation scores tended to have ulcers that never heal and that loneliness may cause the patient to actively interfere with treatment so as to continue the nurse's visits for ulcer treatment. It is important to ascertain the patients' understanding of their ulcer, how it might have been caused, how the ulcer is affecting their life, whether they believe it can be healed, and how willing they are to participate in the treatment programme.

The patient's occupation (or previous occupation) may have a bearing on the ulcer. Occupations that involve prolonged standing, especially in warm conditions (eg. hairdressers and shop assistants), might contribute to the ulcer pathology (Morison and Moffatt, 1994). Smoking exacerbates arterial constriction and is thus linked directly to arterial ulceration (Fowkes, 1989).

Depression generally reduces activity and interest in the future, both of which are necessary for the successful healing of ulcers. The patient's active participation in his/her treatment has been shown to improve results (Eagle, 1990).

Age, sex and parity

Up to the age of 50 years the incidence of leg ulceration is evenly distributed between the sexes; however, over this age the preponderance of ulceration among women increases, reaching a ratio of 7:1 in the very elderly (Cornwall *et al*, 1986). Parity is important as some women may have developed deep vein thrombosis or varicose veins during pregnancy as a result of pressure from the increased abdominal load (Arnoldi, 1957; Abramson *et al*, 1981).

Mobility

Assessment of the patient's mobility facilitates the setting of realistic goals and enables improvement or deterioration to be detected. Limited ankle movement will lead to poor use of the calf muscle pump, which is important for improving venous return (Cullum and Roe, 1995b). A walking aid or alternative footwear may need to be provided.

Nutritional status

Obesity leads to reduced mobility and strain on the ulcerated limb, while wounds in the malnourished patient are notoriously slow to heal. David (1986) and Roberts (1988) both identify the need for a high protein intake to aid wound healing. Roberts (1988) also noted the importance of vitamins A and C, and the trace element zinc, in the healing process.

Medical history

Diabetes mellitus

Diabetics are 11 times more prone to peripheral vascular disease than the general population and have a higher incidence of atherosclerosis (Berklow and Fletcher, 1987). Consequently, arterial ulcers are more common in this group of patients (Fowkes, 1989). Diabetics are also more prone to chronic infection and because neuropathic changes reduce sensitivity to pain, they are vulnerable to trauma and pressure damage from ill-fitting footwear. Diabetic ulcers are commonly found on the foot, often over bony prominences, and are usually sloughy or necrotic in appearance (Cullum and Roe, 1995a). All patients with leg ulceration should be routinely screened for diabetes, either by urinalysis or by random blood glucose monitoring.

Circulatory disorders

A history of hypertension, cardiovascular disease or cerebrovascular disease is a cautionary indicator that may coexist with venous incompetence, whereas a history of intermittent claudication is almost always associated with poor peripheral perfusion (Callam *et al*, 1987b).

Rheumatoid arthritis

The reason why patients with rheumatoid arthritis often develop leg ulcers is not fully understood; it may be that the combination of local vasculitis, poor venous return due to immobility of the ankle joint and the debilitating effect of prolonged steroid therapy on the skin greatly increases the risk of ulceration in these patients (Cullum and Roe, 1995a). Long-term steroid use can also delay healing (Morison, 1992). Patients with a history of rheumatoid arthritis may have straightforward venous ulcers; however, the widespread inflammatory changes that occur can lead to the development of vasculitic ulcers, which are painful and highly resistant to treatment (Ertl, 1993a). Rheumatoid arthritis can be confirmed or eliminated by routine blood screening.

Deep vein thrombosis

Whether known or silent, deep vein thrombosis is a major contributor to valvular incompetence, which can lead to venous ulceration. A possible history of deep vein thrombosis is indicated by previous ulceration, phlebitis, cellulitis, pregnancy, trauma, fractures, and abdominal, vascular and/or orthopaedic surgery (Ertl, 1993b).

Varicose veins

Varicose veins are a common problem, occurring in 10–20 % of the population. They are a sign of chronic venous hypertension in the lower limb which is usually due to damage of the valves in the leg veins (Morison and Moffatt, 1994). Factors that are thought to predispose to the development of varicose veins include a family history of varicose veins, female gender, occupations involving prolonged standing, pregnancy, obesity and a low fibre diet (Moffat and Franks, 1994). Approximately 3% of patients with varicose veins develop leg ulcers; however, as not all patients with venous leg ulcers have varicose veins, it is not clear whether they are associated diseases with a common aetiology or whether varicose veins predispose to the development of venous ulcers (Morison and Moffatt, 1994).

Clinical examination

Before assessing the wound itself, it is important to examine both the legs for signs that may assist in classifying the type of ulcer.

Oedema

Measurement of foot, ankle and calf circumferences repeated at weekly intervals will identify the extent of oedema and subsequent success in reducing it. Oedema is often generalised with venous ulceration, possibly worsening over the course of the day, whereas oedema associated with arterial disease is more likely to be localised or absent.

Appearance of surrounding skin

Staining of the skin in the gaiter region is often present in venous ulceration. It results from distension of the blood capillaries, leading to leakage of red blood cells and large protein molecules, the destruction of which causes pigmentation of the skin. Local areas of capillary infarction can also cause loss of pigment in the skin, giving an appearance known as 'atrophie blanche'. Woody induration of the tissues and ankle flare, the distension of the network of small veins on the medial aspect of the foot just below the malleolus, are sure signs of venous insufficiency. Oedema contains proteins which are irritant and often lead to eczema. Patients with unresolved eczema should be referred for a dermatological opinion.

The ischaemic limb, on the other hand, is often pale, shiny and hairless with evidence of muscle wasting. It may be cold unless infection is present, in which case it will be hot and red. The foot may be white on elevation and bluish on dependency, with atrophic toenails. Capillary filling can be assessed by pressing gently on the patient's great toenail and causing the nailbed to blanche. When the pressure is removed the colour should return instantly. In the ischaemic leg the colour will take longer to return to normal (Cullum and Roe, 1995a). As skin colour and capillary filling can be affected by cold, this test should be undertaken in a warm room.

Site

Although venous ulcers are commonly found in the gaiter region, particularly the medial malleolar area, and arterial and diabetic ulcers are commonly found on the foot, the site alone should not be used as an indicator of origin as mixed disease may be present.

Pain

Venous ulcers are generally not thought to be excessively painful unless oedema is not controlled or bacterial infection gives rise to cellulitis or lymphangitis. However, Franks *et al* (1994) found that 80% of patients with venous ulcers had pain and that the limb is often more comfortable in the elevated position.

Arterial ulcers, conversely, are often extremely painful, particularly at night when the patient is in bed, but are likely to be less so in the dependent position because gravity assists the flow of blood to the foot.

Pain should be assessed regularly to ensure that adequate analgesia is given. Patients should also be advised correctly about whether to elevate or lower their limb to assist with pain relief.

The ulcer

Assessment of the ulcer itself should take into account the size and duration of the wound. The appearance of the edges of the wound may aid diagnosis of the ulcer origin, often being shallow and rolled in a venous ulcer and cliffed and deep in an arterial ulcer. The colour of the wound bed will indicate whether necrosis, slough or infection is present and whether there are signs of granulation or epithelialization

Careful note should be taken of previous treatments used and their effectiveness and acceptability to the patient. A wound tracing should be taken at initial assessment and at monthly intervals thereafter to monitor progress.

Photography is also a useful monitoring tool, especially when shared with the patient.

Palpation of foot pulses

Historically, the presence of pedal pulses has been taken as a sign of unimpaired arterial circulation and the absence of the pulses as indicative of arterial impairment; Moffat and O'Hare (1995) highlight the unreliability of this assumption. It is important to note that the dorsalis pedis pulse is congenitally absent in up to 12% of the population (Barnhorst and Barner, 1968) and that oedema can make pulses hard to feel. However, palpable pedal pulses should still be noted in the assessment documentation (*Figure 4.1*).

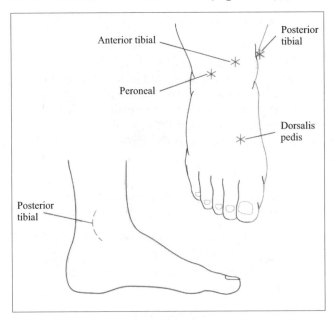

Figure 4.1: Pedal pulses

Doppler ultrasound

Accurate ulcer classification cannot be made solely by clinical examination. Although major pointers to the appropriate aetiology can be gleaned from such an assessment, clinical assessment alone has proved inadequate in approximately one third of cases (Cornwall *et al*, 1986). The introduction of hand-held Doppler ultrasound to measure the ankle:brachial pressure index (ABPI) has greatly assisted in the correct diagnosis and appropriate treatment of ulcer patients. It must be noted that Doppler alone cannot diagnose the ulcer origin, but it can assist in making a holistic assessment which includes all of the aforementioned factors.

Procedure

The patient should be lying flat, or as flat as possible, for 15–20 minutes to eliminate the effects of previous exercise on the blood pressure. After the procedure has been explained to the patient the sphygmomanometer cuff is secured around the arm. Ultrasound gel is applied over the brachial pulse and the Doppler probe is held over the pulse at a 45 angle. Gentle movements may be required to locate a clear, pulsatile signal. The cuff is inflated until the pulse signal disappears and then slowly deflated. The pressure at which the signal returns is the brachial systolic pressure. A measurement should be taken on both arms and the highest reading used (Moffatt and O'Hare, 1995).

The cuff is then applied just above the ankle, covering the ulcer with a non-adherent dressing if necessary. Following application of ultrasound gel, the posterior tibial, anterior tibial, peroneal and dorsalis pedis pulses are located and readings taken using at least two of these pulses in the same way as for the arm, again recording the highest reading (Moffatt and O'Hare, 1995). This will give the ankle systolic pressure. Readings should be taken from both legs to ascertain risk factors for future ulceration. An abnormally high reading may be an indicator of calcified arteries, resulting in an inability of the cuff to compress the artery. This reading must be considered unreliable.

Using a calculator, the ankle systolic pressure is divided by the brachial systolic pressure to obtain ABPI or resting pressure index (RPI) (Morison and Moffatt, 1994).

$$ABPI = \frac{\text{ankle systolic pressure}}{\text{brachial systolic pressure}}$$

The reading can thus indicate the presence and extent of arterial disease (*Table 4.2*).

Table 4.2: Interpreting Doppler readings	
1	Normal arterial flow
0.9	Mild degree of arterial involvement
0.8	The lowest level at which high compression can be safely applied
0.7	Significant arterial disease is present and full compression should not be used. A vascular opinion should be sought
0.5	The limb is greatly at risk and an urgent vascular opinion must be sought
Source: Moffatt (1993)	

Conclusion

This chapter highlights all the important factors that should be considered when assessing any patient who presents with leg ulceration, a history of past ulceration or who appears to be at risk of developing future ulceration. During the past 10 years, the profile of leg ulceration has been raised by practitioners in various parts of the country (Callam *et al*, 1987a; Moffatt and Stubbings, 1990). As a result of their efforts, clinical guidelines on the management of leg ulcers have been drawn up by the NHS executive (1994). All patients can now expect professional nurses to carry out a thorough, holistic assessment of their ulcer and involve other healthcare professionals in their treatment and care as appropriate.

Key points

* Ulcer origin must be determined before treatment is commenced.
* Doppler assessment is essential to determine the status of arterial blood flow to the foot.
* Compression bandaging must not be used when significant arterial disease is present.
* Past medical and social history are an important part of the assessment process.
* The dermatology and vascular departments should be involved in the treatment programme when appropriate.

References

Abramson JH, Hopp C, Epstein CM (1981) The epidemiology of varicose veins: a survey in western Jerusalem. *J Epidemiol Community Health* **35**: 213–17

Arnoldi CC (1957) Aetiology of primary varicose veins. *Dan Med Bull* **4**: 102–7

Barnhorst DA, Barner HB (1968) Prevalence of congenitally absent pedal pulses. *N Engl J Med* **278**: 264–5

Berklow R, Fletcher AJ (1987) *The Merck Manual*. 15th edn. Merck, Sharp and Dohme Research Laboratories, New Jersey

Blair SD, Wright DDI, Backhouse CM *et al* (1988) Sustained compression and healing of chronic venous ulcers. *Br Med J* **297**: 1159–61

Callam MJ, Ruckley CV, Dale JJ *et al* (1987a) Hazards of compression treatment of the leg: an estimate from Scottish Surgeons. *Br Med J* **295**: 1382

Callam MJ, Ruckley CV, DaleJJ *et al* (1987b) *Lothian and Forth Valley Leg Ulcer Survey*. Buccleuch Ltd, Hawick

Callam MJ, Harper DR, Dale JJ *et al* (1988) Chronic leg ulceration: socio-economic aspects. *Scott Med J* **33**: 358–9

Cherry G, Cameron J, Ryan T (1991) *Blueprint for the Treatment of Leg Ulcers*. Convatec, Uxbridge

Cornwall JV, Dore CJ, Lewis JD (1986) Leg ulcers: epidemiology and aetiology. *Br J Surg* **73**: 693–6

Cullum N, Roe B (1995a) Leg Ulcers Nursing Management — A Research-based Guide. Scutari Press, Harrow

Cullum N, Roe B (1995b) Nursing assessment of patients with leg ulcers. *Primary Health Care* **5**(5): 22–4

David J (1986) *Wound Management: A Comprehensive Guide to Dressing and Healing*. Martin Dunitz, London

Department of Health (1989) *Gravitational (Varicose) Ulcers: The Problem, What We Know and What we Need to Know and Do*. Seminar 30 November, DOH, HMSO, London

Eagle M (1990) The quiet epidemic below the knee. *Nurs Stand* **4**(15): 32–6

Ertl P (1993a) The multiple benefits of accurate assessment — effective management of leg ulcers. *Prof Nurse* **9**(2): 139–44

Ertl P (1993b) Planning a route to treatment — a framework for leg ulcer treatment. *Prof Nurse* **8**(10): 675–9

Fowkes FGR (1989) Aetiology of peripheral atherosclerosis. *Br Med J* **298**: 405–6

Franks PJ, Moffatt CJ, Connolly MJ et al (1994) Community leg ulcer clinics: effect on quality of life. *Phlebology* **9**: 83–6

Kenrick M, Luker K, Cullum N *et al* (1993) The management of leg ulcers in the community. Clinical Information Pack, number 1. University of Liverpool

Moffatt C (1993) Doppler ultrasound can be a useful tool when treating leg ulceration. *Pract Nurs* 21 September –4 October: 8–10

Moffatt C, Franks P (1994) A prerequisite underlining the treatment programme: risk factors associated with venous disease. *Prof Nurse* **9**(9): 637–642

Moffatt C, O'Hare L (1995) Ankle pulses are not sufficient to detect impaired arterial ciruclation in patients with leg ulcers. *J Wound Care* **4**(3): 14–18

Moffatt C, Stubbings N (1990) The Charing Cross approach to venous ulcers. *Nurs Stand* **5**(12): 6–9

Morison M (1992) *A Colour Guide to the Nursing Management of Wounds*. Wolfe Publishing Ltd, London

Morison M, Moffatt C (1994) *A Colour Guide to the Assessment and Management of Leg Ulcers*. 2nd edn. Mosby, London

NHS Executive (1994) *Consensus Strategy for Major Clinical Guidlelines — The Management of Leg Ulcers*. Consensus Conference, Liverpool

Roberts G (1988) Nutrition and wound healing. *Nurs Stand* (Special suppl) **2**(51): 8–12

Ross F (1987) District nursing. In: Littlewood J, ed *Community Nursing. Recent Advances in Nursing*. Churchill Libingstone, London: 132–60

Wise G (1986) The social ulcer. *Nurs Times* **82**(21): 47–9

5

Role of the cardioprotective diet in preventing coronary heart disease

Carol Wasling

Diet is a significant feature in the prevention of primary and secondary coronary heart disease (CHD). Obesity management is crucial because of its direct influence on many CHD risk factors, angina symptoms and capacity to exercise. Much evidence is available on the best dietary and nutritional intake for maximum cardiac protection. The dietary habits enjoyed by the Mediterranean countries appear to confer the best health benefits. These involve eating plenty of fruit, vegetables, pulses, nuts, cereal products, olive oil and fish and only small amounts of meat and dairy foods. The Mediterranean diet does not contain the amounts of animal fats, margarines, cakes, sweets, biscuits and manufactured foods that are characteristic of the British diet. Nurses, in their professional capacity, can motivate and support patients to change their eating habits.

The development of coronary heart disease (CHD) is dependent on many risk factors which have a dietary link. These include hyperlipidaemia, hypertension, obesity, diabetes and thrombogenic factors. Cardioprotective dietary advice should form part of any lifestyle education, whether it is primary or secondary intervention of CHD. Indeed, there is evidence to show that before we are even born, what a mother eats during pregnancy may affect the risk of her child developing CHD in adult life (Barker *et al*, 1993).

Undernutrition can trigger the growing fetus to adapt its physiology and metabolism in an effort to survive, but these changes are permanent and may increase the risk of CHD later. So, it seems that good nutrition for cardiac protection starts in the womb. This chapter offers practical information and highlights the food and nutrients needed for a cardioprotective diet.

How diet affects coronary heart disease

Fat

There are three main kinds of fat present in the diet: saturated, polyunsaturated and monounsaturated. If a food contains fat it is always a mixture of these three types. The Health of the Nation (Department of Health [DoH], 1992) target for total dietary fat is that it should provide less than 35% of our total calories by

2005, rather than the current UK average of 39.1% (Ministry of Agriculture, Fisheries and Foods [MAFF], 1998).

Levels of cholesterol in the blood are influenced by dietary fat and other factors including physical activity, smoking, body weight and genetics. Cholesterol circulates round the blood in lipoprotein particles. About two thirds of cholesterol is transported as low density lipoprotein (LDL) cholesterol. A high LDL cholesterol is potentially atherogenic and is linked to CHD. High density lipoprotein (HDL) cholesterol amounts to 15–25% of total cholesterol and is important in removing cholesterol from tissues. HDL cholesterol is protective and is inversely related to the incidence of CHD. Each type of fat plays a different role in CHD (*Table 5.1*).

Table 5.1: Summary of the effects of dietary fatty acids	
Fats	**Effects**
Saturated	Raises LDL and HDL cholesterol
n-6 polyunsaturated	Lowers LDL and HDL cholesterol
n-3 polyunsaturated	Lowers triglycerides Anti-thrombotic properties
Monounsaturated	When substituted for saturated reduces only LDL cholesterol and not HDL cholesterol
Trans fatty acids	Raise LDL cholesterol and lowers HDL cholesterol
LDL=low density lipoprotein; HDL=high density lipoprotein	

Saturated fatty acids (SFA)

These raise LDL cholesterol. Animal products such as meat, milk, cheese, butter and lard contain high proportions of SFA. The Health of the Nation (DoH, 1992) target for SFA is to achieve a reduction from the current 15.3% (MAFF, 1998) to an intake of 11% or less of our total calories.

Polyunsaturated fatty acids (PUFA)

There are two types of PUFA: n-6 PUFA and n-3 PUFA.

n-6 PUFA: The body is unable to make n-6 PUFA and so small amounts are essential in the diet. When substituted for saturated fatty acids, n-6 PUFA reduces both LDL and HDL cholesterol levels. Large amounts of n-6 PUFA also pose a theoretical risk involving the initiation of atherosclerosis. Until more evidence emerges, the Committee on Medical Aspects of Food Policy (COMA) report advises that diets should not provide more than 6% of energy as n-6 PUFA (DoH, 1994). Current average intakes are 6.5% (MAFF, 1998). Corn, safflower, sunflower and soya bean oil are rich sources of n-6 PUFA.

n-3 PUFA (omega 3 PUFA): It is also essential to eat small amounts of n-3 PUFA. Rich sources include oily fish. The n-3 series of PUFA do not affect blood cholesterol significantly but they reduce plasma triglyceride. In addition, fish oils have anti-inflammatory and antithrombotic properties. In a trial on men who had had one myocardial infarction, some followed a standard healthy diet and others ate a healthy diet and oily fish at least twice a week (Burr *et al*, 1989). There was a 29% reduction in death after 2 years in the group eating oily fish.

We await the results of further studies to confirm the precise mechanisms by which the oil in fish work and also to define the amounts required to produce an effect. In the meantime, it seems reasonable to advise regular (at least one 200–400g portion a week) consumption of oil rich fish. For those people who wish to take fish capsules instead, the capsules should contain rich amounts of long chain n-3 PUFA, such as EPA (eicosapentaenoic acid) or DHA (docosahexaenoic acid). The intake of n-3 PUFA in the study by Burr *et al* (1989) was about 430 mg/day.

Monounsaturated fatty acids (MUFA)

Substituting a diet rich in saturated fats for one with less SFA and higher levels of MUFA reduces the total blood cholesterol. Current thinking suggests that this effect is due to the reduction in saturates rather than the increase in MUFA (DoH, 1994). The Committee on Medical Aspects of food policy (DoH, 1994) advises swapping saturated fats with MUFA rather than with PUFA because (a) there is no reduction in the beneficial HDL cholesterol as seen with PUFA and (b) as previously mentioned, there is a theoretical risk with high dietary intakes of PUFA.

Olive and rapeseed oils are low in saturates and are rich sources of MUFA. A diet high in MUFA is enjoyed by Mediterranean countries, which traditionally have a very low incidence of CHD. A recent International Consensus Statement by the European Commission (1997) advocates the Mediterranean diet and a MUFA rich oil because of its beneficial effects on health. *Table 5.2* highlights the main foods contained in such a diet. Any manoeuvre to eat foods containing a high proportion of MUFA should accompany a reduction of SFA richfoods.

Trans fatty acids

When food manufacturers turn liquid oils into solids (known as 'hydrogenation'), the chemical makeup of PUFAs is sometimes changed. These altered fats are known as trans fatty acids. Trans fats raise LDL cholesterol to about the same extent as SFA but, unlike SFA, they also lower HDL (British Nutrition Foundation Task Force, 1995). The main sources of trans fat in the diet are margarines (often those used for baking), spreads, partially hydrogenated oils and bakery products. They are also contained in ruminant meat fats, milk fats and dairy fats.

Advise those eating frequent amounts of biscuits, cakes, confectionery, pastry items and foods containing partially hydrogenated oils/fats to have these foods only occasionally.

Table 5.2: Features of the Mediterranean diet

Foods eaten	Food qualities
Plenty of fish, especially oily fish	Low in saturated fat High in n-3 polyunsaturates Eating more fish means eating less meat therefore there is the added benefit of reducing saturated fat
Lots of fruit and vegetables (at least five servings a day)	Vitamins and minerals Fibre Antioxidant vitamins Very low fat No cholesterol Unknown benefits
Low in dairy products	Contributes less saturated fat to diet
More pulses (includes beans, peas and lentils)	Low in fat Good protein sources Vey high in fibre High carbohydrate Vitamins and minerals No cholesterol
More nuts (unsalted)	Vitamins and minerals Very good for fibre No cholesterol Most are high in fat but are not high in saturated fat Good source of protein
Olive oil (or choose rapeseed oil instead)	Low in saturates Rich in monounsaturates Antioxidants (eg. vitamin E and polyphenols) used instead of animal fats (eg. butter or lard) and margerine
More cereals, pasta and rice	Low in fat Low in cholesterol Good sources of fibre, vitamins and minerals
1–2 units alcohol/day	Alcohol in small amounts regularly seems to have beneficial effects, either because of the alcohol or other substances (eg. antioxidants). Evidence for how it works is still inconclusive
Garlic	Allium — the active substance which has putative cholesterol lowering effects: good trial evidence is awaited to prove this and the dosages required
Very little cakes, biscuits, chocolate, puddings — fruit is eaten routinely as a dessert	These are high in calories, total fat, high in saturated fat, often high in sugar, and are of poor nutritional value in terms of providing very little in the way of vitamins, minerals and fibre. Eating few of these foods clearly has many benefits on total dietary intake

Fibre

The chemical definition of dietary fibre is non-starch polysaccharide or NSP. There are two types of NSP: insoluble and soluble. Both play a part in healthy eating, although only soluble NSP has a role in cardiac protection.

Insoluble NSP

- helps prevent constipation and diverticular disease
- present in unrefined cereal products such as wholemeal bread, wholemeal pasta and wholewheat or bran breakfast cereals.

Soluble NSP

- may help lower LDL cholesterol and blood glucose
- present in oats, beans, fruit and vegetables.

Antioxidants

Free radicals are highly unstable agents that damage all classes of biological compounds. Free radical damage has been implicated in several processes such as ageing and coronary heart disease. Free radicals are produced inside the body naturally but are also generated by outside agents such as smoking. One free radical can interact with another chemical component to produce yet more free radicals, thus starting a chain reaction. In health, there is a balance between free radical production and the activity of preventive antioxidants.

Antioxidants are the body's defence mechanism. They can either prevent a free radical cascade from starting or stop the chain reaction (Khan and Butler, 1998). Antioxidants present in the diet include: trace elements such as selenium, zinc, manganese; vitamins A (beta-carotene), C and E; and flavanoids. Greater evidence exists for the beneficial effects of these foods in epidemiological studies compared with vitamin supplements in trials. These studies suggest that low intakes of antioxidants are associated with high risk of CHD (Gey *et al*, 1991), and that Mediterranean countries that consume large amounts of antioxidant foods have low incidence of CHD (Riemersma *et al*, 1990). However, randomised controlled trials have shown no cardiovascular benefit for antioxidant therapy (Alpha Tocopherol, Beta Carotene Cancer Prevention Study Group, 1994; Waldius *et al*, 1994). The Cambridge Heart Antioxidant Study (CHAOS) suggested that while vitamin E supplementation could reduce heart attacks, it did not reduce mortality (Stephens *et al*, 1996).

It is not yet known whether antioxidant rich foods are markers for unknown components that are themselves beneficial (which could explain why vitamin supplementation is inconclusive), or whether it is combinations of antioxidants that offer the best protection for the heart. At this stage, supplements are not advised: we await the results of larger, controlled trials to determine the true effects of supplementation. It is best to recommend a diet rich in fruit and vegetables, fish, nuts, seeds, wholegrain breads, cereals and vegetable oils that is in line with the Mediterranean style of eating.

Sodium

A high sodium intake can influence blood pressure. Salt is the commonest source of sodium (as sodium chloride). In the UK diet, between 65% and 85% of sodium chloride comes from manufactured foods (Sanchez-Castillo *et al*, 1987; Gregory *et al*, 1990). It follows that a reduced sodium diet is one low in processed foods. The trend of simply avoiding salt at the table or using a 'salt substitute', ie. one that claims to be lower in sodium than standard table salt, will have little impact on total sodium intake if large amounts of processed foods continue to feature in the diet. The COMA report recommends a 33% reduction in salt from the current average of 9g/day. One researcher estimated that an average reduction of 3g of salt could decrease systolic blood pressure by about 3.5mmHg (Law *et al*, 1991).

Alcohol

Excessive alcohol intake is a risk factor for heart disease. At high levels it increases the risk of cardiac arrhythmias, cardiomyopathy and sudden heart attacks. However, unlike cigarette smoking, there are levels of alcohol consumption which are considered beneficial to health. A report by the DoH (1995) concluded that there is evidence to show that in men over 40 years and postmenopausal women, drinking 1–2 units of alcohol a day can offer protection from CHD mortality. At these low levels of intake, protective mechanisms put forward include: raising HDL cholesterol and reducing LDL cholesterol; reducing platelet stickiness and aggregation; and inhibiting the formation of coronary artery atheroma.

Obesity

The Body Mass Index (BMI) (BMI=weight (kg)/height (m)^2) defines grades of undernutrition and obesity. Weight begins to influence CHD risk somewhere between a BMI of 25 and 30 and increases dramatically above a BMI of 30. Linked to obesity are other risk factors: hypercholesterolaemia; hypertension; and poor blood glucose control in diabetes. Reduced physical activity often plays a part in its causation.

There is also evidence to suggest that regular physical activity, even in the obese, substantially improves an individual's risk profile (Blair *et al*, 1995) as well as benefiting his/her general psychological well-being (Martinson and Morgan, 1997), which is frequently poor in the obese population.

A BMI of between 20 and 25 denotes a healthy weight (Garrow and Webster, 1985). However, *Obesity in Scotland* (Scottish Intercollegiate Guidelines Network [SIGN], 1996) recommends that those with a high BMI to aim for 10% weight loss as this is associated with significant health benefits (*Table 5.3*). It goes on to suggest that the next step is to maintain this 10% weight loss for at least two years, regaining no more than 3kg over this period.

Table 5.3: Health benefits of 10% weight loss	
Condition	**Benefits of 10% weight loss**
Mortality	> 20% fall in total mortality >30% fall in diabetes-related deaths >40% fall in obesity-related cancer deaths
Blood pressure	Fall of 10 mmHg systolic Fall of 20 mmHg diastolic
Diabetes	Reduces risk of developing diabetes by >50% Fall of 30–50% in fasting glucose Fall of 15% in HbA1c
Angina	Reduces symptoms by as much as 90% 33% increase in exercise tolerance
Lipids	Fall by 10% in total cholesterol Fall by 15% in LDL cholesterol Fall by 30% in triglycerides Increase by 8% in HDL cholesterol
Reproduced by kind permission of Royal College of Physicians (Edinburgh) (SIGN, 1996)	

In a review by Perri *et al* (1993), regular contact with a health professional seems to aid long-term success. This means that a continuous care model (such as that we currently offer for hypertensive and diabetic patients), rather than one or two single consultations is required for obesity management. Setting up a group class may be an effective means of achieving this level of care.

In addition to obesity per se, the body shape of a person can influence the risk of developing CHD. Central obesity or the apple shape, poses greater risks to health compared with femoral obesity (the pear shape), by contributing to the metabolic syndrome which includes hyperinsulinaemia, hypercholesterolaemia, and hypertriglyceridaemia (Bjorntorp, 1991). It is possible for central obesity to occur with a healthy BMI between 20 and 25: this still requires a weight loss effort. A simple measurement of waist circumference — the midway point between the lowest rib and the iliac crest with the subject standing at the end of a gentle expiration — can be used to indicate the risk to health (Lean *et al*, 1995).The guidelines for action are as follows:

There is no need to lose weight if:

- men have a waist circumference of 94 cm or less
- women have a waist circumference of 80 cm or less.

Advise weight reduction if:

- men have a waist circurnference of 102cm or more
- women have a waist circumference of 88cm or more.

Giving dietary advice

For a balanced diet encourage a variety of foods. Healthy eating does not mean 'perfect eating' but certainly the emphasis is on plenty of fruit, vegetables and starchy foods, in line with Mediterranean dietary habits, rather than the high fat foods we currently eat.

The Balance of Good Health

The Balance of Good Health leaflet was developed by the Health Education Authority. This model is an excellent educational tool which has been validated as an effective way of putting across the healthy eating message. It represents the relative proportions of the main food groups that comprise healthy eating. Leaflets are available from local health promotion units. The pictorial representation gives a strong visual impact. It also represents foods rather than nutrients, which are more readily understood by the public.

Fruit and vegetables: five a day

A daily intake of 400 g of fruit and vegetables (equivalent to five portions) or more helps reduce the risk of developing heart disease and cancer (World Health Organization [WHO], 1990; Block *et al*, 1992). For example, the risk of developing cancer is twice as high in people who consume less than this intake. This consumption excludes potatoes and assumes that the five portions are different. For example, one portion of fruit is equivalent to one apple, orange, banana, one slice of large fruit or two smaller fruits like kiwi or plums. For vegetables, 2–3 spoonfuls amount to one portion and for salad vegetables one dessert bowlful counts as one portion (Williams, 1995).

It does not matter whether the fruit or vegetable is fresh, frozen, tinned or dried. However, tinned fruit in juice is recommended rather than in syrup and tinned vegetables in unsalted water. Encourage people to think about how they could include fruit or vegetables at every meal.

Bread, potatoes, rice, pasta and cereals

These foods provide bulk, vitamins and minerals and form an important part of the diet. They are naturally very low in fat. However, the way they are cooked and the foods they are eaten with (eg. bread with an inch thick layer of butter), can significantly increase their fat content. Encourage a wide variety of products, especially the less refined foods as these are good sources of dietary fibre — wholemeal bread and wholewheat pasta.

Dairy foods

These are excellent sources of calcium, vitamins and minerals. However, because they can be high in fat, encourage the lower fat versions. For example, skimmed or semi-skimmed milk, low fat yoghurts and lower fat cheeses such as reduced fat cheddar, Edam, feta, Brie, Camembert, mozzarella and cottage.

Meat

Advise small amounts of lean meat or chicken/turkey without skin. Discourage meat products that are high in fat and salt such as sausages, burgers, pies.

Fish

Encourage fish in place of meat as the main meal at least twice a week. Advise oily fish (fresh, frozen or tinned) at least twice a week. Examples of oily fish include mackerel, sardines, herring, pilchards, trout and kippers. Suggest tinned fish, in water, brine, tomato or mustard sauce, rather than in oil. Good cooking methods for fish include: poaching, grilling, baking, and eaten coated in breadcrumbs oven-baked or grilled. Fish fingers or fish cakes are good, quick alternatives.

Nuts

Nuts are good sources of protein, fibre, vitamins, minerals and antioxidants. Most nuts are high in fat but the types of fat they contain are mostly MUFA and PUFA. In the Adventist Health Study (Fraser *et al*, 1992), nut consumption has consistently been found to protect against the risk of CHD in a dose response manner. Unsalted nuts are acceptable as a replacement for meat or fish, but calories and fat may add up if eaten as an extra in the form of a snack.

Fats and oils

Advise restricted use of all fats and oils. Recommend a reduced fat spread that is rich in MUFA or PUFA and low in saturates for spreading on bread, such as one of the many olive oil based spreads now available. For baking, recommend a margarine which is low in saturated and trans fats. For frying, opt for an oil rich in MUFA such as olive or rapeseed oil. Many of the oils labelled simply as 'vegetable oil' contain a large amount of rapeseed oil.

Eggs

Eggs are a good source of protein. They also contain dietary cholesterol. One or two eggs eaten in place of meat or fish is acceptable as part of a varied diet.

Fatty and sugary foods

Fatty and sugary foods include biscuits, chocolate, cakes, puddings, pies and pastry items. It is not necessary to avoid any food for healthy eating. However, if a patient eats a food or a number of high fat foods regularly they can significantly add up. Tackle such habits as a daily intake of chocolate or a biscuit with every cup of tea. For a healthier snack suggest fruit or a starchy based alternative.

Sugary drinks

Encourage people to drink sugar-free drinks. If people find cutting out sugar difficult, suggest a sweetener instead. When choosing squashes or fizzy drinks opt for the diet versions or the 'no added sugar' versions.

Patients within a healthy weight range

If patients do not need to lose weight but do need to reduce their intake of fat then it is important to encourage a greater intake of starchy foods to prevent unnecessary weight loss.

Putting healthy eating into practice: advising change

While many people understand the main healthy eating messages in terms of eating less saturated fat and more fibre, people are not always sure how to put this into practice. From experience of working on cardiac rehabilitation programmes, many patients seem just to focus on fat reduction, while failing to recognise the need or the importance of increasing fruit and vegetables. At the start of a consultation establish what the patient understands by 'healthy eating' and what changes he/she has made already.

When advising patients on what to eat refrain from using technical words; speak in terms of foods and try to give examples. Keep your messages simple and positive, eg. 'choose semi-skimmed milk to help reduce your fat intake'. This also helps to avoid negative, eg. 'don't eat', or guilt-provoking, eg. 'eating chips causes a high cholesterol', messages as these are less likely to be persuasive (Murphy *et al*, 1993).

To help motivate your patients, begin and end the session with positive statements about food and the reasons for change. The use of visual aids such as posters, food packets, flip charts and diet sheets are extremely useful in maintaining interest and reinforcing any verbal messages you give. Remember that achieving dietary change is often difficult because many factors, such as income, cookery skills, time and the home situation influence food choice.

To assess a patient's diet it might be useful to have a checklist under the main headings used in *The Balance of Good Health* plate model. *Table 5.4* offers an example of how you may set this out. Look at the frequency and amounts of foods eaten in a week and then at any one time. Afterwards, try to assess what needs to be done to achieve a healthier intake and then agree with the patient a few targets to achieve by his/her next visit.

Table 5.4: Dietary assessment checklist

Food group	Current habits	Advice	Patient targets
Fruit and vegetables	Fruit	Aim: at least five different servings of fruit and vegetables per day	
	Vegetables	Include fresh, frozen, canned and dried	
Starchy foods	Bread	Eat plenty. Wholemeal bread most often	
	Potatoes	Eat plenty. Eat potatoes boiled, baked or mashed (with milk) rather than fried	
	Cereal	Eat daily high fibre breakfast cereal, eg. branflakes, wheat biscuits, porridge	
	Pasta/rice	Eat mostly wholemeal pasta and brown rice	
Dairy	Milk	Skimmed or semi-skimmed (0.5–1 pint per day)	
	Cheese	Eat mostly lower fat types, eg. cottage, Edam, Brie, reduced fat cheddar	
	Yoghurt	Eat low fat, low sugar types	
Meat/fish and alternatives	Meat/poultry	Small amounts, include lean meat, chicken, turkey	
	Meat products	Reduce sausages and burgers to a minimum	
	Fish	Eat fish at least once a week, eg. mackerel, sardines, pilchards, tuna, salmon, kippers. Also white fish and fish products (not fried) instead of meat	
	Eggs	Not fried	
	Nuts	In place of meat if desired, not salted	
	Beans/pulses	Encourage in place of meat	
Fat-containing/ sugar-containing foods	Fats and oils (for spreading, baking and frying)	Use all sparingly Choose those rich in monounsaturates and low in saturates, eg. olive and rapeseed oil	
	Biscuits, crisps, chocolate/sweets, pastry, cakes/ puddings	Reduce all of these foods, especially if eaten habitually. Encourage fruit or starchy based snack instead	
	Sugary drinks	Choose diet or sugar-free drinks instead	

Conclusions

A diet rich in fruits, vegetables, starchy foods, vegetable oils, nuts and fish will not only benefit general health, but also help protect against the development of cardiovascular disease and other major diseases such as cancer. New evidence continues to emerge and reveals the mechanisms by which foods and nutrients exert their effects on health but there is still much to understand. Patients should curtail smoking and do more exercise.

A poster, diet sheet or leaflet alone is unlikely to give patients the help and support they need to make and maintain healthy eating habits. While government policies, mass media campaigns, the food industry and efforts from other organisations can contribute to public awareness of the changes required to the nation's diet, the healthcare professionals, in particular those in primary care, are best suited to discuss eating habits and help individuals and families change.

For some patients referral to a state registered dietitian may be appropriate. Check to see if your health authority or local dietetic department has a protocol for appropriate dietetic referrals. Due to the relatively small number of dietitians in the UK it is obviously not feasible to refer everyone with CHD risk factors because such a large proportion of the population are affected.

Your role as nurses, whether in the hospital or community setting, is therefore crucial in helping to change the nation's eating habits. Implicit in this role is the requirement to keep abreast of current advice on diet, so that the public receive consistent food messages: do keep in regular contact with your local state registered dietitian for any new developments and updates.

Recommendations

Your knowledge of food

Ensure you have a good grasp of the main features of the cardioprotective diet and how food affects the heart; this means going beyond what you know about dietary fat and blood cholesterol, and considering the role of fruit, vegetables, nuts, oily fish and monounsaturated fats. It is essential to think ahead about how you can explain these issues in a simple way to patients.

Giving advice

Build on a patient's existing knowledge. Assess his/her readiness to change. Individualise advice and negotiate key targets. Give as many food examples as possible — this may include tips on cooking, shopping and menu planning. Consider involving the whole family. Ensure you are happy that the leaflets you hand out are up to date and helpful.

Obesity management

Use the waist circumference measures as a guide to assessing who needs to lose weight. Set a 10% weight loss target, with the aim of losing 0.5–1kg a week. See patients as often as possible (consider group work) during the weight loss phase — but do not then stop. It is vital that some kind of weight maintenance programme follows this initial support so that ongoing contact in line with other continuous care models is provided.

Key points

* A Mediterranean diet seems to offer protection for the heart. This means eating more fruit, vegetables, pulses, nuts, cereal products, mono-unsaturated oil and fish and less meat, animal fats, margarines, cakes, biscuits, confectionary and dairy foods.
* Education, positive food messages and negotiation of specific targets can encourage and support patients making dietary changes.
* A 10% weight loss in those who are obese can have substantial effects on CHD risk factors.

References

Alpha Tochopherol, Beta Carotene Cancer Prevention Study Group (1994) The effect of vitamin E and beta carotene on the incidence of lung cancer and other cancers in male smokers. *N Eng J Med* **330**: 1029–35

Barker DJP, Gluckman PD, Godfrey KM *et al* (1993) Fetal nutrition and cardiovascular disease in adult life. *Lancet* **341**: 938–41

Bjorntorp P (1991) Coronary disease and obesity. *Medicographia* **13**(2): 15–47

Blair SN, Kohl HW, Barlow C *et al* (1995) Changes in physical fitness and all cause mortality: prospective study of healthy and unhealthy men. *J Am Med Assoc* **273**: 1093–8

Block G, Patterson B, Suhar A (1992) Fruit, vegetables and cancer prevention: review of the epidemiological evidence. *Nutr Canc* **18**(1): 1–30

British Nutrition Foundation Task Force (1995) Trans Fatty Acids. British Nutrition Foundation, London

Burr ML, Gilbert JF, Holliday RM *et al* (1989) Effects of changes in fat, fish and fibre intakes on death and myocardial reinfarction: diet and reinfarction trial (DART). *Lancet* **334**: 757–61

DoH (1992) *The Health of the Nation: A Strategy for Health in England*. HMSO, London

DoH (1994) *Nutritional Aspects of Cardiovascular Disease: Report of the Cardiovascular Review Group, Committee of Medical Aspects of Food Policy.* HMSO, London

DoH (1995) *Sensible Drinking: Report of Interdepartmental Working Group.* HMSO, London

European Commission (1997) Olive oil and the Mediterranean diet: implications for health in Europe. International consensus statement following meeting at the Italian Research Council in Rome, 11 April (details available from: Dr Martin Godfrey; tel: 0171 413 3027; fax: 0171 413 3010; e-mail:mgodfrey@hillandknowlton.com

Fraser GE, Sabate J, Beeson WL, Strahan TM (1992) A possible protective effect of nut consumption on risk of coronary heart disease: the adventist health study. *Arch Intern Med* **152**: 1416–24

Garrow JS, Webster J (1985) Quetelet's index (W/H) as a measure of fatness. *Int J Obesity* **9**(2): 147–53

Gey KF, Puska P, Jordan P *et al* (1991) Inverse correlation between plasma vitamin E and mortality from ischaemic heart disease in a cross-cultural epidemiology. *Am J Clin Nutr* **53**: 326–4

Gregory J, Foster K, Tyler H *et al* (1990) *The Dietary and Nutritional Survey of British Adults: A Survey of the Dietary Behaviour, Nutritional Status and Blood Pressure of Adults Aged 16 to 64 Living in Great Britain*. HMSO, London

Khan F, Butler R (1998) Free radicals in cardiovascular disease. *Proc Royal College Physicians Edinburgh* **28**: 102–10

Law MR, Frost CD, Wald NJ (1991) By how much does dietary salt reduction lower blood pressure? I-III analysis of observational data among populations. *Br Med J* **302**: 811–24

Lean MEJ, Han TS, Morrison CE (1995) Waist circumference as a measure for indicating need for weight management. *Br Med J* **311**: 158–61

MAFF (1998) *The National Food Survey 1997*. HMSO, London

Martinson EW, Morgan WP (1997) Antidepressant effects of physical activity. In: Morgan WP, ed. *Physical Activity and Mental Health*. Taylor and Francis, Washington DC

Murphy M, Wise A, McLeish A (1993) Persuasiveness of nutritional messages. *J Human Nutr Dietet* **6**(1): 3–11

Perri MG, Sears FS, Clark JE (1993) Strategies for improving maintenance of weight loss: towards a continuous care model of obesity management. *Diabetes Care* **16**(1): 200–9

Riemersma RA, Oliver MF, Elton RA *et al* (1990) Plasma antioxidants and coronary heart disease: vitamins C, E and selenium. *Eur J Clin Nutr* **44**(2): 143–50

SIGN (Scottish Intercollegiate Guidelines Network) (1996) *Obesity in Scotland; Integrating Prevention with Weight Management. A National Clinical Guideline Recommended for Use in Scotland by the Scottish Intercollegiate Guidelines Network SIGN*. SIGN, Edinburgh

Sanchez-Castillo CP, Warrender S, Whitehead TP *et al* (1987) An assessment of the sources of dietary salt in a British population. *Clin Sci* **72**: 95–102

Stephens NG, Parsons S, Schofield PM *et al* (1996) Randomized controlled trial of vitamin E in patients with coronary heart disease: Cambridge Heart Antioxidant Study (CHAOS). *Lancet* **347**: 781–6

Waldius G, Erikson V, Olsson AG *et al* (1994) The effect of probucol on femoral atherosclerosis: the Probucol Quantitative Regression Swedish Trial (PQRST). *Am J Cardiol* **74**: 875–83

WHO (1990) *Diet, Nutrition and the Prevention of Chronic Diseases*. WHO, Geneva

Williams C (1995) Healthy eating: clarifying advice about fruit and vegetables. *Br Med J* **310**: 1453–5

Section two: Nursing management of clients suffering from cardiovascular disorders

6
Understanding shock

Renee Adomat

Shock is a life-threatening condition requiring skilful observation and intervention. It is therefore essential for nurses to understand the physiological processes associated with different types of shock and the nursing management of shocked patients.

Shock is a progressive state of circulatory failure which, if left untreated, can result in death. It is really a syndrome rather than a disease as it comprises a collection of physiological responses. For all types of shock, except septic shock, the circulatory dysfunction causes inadequate perfusion of vital organs and an abnormal metabolism. In septic shock there is a generalised peripheral vasodilation and a concomitant loss of circulatory volume. The serious nature of shock can be very distressing for both patients and relatives and, once the patient is stable, the nurse must provide support during the period of recovery. Patients and relatives need clear honest information and time to express anxieties. The suddenness of death can be very difficult to understand and nurses need to develop their skills in order to help relatives and friends cope with their loss.

Resulting overall cellular effects

When cells are deprived of oxygen the mitochondria are unable to carry out their aerobic functions. The fall in intracellular oxygen over an extended period results in cell membrane damage. The cell walls of lysosomes also become damaged and proteolytic enzymes are released into the cell and finally the bloodstream. This results in the conversion of inactive kininogens into vasoactive kinins leading to increased capilliary permeability and vasodilation. Histamine is also released as a response to cellular damage and is an additional vasodilator. Histamine also causes separation and swelling of the capillary endothelium, resulting in passage of white blood cells and acute phase proteins into the extracellular fluid. The ichaemic and cellular damage in shock are shown in *Figure 6.1*.

Lysosomal proteases may also activate the coagulation system, causing disseminated intravascular coagulation (DIC). Anaerobic metabolism leads to an accumulation of lactic acid which increases metabolic acidosis.

In an attempt to compensate for the metabolic acidosis, hyperventilation occurs early causing respiratory alkalosis. This may result in a fall in partial pressure of carbon dioxide (pCO_2), reduced cerebral blood flow and a reduced conscious level. As shock persists release of noradrenaline and adrenaline cause further vasoconstriction which leads to decreased pulmonary blood flow, hypoxia and respiratory shunting. The kidneys are particularly susceptible to reduced blood flow and acute tubular necrosis may occur which leads to oliguria. Blood flow is further reduced by intravascular coagulation. Unless shock is aggressively treated within three hours of onset, it is usually irreversible.

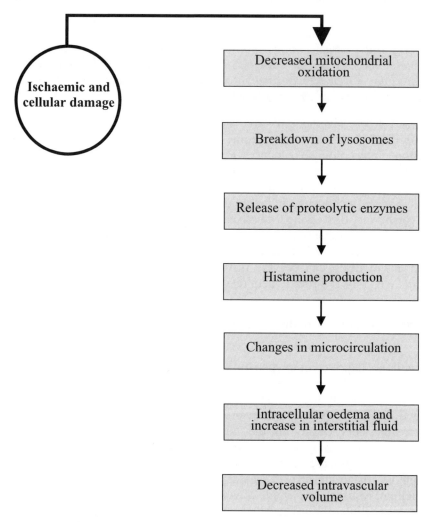

Figure 6.1: Ischaemic and cellular damage in shock

The types of shock and their clinical symptoms are shown in *Figure 6.2.*

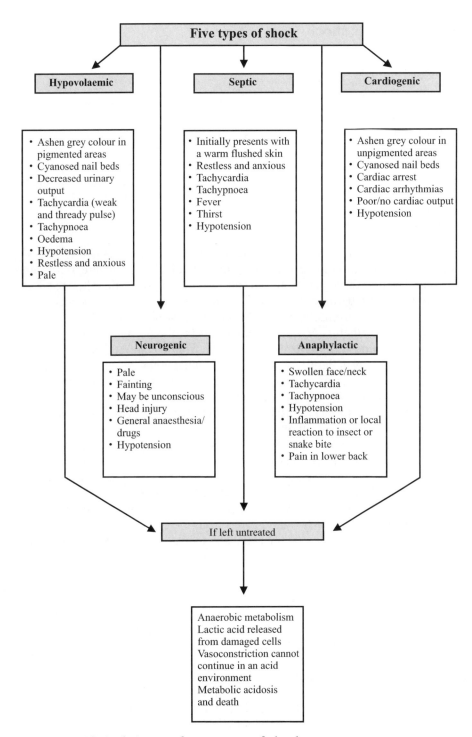

Figure 6.2: Clinical signs and symptoms of shock

Classification of shock

Cardiogenic shock

Cardiogenic shock is often referred to as 'pump failure' and is characterised by low cardiac output, eg. from myocardial damage or cardiac arrhythmias. The result of too little blood being pumped into the arteries is inadequate tissue perfusion of vital organs and unless the basic disorder is corrected the cardiogenic shock will lead to the heart being unable to supply its own coronary vessels. The resulting myocardial hypoxia can result in serious damage or death. Respiratory function may also be compromised due to pulmonary oedema.

Hypovolaemic shock

Haemorrhage is the most common cause of hypovolaemic shock although body fluid can be lost through excessive vomiting, diarrhoea, severe burns and sweating. The decreased venous return caused by the blood or fluid loss results in the stimulation of baroreceptors in the aorta and carotid arteries leading to stimulation of the vasomotor centre in the medulla oblongata. This serves to activate the sympathetic nervous system to release the hormone adrenalin from the adrenal medulla and indirectly aldosterone from the adrenal cortex.

The increased osmolarity of the blood stimulates the posterior pituitary to secrete anti-diuretic hormone (ADH). These hormones cause vasoconstriction, increasing cardiac output and decreasing urinary output. The resulting constrictions will also increase the venous return to the heart, but this cannot successfully compensate if fluid loss continues.

Slow fluid loss can result in the blood volume being reduced as much as 10–20% without cellular anoxia resulting. If the loss is greater, or continues, sudden cardiovascular taxation or cardiac arrest will ensue (Drake and Kidd, 1989). Electrolyte imbalance can occur due to reduced synthesis of cellular adenosine triphosphate (ATP). As a result the sodium pump fails, allowing an influx of sodium and water into the cells. Potassium escapes from the cell causing hyperkalaemia. Combined with sodium pump failure and the vasodilating effects of bradykinin and histamine, the whole situation becomes a cascade (Walsh, 1990).

Septic shock (endotoxic shock)

Septic shock is usually caused by an overwhelming bacterial infection. The bacteria most commonly responsible are Gramnegative enteric bacilli. The bacteria may invade phagocytes causing damage or even death of the cell thereby releasing histamine and proteolytic enzymes leading to vasodilation and increased capilliary permeability. Endotoxin release from the bacteria leads to complement activation, chemotaxis of white cells, membrane damage and pyrexia. Histamine is thought to interfere with normal reactivity of the blood vessels if it is released in large quantities (Budassi and Barber, 1981).

The severe vasodilation and resulting hypotension of septic shock may cause a fall in the glomerular filtration rate, resulting in acute tubular necrosis, oliguria and an inability to concentrate urine effectively. Other features of sepsis are DIC, respiratory failure and glucose intolerance.

Anaphylactic shock

Anaphylaxis is the result of an antigen-antibody reaction. This may occur from the infusion of incorrectly cross-matched blood products, drugs (mainly penicillin), cheese, investigative dyes, or insect and snake bites. The result is the degranulation of mast cells and the release of large amounts of histamine and bradykinin which can result in laryngeal oedema and bronchospasm leading to asphyxiation. The resulting agglutination from a transfusion of mismatched blood products may ultimately result in poor tissue perfusion caused by intravascular haemolysis especially in the kidneys.

Toxic shock syndrome also falls into the category of anaphylaxis and is commonly due to toxins released following *Staphylococcus aureus* infection of the genital tract in association with tampon use.

Neurogenic shock

Neurogenic shock is the result of loss of both sympathetic and parasympathetic control that can lead to the dilation of venules, capillaries, and arterioles (Beland and Passos, 1981). Common causes are severe head injury, neurogenic illness, eg. Guillain-Barré syndrome, drugs and anaesthetics. However, fright can cause a degree of hypotension, which is produced by central or peripheral vasomotor activity associated with a decrease in the contractility and capacity of blood vessels.

Nursing responsibilities

Most patients in shock will be admitted to an intensive therapy unit (ITU) or a high dependency ward (*Table 6.1*). As shock is life-threatening, the nurse must be aware of the following responsibilities.

Table 6.1: Initial investigations for shock	
1.	Diagnose the cause of the shock.
2.	Blood gas analysis.
3.	X-ray.
4.	Haemoglobin and haematocrit levels.
5.	Crossmatch for blood if haemorrhage is suspected.

Observations

Although complicated equipment is attached to the patient in the ITU to monitor progress, the nurse will need to observe the general condition of the patient and not merely the readings from the machinery. Any changes in skin colour, excessive oozing from a wound, restlessness and confusion should be reported urgently.

Patients should have their blood pressure measured at least every 30 minutes until their condition stabilises. The nurse should watch for decreasing blood pressure and measure any change in heart rate. The strength of the pulse along with any irregularities should also be recorded. A monitor is useful for measuring heart rate as there is less likelihood of errors in calculation.

The patient's core and peripheral temperatures will need to be recorded to ensure that there is no loss of peripheral circulation. Shocked patients will need to be warmed slowly to prevent peripheral vasodilation. A peripheral temperature probe placed on the patient's toe is ideal for measuring peripheral temperature. The core temperature can be recorded with a rectal probe which can be left in place until the nurse is satisfied that the patient's condition is stabilising (*Table 6.2*).

The patient may be attached to a cardiac monitor; cardiac arrhythmias or general pump failure can be seen in the initial stages of shock and should be reported immediately. The central venous pressure should be measured regularly, especially if blood or fluids are being replaced. Any fluctuation of more than +3 or –3 mmHg should also be reported (*Table 6.2*). Some patients may need to have their pulmonary artery wedge pressure (PAWP) measured. Any increase in the PAWP could indicate fluid overload and should be recorded regularly.

Table 6.2: Intervention and management for shock	
1.	Restabilise blood and body fluid volumes.
2.	Insert one or more intravenous cannulae for infusions.
3.	Swan-Ganz catheterisation.
4.	Encourage a diuresis and monitor urine output by catheterisation.
5.	Give oxygen at a concentration of 40% at 4–6 litres/minute (initially). Mechanical ventilation if necessary.
6.	Replace lost fluid.
7.	Insert a CVP (central venous pressure) line.
8.	Correct metabolic disturbance.
9.	Treat any underlying infection.
10.	Take temperature two-hourly at first.

Fluid balance

No fluids or food will be given orally until the patient's condition improves sufficiently for bowel sounds to be heard. Therefore, frequent mouth care is essential to ensure that the patient's mouth remains moist, clean and free from infection. Large amounts of fluid that have to be transfused in a hurry should be warmed. Intravenous pumps are often used and it is the nurse's responsibility to ensure that they are correctly set, checked and labelled. Some ITU beds have machines that allow the patient to be weighed while still in bed. This can be useful in determining fluid balance.

The increase in the secretion of aldosterone and ADH is a compensatory measure in shock, and this activates the renin angiotensin system, which assists in conserving body fluid and supporting the blood pressure. Patients usually have a urinary catheter inserted on admission and a burette type of urine bag can be used to measure hourly urine output. Volumes of 1 ml/kg/h or less should be reported (*Table 6.2*). Catheter care must be done at regular intervals. Low-dose inotropes, eg. dopamine may be used to optimise renal blood flow and diuretics such as frusemide or mannitol may be necessary to maintain a diuresis.

The patient in bed

The patient should lie fairly flat, and must be turned at least every two hours to prevent fluid accumulation in the lungs. A minimal amount of personal hygiene and care should be performed by the patient.

Respiratory assistance

The patient will probably be given oxygen. This may be delivered for a short period via nasal cannulae or a properly fitted face mask; however, in the long term, humidified oxygen should be used to prevent damage to the bronchial mucosa and cilia and to help promote expectoration of secretions. Some patients need the assistance of mechanical ventilation, and a volume cycled ventilator is usually used (*Table 6.2*). Respiratory rate and depth must be recorded and regularly assessed if the patient is breathing unaided. Tachypnoea may be a sign that the patient is distressed and will need assistance mechanically. If the patient is ventilated, regular machine readings, endotracheal suction and physiotherapy will be required.

Dealing with relatives and friends

Relatives and friends should always be informed of the patient's progress. This will allow them to express their anxieties and fears. Often there is little time to prepare relatives and friends for either a critical intervention or death. Indeed, 80–85% of patients with cardiogenic shock die. It is important that when the outlook is bleak nurses do not give people undue optimism. Even though relatives may be expecting the worst, they are usually greatly shocked when the patient deteriorates or dies.

It is often argued that doctors should inform relatives of the patient's prognosis. However, it is increasingly felt that as nurses spend more time forming relationships with the patient and their relatives, they are in the best position to do so. It should be noted that the next of kin is not always the person closest to the patient, eg. a homosexual, unmarried couple may be cohabiting, but the relationship is not recognised in law. Nurses need to develop a sensitivity concerning such relationships, in the same way as they would with cohabiting heterosexual partners (Dyer, 1991). Many patients who suffer from shock are admitted to ITU where, sadly, the facilities to break bad news are often not very private (*Table 6.3*).

Table 6.3: Step-by-step guide to giving progress reports or bad news
1.   Find a private room to take relatives or friends.
2.   The nurse or doctor should be someone that the relatives or friends have met or spoken to before.
3.   Inform them of the progression of the patient's condition to a state of shock or death.
4.   Describe the resuscitation employed or attempted.
5.   Explain the main physiological problems in clear simple language.
6.   Explain how the patient responded to any resuscitative measures and any outstanding physiological problems.
7.   Explain the extent of the seriousness of the patient's physiological instability or why you think they died.

Complications of shock

If the shock is not treated patients will not be able to physiologically compensate and the condition will become irreversible, resulting in death. Disseminating intravascular coagulation (DIC) is a serious complication of shock, particularly in septic shock. Diffuse haemorrhage and thrombosis are often seen with Gram-negative septicaemia. The nurse must observe for pupura, petechiae, sacral cyanosis, haemorrhagic bullae and excessive bleeding. If the metabolic state is not stabilised, metabolic acidosis and death will follow.

Key points

* Shock is a life-threatening condition requiring sound physiological knowledge in its management.

* Different types of shock can be classified according to the cause: cardiogenic, hypovolaemic, septic, anaphylactic and neurogenic.
* Relating the nursing responsibilities to physiological events is essential.
* A clear understanding of the nursing/medical interventions and management can save lives and prevent serious tissue damage.

My thanks to Michael Wilkes (School of Communication, Birmingham Polytechnic) for his help with producing the art work, and to Judy Hubbard and Dr Roy Smith (School of Health Sciences, Birmingham Polytechnic) for their physiology advice.

References

Beland IL, Passos JY (1981) *Clinical Nursing — Pathophysiological and Psychosocial Approaches*. 4th edn. Macmillan Publishing Company, London

Budassi SA, Barber JM (1981) *Emergency Nursing — Principles and Practice*. CV Mosby, London

Drake M, Kidd JR (1989) Infection, shock and trauma. In: Game C, Anderson E, Kidd JR, eds *Medical Surgical Nursing — A core text*. Churchill Livingstone, London

Dyer ID (1991) Meeting the needs of visitors — a practical approach. *Intensive Care Nurs* **7**: 135–47

Walsh M (1990) *Accident and Emergency Nursing — A New Approach*. 2nd edn. Heinemann Nursing, Oxford

7

Treatment of venous leg ulcers: one

Clare Williams

The management of venous ulcers is an important issue for many healthcare professionals. If treatment is to be successful, it is vital that clinicians understand the physiology and disease processes of the venous system in general, and of venous ulceration in particular. This chapter presents an outline of the normal physiology of the venous system in the lower limb followed by a brief history of venous leg ulcers and an in-depth analysis of the way in which venous disease can lead to ulceration. The analysis compares traditional theories of leg ulcer development with current hypotheses.

A diverse range of disease processes, including metabolic disorders and deficiencies, can result in the formation of an ulcer on the leg or foot. However, most ulcers are associated with venous and/or arterial insufficiency.

Two studies in Britain have estimated the prevalence of leg ulcers at between 0.15% (Callam *et al*, 1985) and 0.18% (Cornwall *et al*, 1986) of the total population. It is estimated that 70% of venous ulcers are the result of chronic venous hypertension (Morison and Moffatt, 1994).

Venous disease is known to affect approximately one quarter of the adult population in the UK (Franks *et al*, 1992). This means that the estimated £400 million that is currently spent per annum on largely ineffective leg ulcer care (Bosanquet, 1992) looks set to rise.

Anatomy and physiology

An understanding of the aetiology of venous ulceration requires anatomical and physiological knowledge of the venous system of the lower limb and the mechanics of its blood flow.

Veins convey blood from the tissues back to the heart. Blood is collected from the capillaries by small veins, termed venules, which then drain the blood into the veins. Veins are composed of three layers of tissue surrounding a hollow core, the lumen.

1. The inner layer is the tunica intima which is composed of endothelium, a subendothelial layer and an internal elastic lamina.

2. The middle layer is the tunica media which is composed of endothelium.

3. The outer layer is the tunica adventitia (*Figure 7.1*).

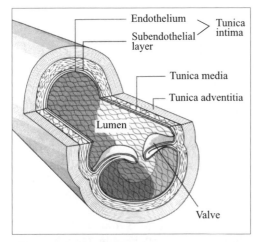

Endothelium — Tunica intima
Subendothelial layer
Tunica media
Tunica adventitia
Lumen
Valve

Figure 7.1: Structure of the vein. Adapted from Marieb (1992)

Veins have considerably less elastic tissue and smooth muscle than arteries but more white fibrous tissue.

The pressure of blood flowing through veins is considerably lower than that in arteries, and this accounts for the difference in their structures. The low blood pressure in veins has disadvantages. When a person is standing up, the pressure pushing blood up the veins in the lower limbs is barely enough to balance the force of gravity pushing blood back down. For this reason, many veins, especially those in the lower limbs, contain valves to prevent the backflow of blood. Blood flows through this system of closed vessels because of the continuous drop in pressure.

Although blood pressure is constantly decreasing from the aorta to the inferior vena cava, the velocity of the blood flow decreases as blood flows through the aorta, arterioles and capillaries, but then increases as it passes into the venules and veins. This is important as it allows the exchange of materials between blood and body tissues.

The movement of water and dissolved substances, except proteins, through the capillary wall is dependent on several opposing forces or pressures. Some forces push fluid out of the capillaries into the surrounding interstitial spaces, resulting in filtration.

Not all of the fluid filtered at one end of the capillary is reabsorbed at the other end. Some of the filtered fluid, together with any proteins that escape from the blood into the interstitial fluid, is returned via the lymphatic system.

Venous system and mechanics of blood flow

The lower limb contains both superficial and deep veins (*Figure 7.2*). The superficial long and short saphenous veins are designed to carry blood under low pressure and have many valves to prevent the backflow of blood. They lie outside the deep fascia and drain into the deep venous system, ie. the popliteal and femoral veins. The deep veins are designed to carry blood back to the heart under much higher pressure, and have fewer valves. The superficial and deep systems are connected by perforating veins which pass through the fascia.

Blood is returned to the heart from the periphery via the venous system by a combination of mechanisms acting together. These include compression of the veins by muscle contraction and variations in intraabdominal and intrathoracic pressures.

Active calf muscles in their semi-rigid fascial envelope act as a pump, forcing deep venous blood upwards towards the heart. When the valves in the perforating veins are healthy and intact, they prevent the backflow of blood to the superficial system (*Figure 7.3*). During periods of muscle relaxation, blood flows from the superficial veins to areas of temporarily lower pressure in the deep veins beneath the closed valves, before the calf muscle pump acts again to force this blood away from the extremities.

If valves in the perforating veins become incompetent, the back pressure is transmitted directly to the superficial venous system, reversing the flow, damaging more distal valves and eventually leading to varicose veins (*Figure 7.4*). Damaged valves in the deep and perforating veins are one cause of chronic venous hypertension in the lower limb, with high back pressure causing venous stasis and oedema.

The ankle movement produced by walking is also important, as the contraction and relaxation of the Achilles tendon alternately stretches and relaxes the calf muscle independently of calf muscle contraction, further aiding venous return. Emptying of the veins of the foot is facilitated by external pressure as the heel strikes the ground during walking. In patients who are immobile for long periods, neither the foot pump nor the calf muscle pump can operate and the efficiency of venous return is markedly impaired.

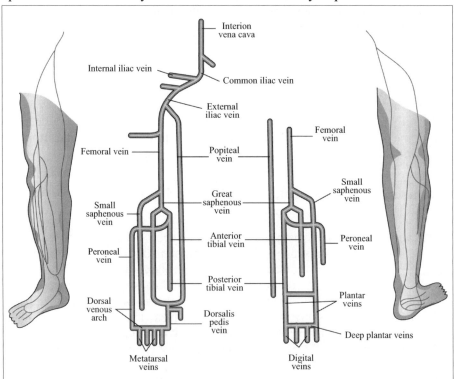

Figure 7.2: Veins of the right lower limb. Adapted from Marieb (1992)

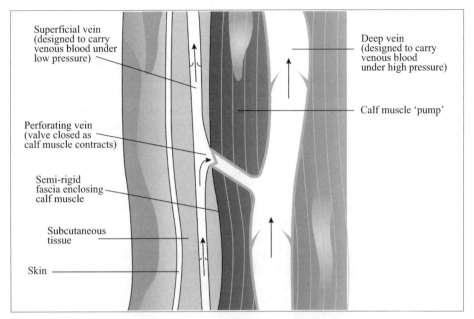

Figure 7.3: Healthy intact valves prevent the backflow of blood from the deep to the superficial veins. Adapted from Morison and Moffatt (1994)

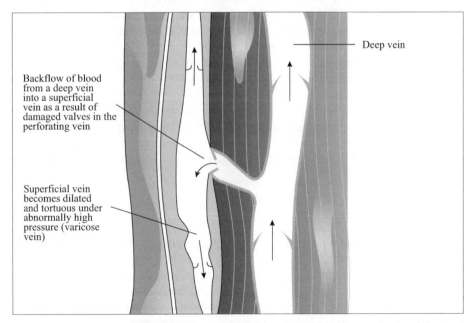

Figure 7.4: An incompetent valve in a perforating vein allows the backflow of blood from the deep to the superficial venous system. Adapted from Morison and Moffatt (1994)

History of venous disease and ulceration

Ulceration of the legs was much more common in the eighteenth and early nineteenth centuries and occurred in much younger people. The evidence for this has been found mainly in hospital records and dispensary and medical records of the armed forces. It is likely that the underlying pathology was much more varied in the past and it is possible that ascorbic acid deficiency may have played a significant part in the high frequency of leg ulcers (London, 1981; Bruijn and Bruijn, 1991).

Today, leg ulcers are regarded as a disease of elderly female patients. During the eighteenth and early nineteenth centuries, however, they were much more common in men than in women. By the early twentieth century the incidence of leg ulcers had fallen and a complete reversal of both age and sex ratios had occurred (*Journal of the Royal College of General Practitioners*, 1981).

Scott (1992) reviewed the literature on venous diseases through the ages and reported that a large number of old theories were based on both science and conjecture. There was a good understanding of venous ulceration even in ancient times, despite the lack of knowledge of fundamental mechanisms of physiology and pathology.

Until recently, estimates of the prevalence of chronic leg ulceration were based on a small amount of data from selected populations. In the last decade, however, several detailed studies into the epidemiology of chronic leg ulceration and its association with venous disease have been undertaken.

Information on the true prevalence of this condition is essential for the planning and provision of appropriate resources. Callam (1992) reviewed the prevalence of chronic venous ulceration in western countries and concluded that active chronic leg ulceration has a point prevalence of 0.1–0.2% of the adult population.

Thus 1–2% of the population will suffer from leg ulceration at some point in their lives. Women appear to be slightly more prone to this condition and there is a marked increase in the prevalence of chronic leg ulceration with age. Evidence of venous disease will be found in 60–80% of ulcerated legs.

Pathogenesis of venous ulceration

There is now general agreement that venous ulceration results from failure to lower the venous pressure in the veins of the lower limb on exercise. This may be due to disease of the deep veins, the superficial veins or the communicating veins (Scurr and Coleridge Smith, 1992a; Loosemore and Dormandy, 1993; Burton, 1994). At cellular level, the sequence of events between raised venous pressure and venous ulceration is unclear and remains controversial.

Although venous disease is rarely life-threatening, it represents a considerable drain on health resources. The identification of risk factors is therefore essential in order to counteract this (Coleridge Smith, 1992; Moffatt and Franks, 1994) (*Table 7.1*).

Deep vein thrombosis (DVT) is important in the development of varicose veins and venous ulceration. Long periods of prolonged bed rest are associated with an increased rate of DVT, and the type and length of surgical operations also affect the outcome.

The exact mechanism whereby chronic venous hypertension causes trophic skin changes which result in chronic ulceration is not fully understood. Morison and Moffatt (1994) described the clinical signs of chronic venous hypertension.

Varicose veins are a sign of chronic venous hypertension. In this condition, the superficial venous network is exposed to much higher pressures than normal and the thin-walled superficial veins become dilated, lengthened and tortuous. It is not clear whether varicose veins and venous ulcers are merely associated conditions with a common aetiology, or whether varicose veins are a predisposing factor for venous ulceration.

Table 7.1: Risk factors for venous disease	
Varicose veins	The presence of any dilated, elongated or tortuous vessels
Age and sex	A number of studies have demonstrated an increase in prevalence with age and significant differences between the sexes. Women are over three times more likely to suffer from varicose veins than men
Race	Non-whites are reported to be less susceptible to venous disease
Social factors	Anecdotally, venous disease is reported to be a disease of the lower social classes
Body shape	Increased body weight has been consistently associated with the development of varicose veins. Obesity is also often accompanied by other factors such as immobility, menarche and menopause. It has long been recognised that varicose veins have been associated with pregnancy, the risk doubling in women who have had two or more pregnancies. Increasing age at menarche together with age at menopause give an increased risk of varicose veins
Reduced physical activity	Has also been associated with venous disease. Functional changes occur in immobile patients as a result of reduced calf muscle pump function and a rise in venous pressure which is exacerbated on dependency
Source: Moffatt and Franks (1994)	

Staining of the skin in the gaiter area is caused by chronic venous hypertension leading to distention of blood capillaries, which results in damage to the endothelial walls and leakage of red blood cells and large protein molecules into the interstitial fluid. Destruction of the red blood cells releases the breakdown products of haemoglobin, causing pigmentation.

Ankle flare, or distension of the tiny veins on the medial aspect of the foot, is particularly noticeable when the valves in the perforating veins of the ankle and lower calf are incompetent. Atrophy of the skin or thinning of the dermis is associated with a poor blood supply and makes the skin very susceptible to trauma. Eczematous changes in the skin are often linked with venous insufficiency, but can also be aggravated by a number of wound care products through irritation and allergy. Lipodermatosclerosis is a 'woody' induration of the tissues in which fat is replaced by fibrotic tissue; it is often seen as an end-stage phenomenon.

The precise mechanisms leading to ulceration are not fully understood and are still the subject of intense debate. They can be described in terms of either macrocirculatory changes or microcirculatory changes.

Macrocirculatory changes

Loosemore and Dormandy (1993) reviewed the macrocirculatory changes associated with venous ulceration. They described these broadly as reflux, retrograde flow or obstruction to outflow, leading to ambulatory venous hypertension and reflux. In the past, all venous ulcers were believed to be secondary to deep vein disease. More recently, it has become widely accepted that superficial vein disease alone can result in raised ambulatory venous pressure.

In the superficial veins the cause of reflux is usually primary valve failure. In the deep and perforating veins the valve incompetence may be primary or secondary to DVT.

Microcirculatory changes

Several hypotheses have been proposed to explain the link between raised venous hypertension and the cutaneous microcirculatory changes which can lead to venous ulceration. The two most recent theories are the fibrin cuff and the white blood cell trapping hypotheses. Earlier theories involved stasis (Homans, 1917), arteriovenous shunting (Pinlachs and Vidal-Barraquer, 1953), tissue hypoxia (Holmans, 1917), lymphatic obstruction (Bollinger *et al*, 1982) and macroangiopathy (Fagren, 1982).

Fibrin cuff: The fibrin cuff hypothesis was put forward by Browse and Burnard (1982). Reviews of the hypothesis have been carried out by Scurr and Coleridge Smith (1992a,b), Loosemore and Dormandy (1993) and Burton (1994). Browse and Burnard (1982) proposed that oxygen diffusion into the tissue of the skin is restricted by a pericapillary fibrin cuff (which they had observed histologically). They suggested that increased capillary pressure as a consequence of the raised venous pressure results in an increased loss of plasma proteins through the capillary wall. These proteins include fibrinogen, which polymerises to give the fibrin cuff.

Measurements of protein loss from capillaries showed that fibrinogen was the most important plasma protein leaking into the tissues in patients with venous disease. They also demonstrated reduced fibrinolytic activity in the blood and veins, which might explain why the fibrin cuff persists. In this theory of ulceration, the fibrin cuff has a central role in restricting the supply of oxygen to the tissues.

There is, however, no published evidence that fibrin provides a barrier to oxygen diffusion. It has been calculated that a fibrin layer containing 0.5% fibrin, ie. similar to the composition of a fibrin blood clot, would not impair oxygen delivery to the tissues (Scurr and Coleridge Smith, 1992a). Browse and Burnard (1982) had used bovine fibrin for their studies, and it is now thought that it is unlikely to have the same compositions as human fibrin.

After looking for evidence of reduced tissue oxygenation in patients with venous disease, Scurr and Coleridge Smith (1992a) concluded that it was unlikely that patients with chronic venous insufficiency would have an abnormality in the delivery of oxygen to the tissues. Many workers now question this hypothesis in the light of new evidence (Scurr and Coleridge Smith, 1992b; Loosemore and Dormandy, 1993).

Following their major clinical trial, Herrick *et al* (1992) described the changing patterns of tissue architecture and extracellular matrix synthesis during healing. Initial biopsies indicated prominent fibrin cuffs. These were highly organised structures composed of laminin, fibronectin, tenacin, collagen, trapped leucocytes and fibrin (*Table 7.2*). After two weeks of pressure bandaging therapy, haemosiderin, acute inflammation and granulation tissue with the deposition of fibronectin had all increased. Complete epithelialisation was frequently seen by the fourth week of treatment. By this time, haemosiderin and red blood cell extravasation had decreased and fibrin cuffs were virtually absent, although chronic inflammation remained. Herrick *et al* (1992) concluded that fibrin cuffs may inhibit angiogenesis in addition to their previously ascribed role in causing tissue ischaemia.

Table 7.2: The functions of proteins involved in the fibrin cuff theory of venous ulceration	
Laminin	Present in the basement plasma membrane along with collagen
Fibronectin	A chemotactic factor released by macrophages which attract fibroblasts to the wound
Fibrin	A substance (threads) formed in the blood as it clots. The threads then form a close meshwork
Collagen	Forms a framework during granulation for migration and re-epithelialisation
Leucocytes	White blood cells that play an important role in the defence mechanism against infection
Tenacin	A protein involved in cell adhesion
Haemosiderin	The breakdown product of red blood cells

The white blood cell trapping hypothesis: This hypothesis proposes that at reduced perfusion pressure, white blood cells are trapped in the microcirculation.

These trapped cells become activated and release proteolytic enzymes, superoxide radicals and chemotactic substances. Thus a vicious cycle of endothelial and tissue cell damage is established, with further white blood cell and platelet recruitment.

Leucocytes have been shown to accumulate in the dependent limbs of healthy subjects, and to accumulate to a greater extent in patients with chronic venous insufficiency. These acute changes are reversible when the leg is elevated (Coleridge Smith, 1992). Free radicals are released following activation of white blood cells and are known to be involved in the mechanism of injury following ischaemia. It seems that much of the tissue damage is due to active destruction rather than cell death from hypoxia alone (Scurr and Coleridge Smith, 1992b).

Scott *et al* (1989) demonstrate white blood cells trapping in the legs of patients with chronic venous insufficiency in response to raised venous pressure. Capillary microscopy confirmed that the number of functional capillaries fell in response to an increase in venous pressure.

Scott *et al* (1991) also demonstrated an increased number of white blood cells in the skin of patients with venous disease resulting in lipodermatosclerosis. Those patients whose disease was sufficiently severe to result in ulceration had significantly more white blood cells than those in whom ulceration had never occurred. This study could not establish whether the increased white blood cell content of the skin was a cause or a result of the skin changes.

It is not known whether the mechanisms described in these two hypotheses are sufficient to result in skin necrosis. It is certainly the case, however, that when an inflammatory skin response is later followed by an additional stimulus that activates the cells present in the tissues, rapid necrosis of the skin results. In patients with venous disease, the skin conditions that are present might permit such a reaction to progress. The inflammatory infiltrate is already available and only requires some minor trigger to precipitate tissue destruction. This might explain why patients with lipodermatosclerosis are at high risk of ulceration in response to minor trauma of the leg (Scurr and Coleridge Smith, 1992b).

Falanga and Eaglsein (1993) described a new hypothesis for venous ulceration. They proposed that fibrin and other macromolecules leak into the dermis and trap growth factors and other stimulatory or homeostatic substances, rendering them unavailable for the maintenance of tissue integrity and repair. Bradbury *et al* (1993) and Stacey *et al* (1993) also reviewed the role of white blood cells and other forms of trapping.

Conclusion

The microcirculatory changes that result in venous ulceration are not completely understood. The fibrin cuff and white blood cell trapping hypotheses are not mutually exclusive, and together they can explain some of the observations noted in patients with venous disease.

A complete understanding of the pathophysiological process of ulceration might lead to a combination of pharmacological therapy for microcirculatory changes, and compression therapy for macrocirculatory changes. This could result in faster healing and possibly a lower recurrence rate.

Key points

* The estimated prevalence of leg ulcers is between 0.15 and 0.18% of the total population, most of which are venous and/or arterial in origin.
* An understanding of venous ulceration requires an understanding of the anatomy and physiology of the venous system of the lower limb.
* The precise mechanisms leading to ulceration are not fully understood, but can be described as either macrocirculatory or microcirculatory.
* The two main hypotheses are the fibrin cuff and the white cell trapping theories.

References

Bollinger A, Isensing G, Franzeck UK (1982) Lymphatic microangiopathy: a complication of severe chronic venous incompetence. *Lymphology* **15**: 60–5

Bosanquet N (1992) Cost of venous ulcers: from maintenance therapy to investment programmes. *Phlebology* **7**(1): 44–6

Bradbury AW, Murie JA, Ruckley CV (1993) Role of the leucocyte in the pathogenesis of vascular disease. *Br J Surg* **80**: 1503–12

Browse NL, Burnard KG (1982) The cause of venous ulceration. *Lancet* **8282**: 243–5

Bruijn IDR, Bruijn GW (1991) An eighteenth century medical hearing and the first observation of tropical Phagedaena. *Med Hist* **35**: 295–307

Burton CS (1994) Venous ulcers. *Am J Surg* **167** (suppl 1a): 37s–41s

Callam MJ, Ruckley CV, Harper DR *et al* (1985) Chronic ulceration of the leg: extent of the problem and provision of care. *Br Med J* **290**: 1855–6

Callam M (1992) Prevalence of chronic leg ulceration and severe chronic venous disease in Western countries. *Phlebology* **7**(1): 6–12

Coleridge Smith PD (1992) Consensus paper on venous leg ulcers. *Phlebology* **7**: 48–58

Cornwall JV, Dore CJ, Lewis JD (1986) Leg ulcers: epidemiology and aetiology. *Br J Surg* **73**: 693–6

Fagren B (1982) Microcirculatory disturbances — the final cause for venous leg ulcers? *Phlebology* **11**: 101–3

Falanga V, Eaglstein WH (1993) The 'trap' hypothesis of venous ulceration. *Lancet* **341**: 1006–8

Franks PJ, Wright DDI, Moffatt CJ *et al* (1992) Prevalence of venous disease: a community study in West London. *Eur J Surg* **158**: 143–7

Herrick SE, Sloan P, McGurk M *et al* (1992) Sequential changes in histologic pattern and extracellular matrix deposition during the healing of chronic venous ulcers. *Am J Pathol* **141**(5): 1085–95

Homans J (1917) The aetiology and treatment of varicose ulcers of the leg. *Surg Gynaecol Obstet* **24**: 300–11

Journal of the Royal College of General Practitioners (1981) Leg ulcers: past and present. *J R Coll Gen Pract* **31**: 260–1

London ISL (1981) Leg ulcers in the eighteenth and early nineteenth centuries. *J R Coll Gen Pract* **31**: 263–73

Loosemore TM, Dormandy JA (1993) Pathophysiology of venous ulceration. *Vascular Med Rev* **4**: 49–57

Marieb EN (1992) *Human Anatomy and Physiology*. Benjamin/Cummings, California

Moffatt CJ, Franks PJ (1994) A prerequisite underlining the treatment programme: risk factors associated with venous disease. *Prof Nurse* **9**(9): 637–42

Morison M, Moffatt C (1994) *A Colour Guide to the Assessment and Management of Leg Ulcers*. Times Mirror International, London

Pinlachs P, Vidal-Barraquer F (1953) Pathogenic study of varicose veins. *Angiology* **4**: 59–100

Scott HJ (1992) History of venous disease and early management. *Phlebology* **7**(suppl 1): 2–5

Scott HJ, McMullin GMJ, Coleridge Smith PD *et al* (1989) Venous ulceration: the role of the white blood cell. *Phlebology* **4**: 153–9

Scott HJ, Coleridge Smith PD, Scurr JH (1991) Histological study of white blood cells and their association with lipodermatosclerosis and venous ulceration. *Br J Surg* **78**: 210–1

Scurr JH, Coleridge Smith PD (1992a) Pathogenesis of venous ulceration. *Phlebology* **7**(suppl 1): 13–6

Scurr JH, Coleridge Smith PD (1992b) Venous disease: a role for the microcirculation. *Wounds* **4**(6): 236–40

Stacey MC, Burnard KG, Mahmoud-Alexandroni M *et al* (1993) Tissue and urokinase plasminogen activators in the environs of venous and ischaemic leg ulcers. *Br J Surg* **80**: 596–9

8

Treatment of venous leg ulcers: two

Clare Williams

This chapter discusses the treatment options available for venous leg ulceration, and their implications for the nursing profession. Current views on the use of compression therapy, drug therapy, growth factors and surgery are examined. Successful management of patients with venous leg ulcers depends on thorough assessment, effective treatment and prevention of recurrence. Many healthcare professionals lack the necessary knowledge, understanding and training to treat such patients effectively. Improvements in the care of venous leg ulcers will lead to significant reductions in treatment costs.

Compression therapy is the main treatment for venous leg ulceration. Other treatment options include drug therapy, the use of growth factors and surgical management.

The principal aim of any therapeutic regimen for the treatment of venous leg ulcers is reduction of the venous hypertension resulting from valvular incompetence. In ambulatory patients this can be accomplished either by surgical intervention to the superficial and perforating veins or by conservative management with compression bandaging (Cherry *et al*, 1992).

There are a number of non-invasive investigative techniques which allow more precise diagnosis of the extent and type of venous disease (Coleridge Smith, 1992), including photoplethysmography, light reflective rheology and duplex scanning.

Compression therapy

Compression bandaging improves the function of the calf muscle pump and reduces venous hypertension, which in turn leads to healing. The exact pressure needed to provide good compression therapy is disputed. It has been recognised for over 300 years that compression is an essential part of the treatment of venous leg ulcers, but we still do not know the optimal pressure or how to achieve it (Blair *et al*, 1987). According to Blair *et al* the optimal pressure may vary depending on the height and weight of the patient and the degree of venous incompetence. It is generally accepted that 20–40 mmHg pressure at the ankle graduating to the knee is sufficient. Before using compression bandaging it is vital to ensure that the arterial blood supply to the legs is adequate. The effects of graduated compression are shown in *Table 8.1*. Compression can also be applied by means of hosiery, inflatable pneumatic sleeves (Lawrence and Kakkar, 1980), hydrostatic devices or rigid gaiters of various types, including plasters.

Table 8.1: Effects of graduated compression on venous leg ulcers	
Increases	Local interstitial pressure
	Venous flow velocity (deep veins)
	Release of plasminogen activator
	Prostacyclin production
	Expelled calf volume on exercise
	Venous refilling time
	Local capillary clearance
	Transcutaneous oxygen tension
Decreases	Capacity and pressure in superficial veins
	Ambulatory venous pressure
	Oedema
	Lipodermatosclerosis
No change	Calf muscle blood flow
(<18 mmHg)	Subcutaneous blood flow
	Factor VIII activation

Thomas (1992, 1993) and McCollum (1992) divided compression bandages into four groups based on their ability to retain predetermined levels of tension under controlled laboratory conditions (*Table 8.2*). Bandages can also be classed as long-stretch, either single layer or multilayer, or short-stretch.

The perfect bandaging system for venous leg ulcers should have the characteristics shown in *Table 8.3*. It is important to keep in mind the skill of the bandager and the circumference of the patient's leg, as both factors will affect the pressure achieved under the bandage.

Blair *et al* (1988) compared the four-layer bandaging system with the traditional system of adhesive plaster bandaging and concluded that the former achieved sustained compression of 40 mmHg and improved the healing rates of venous leg ulcers. Duby *et al* (1993) compared a short-stretch bandage with the four-layer system in the treatment of venous leg ulcers and concluded that they gave comparable results. These are just two of numerous controlled trials which have compared different bandaging systems. There is still no consensus on which system is best. By elevating their legs during daily leisure time, patients with venous leg ulcers can themselves make an immense contribution to the rate at which their ulcers heal.

Table 8.2: The four groups of compression bandages
Light compression (14–17 mmHg at the ankle)
Moderate compression (18–24 mmHg at the ankle)
High compression (25–35 mmHg at the ankle)
Extra high compression (60 mmHg at the ankle)
Data from Thomas (1993)

Table 8.3: Ideal characteristics of a compression bandaging system
Extends from the base of the toes to the tibial tuberosity without gaps
Provides compression appropriate for the individual
Provides a gradient of pressure diminishing from the ankle to the upper calf
Provides pressure evenly distributed over the anatomical contours
Maintains pressure until the next change of dressing
Capable of remaining in position as originally applied until the next dressing change (usually for at least a week)
Functions in a complementary way with the dressing, providing additional absorptive capacity
Non-irritant and non-allergenic
Comfortable
Washable
Data from Ruckley (1992)

Drug therapy

There has been renewed interest in the use of drug therapy for venous ulcers. Colgan *et al* (1992) divided drug therapy into four main classes:

Fibrinolytics: These drugs are given in an attempt to reverse the effects of pericapillary fibrin cuffs, eg. stanozolol (an anabolic steroid).

Hydroxyrutosides: These drugs are given to restore the barrier properties of the fibre matrix between capillary endothelial cells, eg. praveon.

Prostaglandin E: The properties of this agent include vasodilatation, inhibition of platelet aggregation and inhibition of neutrophil activation.

Methylxanthines: Oxpentifylline has been used for many years. It increases red blood cell deformability, and thus improves oxygen delivery to the tissues. It also reduces white blood cell aggregation and activation and has mild fibrinolytic activity. These properties suggest a possible use for this drug in venous disease.

Colgan *et al* (1992) concluded that all of these agents require further research to establish their role in the management of patients with venous ulcers.

Layton *et al* (1994) reported a reduction in venous ulcer size in 52% of patients treated with aspirin compared with 26% of patients in the placebo group. The patients also received compression therapy. It should be noted, however, that the healing rates in both groups were remarkably poor compared with those in many clinical studies using compression alone.

Growth hormones

Some studies have looked into the effect of growth hormones on venous ulcers, and this therapy appears to have great potential.

Freak *et al* (1994) report the use of biosynthetic growth hormone to treat chronic venous ulcers. This growth hormone has been reported to improve the tensile strength of incisional wounds and to improve epithelialisation. It has also been shown to produce substantial increases in healing rates when applied topically to chronic venous ulcers. Unfortunately, the combination of occlusive dressings and fluid instillation in Freak *et al's* study led to such problems with skin maceration that the project had to be abandoned. The authors commented that they look forward to the development of an adequate delivery system so that the promising effect of low dose human growth hormone can be tested fully.

Falanga (1992) also endorsed the need for more research to test fully the optimal dose and delivery of growth hormone and combination of therapies in the management of venous ulcers.

Surgery

Many venous leg ulcers can be healed by conservative treatment with the use of compression. However, as Defriend *et al* (1992) pointed out, 10–15% of large chronic ulcers may not heal with conservative treatment and many ulcers that do heal will recur unless the underlying venous incompetence is corrected.

Surgery has a role in both skin grafting of larger ulcers to promote initial healing and correction of underlying venous incompetence to prevent ulcer recurrence (Young, 1992).

The results of surgery for venous ulceration, such as skin grafting, repair or replacement of damaged veins, valvuloplasty and valve transplantation, are often conflicting and difficult to assess (Defriend *et al*, 1992). There have been no properly conducted randomised controlled trials of the effects of venous surgery on either venous ulcer healing or recurrence.

It has been estimated that, in the UK, between £1000 and £5200 per patient per year, or a total of £400–600 million per annum, is spent on the treatment of leg ulcers (Podmore, 1994). These costs can be reduced dramatically with effective treatment; however, this treatment has implications for the nursing profession.

Nursing implications

The implications of venous leg ulcer treatment for the nursing profession lie in three areas:

1. Accurate assessment.
2. The development of community-based leg ulcer clinics.
3. Education.

The treatment of venous leg ulcers is very much nursing led, and until recently vast quantities of money were spent on largely ineffective care. In addition, venous leg ulcers have been shown to be principally a community nursing problem, with district nurses spending up to half their time managing leg ulcers (Moffatt *et al*, 1992; Podmore, 1994). Roe *et al* (1993) believe that the onus is on the community nurse to conduct an exhaustive and accurate nursing assessment. Where the diagnosis is uncertain the nurse should ensure that patients are seen by their GP and referred to a consultant where necessary (Phillips *et al*, 1994).

The effective management of venous leg ulcers need no longer be a hit-or-miss affair (Ertl, 1993). Successful management can be divided into three areas:

1. Assessment: looking for predisposing, perpetuating and presenting factors.
2. Effective treatment: treating the underlying cause, eliminating perpetuating factors and allowing the wound to heal.
3. Prevention of recurrence: surgery, compression hosiery and routine checks.

The first of these is, undoubtedly, the most important.

Assessment should encompass the general state of the patient and the specific characteristics of the limb and the lesion. Clinical inspection of the ulcer should include noting its appearance, site, size and depth. Examination of the limb should take into account: varicosities; the presence of local or general oedema; skin signs such as hypertrophic changes, eczema and dermatitis; and whether the limb is cold or warm to the touch. Although these factors alone cannot be relied upon for accurate diagnosis, they may give an indication of the underlying aetiology, as striking differences exist between arterial and venous ulcers. An assessment of the patient's past medical history may help to identify the underlying vascular problems which have led to the development of the ulcer. The blood glucose level should be checked for the possibility of undiagnosed diabetes. Wound swabs are only required where it is necessary to identify the nature and antibiotic sensitivity of organisms causing clinical signs of infection.

Indicators of possible venous problems include previous thrombogenic events such as deep vein thrombosis, thrombophlebitis or a leg or foot fracture in the affected limb. Other indicators are the presence of prominent superficial leg veins with signs of valve incompetence, and any history of varicose vein surgery or sclerotherapy in the affected leg.

The final part of the assessment should be a simple vascular assessment. In the past the presence of palpable foot pulses has been taken as a sign of unimpaired arterial circulation in the lower limb and their absence as a sign of arterial impairment. This is not an entirely fail-safe test and a vascular assessment should always be performed. The non-invasive assessment can give objective significance to the findings detected on clinical examination, the patient's reports of symptoms and any indicators of venous or arterial problems in the patient's past medical history.

Vascular assessment is carried out by means of a hand-held portable Doppler machine. This is a simple technique that can be readily performed by nurses following a period of supervised practice. It enables calculation of the resting pressure index or the ankle:brachial pressure index (ABPI; the ratio of the systolic pressure in the dorsalis pedis or posterior tibial artery of the ankle to that in the brachial artery).

The ABPI should normally be >1.0. Patients with an ABPI of 0.90–0.95 probably have some degree of arterial disease. If the ABPI is <0.8 the arterial blood supply is significantly impaired, and compression bandaging is contraindicated. An ABPI of >1.0 indicates calcification of the arteries. In diabetic patients a falsely high ratio may be obtained as the blood vessels are difficult to compress. Such patients should be referred to a vascular surgeon.

Callam *et al* (1987) found that 21% of 600 patients with chronic leg ulcers had a pressure index of ≤0.9. They concluded that careful assessment for arterial disease is mandatory before instituting compression therapy.

Having acknowledged that leg ulceration is a community problem it follows that the application of research-based treatment is community led. Many areas are now establishing community clinics to provide this care.

Moffatt and Oldroyd (1994) described a pioneering service called the Riverside Community Leg Ulcer Project which is supported by a major grant from the King's Fund. A network of six community clinics were developed in health centres and clinics throughout the district. The training needs of the project were considerable and it was obvious that there was a lack of resources and educational structure to meet this requirement. The Riverside Project highlighted the need for improved quality of care in the community for patients with chronic venous leg ulcers. Moffatt *et al* (1992) achieved substantial improvements in ulcer healing rates by providing a co-ordinated research-based service. Others have also described beneficial effects following the development of leg ulcer clinics (Awenat, 1992).

Future developments

Nurse education has not kept pace with the rapid developments in leg ulcer management. It is vital that nurses have more training in assessment and treatment to enable them to provide effective care for patients with venous leg ulcers.

In order to improve their assessment of venous leg ulcers, nurses require a greater understanding of the underlying anatomy of the venous system and the pathogenesis of venous ulceration. They also need training in the use of Doppler equipment and supervised practice. As regards the treatment of these patients, nurses need a greater understanding of compression bandaging and its application, together with supervised practice.

Moffatt and Karn (1994) reported that nurses received little formal training in the treatment of leg ulcers and persisted in using many unsuitable products; compression bandaging was rarely used. They described the development of a nationally recognised course in leg ulcer management, including both theory and practice. These authors concluded that as health authorities develop new services, they must appreciate that these have to be supported by comprehensive training programmes if they are to achieve improved health outcomes, and that education is not an optional extra.

Conclusion

A great many people are affected by venous disease and venous leg ulcers. As a nation we spend vast quantities of money on ineffective treatment because many healthcare professionals do not have the knowledge, understanding or training to treat these patients successfully. Research-based material is available that shows how the correct treatment can have dramatic effects on the healing rates of venous leg ulcers.

In order to understand how the treatment works, nurses must first understand the anatomy of the venous system of the lower limb and the mechanics of its blood flow. It is also important to have some knowledge of the pathogenesis of venous ulceration, although this area is hotly debated and not completely understood. Many researchers are striving for a complete understanding of the pathophysiological process.

Compression therapy is now a well-established treatment for venous leg ulcers. It is vital that healthcare professionals receive the education and training to enable them to assess their patients correctly and manage their subsequent care effectively. This area has not yet been developed to its full potential.

The future for leg ulcer care is very bright. Health professionals in many areas are involved in consensus meetings, and trust hospitals are at last funding educational and training initiatives. It should not be too long before estimates of the financial costs of leg ulcers are dramatically reduced.

Key points

* The main treatment for venous leg ulcers is compression therapy, but there are other options.

* Compression bandaging improves the function of the calf muscle and reduces venous hypertension.
* The treatment of leg ulcers has many implications for the nursing profession regarding assessment, leg ulcer clinics and education.
* Successful management is achieved by a combination of assessment, effective treatment and the prevention of recurrence.

References

Awenat Y (1992) Leg ulcer clinics: advanced nursing. *Nurs Standard* **4**(7): 4–7

Blair SD, Wright DDI, McCollum CN (1987) Comparison of high and low pressure compression bandages in healing chronic venous ulcers. Swiss Society of Phlebology and Practical Angiology, Swiss Society of Angiology, 2nd International Symposium, 14–16 May, Zurich

Blair SD, Wright DDI, Backhouse CM *et al* (1988) Sustained compression and healing of chronic venous ulcers. *Br Med J* **297**: 1159–61

Callum MJ, Harper DR, Dale JJ *et al* (1987) Arterial disease in chronic leg ulceration: an underestimated hazard? Lothian and Forth Valley Leg Ulcer Study. *Br Med J* **294**: 929–31

Cherry GW, Cameron J, Ryan TJ (1992) Management of leg ulcers: Oxford Dermatology Unit community liaison approach. *Phlebology* **7**(suppl 1): 27–32

Coleridge Smith PD (1992) Investigation of patients with venous ulceration. *Phlebology* **7**(suppl 1): 17–21

Colgan MP, Moore DJ, Shanik DG (1992) Drug therapy for venous ulcers: new methods of treatment. *Phlebology* **7**(suppl 1): 41–3

Defriend DJ, Edwards AT, McCollum C (1992) Treatment of venous ulceration — when is surgical management indicated? *Phlebology* **7**(suppl 1) 33–7

Duby T, Hoffman D, Cameron J *et al* (1993) A randomized trial in the treatment of venous leg ulcers comparing short stretch bandages, four layer bandage system, and a long stretch-paste bandage system. *Wounds* **5**(6): 276–9

Ertl P (1993) The multiple benefits of accurate assessment: effective management of leg ulcers. *Prof Nurse* **9**(2): 139–44

Falanga V (1992) Growth factors and wound repair. *J Tissue Viability* **2**(3): 101–4

Freak L, Simon D, Edwards AT *et al* (1994) The use of topical human growth hormone on chronic venous ulcers. *J Wound Care* **3**(2): 68–70

Lawrence D, Kakkar VV (1980) Graduated, static, external compression of the lower limb; a physiological assessment. *Br J Surg* **67**: 119–221

Layton AM, Ibbotson SH, Davies JA *et al* (1994) Randomised trial of oral aspirin for chronic venous leg ulcers. *Lancet* **344**: 164–5

McCollum C (1992) Extensible bandages. *Br Med J* **304**: 520–1

Moffatt CJ, Karn A (1994) Answering the call for more education: development of an ENB course in leg ulcer management. *Prof Nurse* **9**(10): 708–12

Moffatt CJ, Oldroyd MI (1994) A pioneering service to the community: the Riverside Community Leg Ulcer Project. *Prof Nurse* **9**(7): 486–97

Moffatt CJ, Franks PJ, Oldroyd M *et al* (1992) Community clinics for leg ulcers and impact on healing. *Br Med J* **305**: 1389–92

Phillips T, Stanton B, Provan A *et al* (1994) A study of the impact of leg ulcers on quality of life: financial, social and psychological implications. *J Am Acad Dermatol* **31**: 49–53

Podmore J (1994) Leg ulcers: weighing up the evidence. *Nurs Standard* **8**(38): 25–7

Roe BH, Luker KA, Cullum NA *et al* (1993) Assessment, prevention and monitoring of chronic leg ulcers in the community: report of a survey. *J Clin Nurs* **2**: 299–306

Ruckley CV (1992) Treatment of venous ulceration — compression therapy. *Phlebology* **7**(suppl 1): 22–6

Thomas S (1992) Extensible bandages. *Br Med J* **304**: 984–5: 64

Thomas S (1993) Bandages and bandaging. *Pharm J* 29 May: 744–5

Young RAL (1992) A surgeon's personal view of managing venous ulcers in the community. *Phlebology* **7**(suppl 1): 38–40

9

Acute MI: analysing health status and setting immediate priorities

Neal F Cook and Vidar Melby

This chapter uses a case study approach to demonstrate how awareness of recent research findings and a sound understanding of pathophysiology enable the nurse to become an effective practitioner. A scenario is described in which the nurse is faced with a man admitted to the coronary care unit with a diagnosis of suspected acute myocardial infarction (AMI). Through analysis of the patient's health status, with frequent reference to pathophysiology, the nurse can perform an accurate nursing assessment and so determine immediate priorities for nursing care. The priority objectives were identified as pain control, management of cardiogenic shock, reperfusion of the myocardium, cardiac monitoring for complications of AMI and the effects of treatment, and management of anxiety. Research-based rationales are provided for all objectives.

This chapter sets out to demonstrate how an understanding of pathophysiology and awareness of recent research findings enable the nurse to analyse a patient's health status comprehensively and holistically.

A scenario is described in which the nurse is faced with a man admitted to the coronary care unit with a suspected diagnosis of acute myocardial infarction (AMI) (see *page 89).* The analytical skills of the nurse are crucial for the setting of appropriate objectives for care in the immediate period following admission.

Management of AMI

AMI is the end-product of coronary artery disease (CAD), and the most common cause of serious chest pain seen in the accident and emergency unit (Walsh, 1990). More than 50000 people in the UK die prematurely from CAD every year (Abraham and Wyper, 1995). Over the past 30 years, the approach to care has moved from a 'wait and see' strategy to a dynamic intervention strategy, to reduce the size of the infarct and induce early repair of the changed myocardium (Quinn, 1996).

By analysing the patient profile, the nurse can evaluate clinical features, with reference to pathophysiology, and prioritise subsequent objectives for immediate care on the basis of relevant and recent research.

Case scenario

John, aged 40, is admitted to a coronary care unit with a suspected diagnosis of myocardial infarction. On admission, a full nursing assessment is carried out. This reveals that he is married with three children under the age of 12, and that his wife stays at home looking after the children. He works as a labourer, and enjoys mountaineering in his spare time. He smokes 40 cigarettes a day, but does not drink alcohol. He is not overweight, but tends to be anxious regarding provision for his family. He has no past medical history of angina or myocardial infarction. He arrived at the accident and emergency department, accompanied by his wife, 25 minutes after the onset of symptoms. No medications had been taken by the patient to treat the symptoms.

Clinical features on admission were:

- Pulse: 90 beats/min, weak and irregular
- Blood pressure: 100/75 mmHG
- Respiration: 22 breaths/min
- Temperature: 37.8°C
- Colour: lips slightly cyanosed, oxygen saturation 88% by peripheral oximetry
- Pain: reported central crushing pain radiating to his left arm and to his chin
- Anxiety level: high, scoring 7/10 on a 1–10 anxiety scale.

Health status analysis

Vital sign abnormalites may arise for a number of reasons. *Table 9.1* gives an overview of the potential causes of vital sign aberrations in John's case.

John's pulse of 90 beats/min may be considered mildly tachycardic, depending on his usual baseline value. Normal pulse is generally approximately 70 beats/min (Carver and Mackinnon, 1994). John's heart rate may have been higher earlier in the course of the infarction because of initial compensatory mechanisms, but these mechanisms may now be failing as the cardiovascular problem persists (Barrows, 1996). The rise in pulse rate is a consequence of decreased cardiac output and the subsequent cardiovascular compensatory response which attempts to meet the oxygen demands of the body and myocardium by increasing heart rate (Porth, 1994; Carpenito, 1995; O'Donnell, 1996).

An increase in heart rate is highly undesirable in patients with cardiac problems, as it increases the oxygen demand of the myocardium, decreases the duration of diastole, and results in less time available for coronary filling and myocardial perfusion (Field, 1997). An increase of 5–10 beats/min is regarded as significant in this respect (Field, 1997).

The dysrhythmias are caused by altered electrical conduction through the myocardium as a result of ischaemia and myocardial cell death (Monahan *et al,*

1994). Anxiety will also raise the heart rate, and patients with AMI are often observed to be highly anxious (Fowler, 1996). The crushing chest pain experienced by these patients may also lead to an increase in heart rate (Carver and Mackinnon, 1994). Thus, John's increased pulse rate may have many origins, and his myocardium is at risk of further damage unless these problems are addressed.

Table 9.1: Potential causes of abnormalities in John's vital signs	
Vital signs	**Potential causes**
Pulse 90 beats/min	Anxiety, pain, pulmonary oedema, compensatory mechanisms, early cardiogenic shock, infection, nicotine
Blood pressure 100/75 mmHg	Compensatory mechanisms, early cardiogenic shock, metabolic acidosis
Temperature 37.8°C	Infection, early inflammatory response to myocardial damage
Respiration 22 breaths/min	Anxiety, pain, compensatory mechanisms, early cardiogenic shock, pulmonary oedema, metabolic acidosis, infection, nicotine

John's blood pressure (BP) may be considered mildly hypotensive, depending on his baseline value (Riegel *et al*, 1995). Normal BP is considered to range between 100/60 mmHg and 150/90 mmHg (Carver and Mackinnon, 1994). The nurse should consider the possibility that John's baseline BP may be higher than what is regarded as normal as he smokes and nicotine is a vasoconstrictor (Carver and Mackinnon, 1994).

Because AMI impairs myocardial function, coronary circulation is decreased, further contributing to hypotension (Monahan *et al*, 1994; Porth, 1994). Such hypotension is a further indication of reduced cardiac output (Carpenito, 1995), developing cardiogenic shock (Porth, 1994; O'Donnell, 1996), and an ineffective renin-angiotensin compensatory mechanism (Barrows, 1996).

It may also indicate that the oxygen supply to vital organs is reduced and that further myocardial complications and damage are developing (Carver and Mackinnon, 1994). Indeed, lower systolic pressure in AMI patients is significantly associated with increased mortality (Lee *et al*, 1995). In such patients, BP also falls in an attempt to disperse the acidic molecules developing as a consequence of metabolic and respiratory acidosis (Barrows, 1996).

Respiratory rate normally rises after an AMI (Tsunoda, 1996), and may have either a psychological or physiological aetiology. Normal respiratory rate is 12–20 breaths/min (Hoffman and Manzetti, 1996). An anxious patient with AMI, such as John, may hyperventilate from anxiety, causing his respiratory rate to rise even further (Carver and Mackinnon, 1994).

Left ventricular contractility is impaired because of myocardial ischaemia, resulting in stiffness of the relevant myocardial section (O'Donnell, 1996). This leads to ineffective cardiac contraction and reduced cardiac output, causing a back-up of blood in the pulmonary circulation (O'Donnell, 1996) and hence increased pulmonary venous pressure. The resulting pulmonary oedema impairs gaseous exchange and reduces oxygen saturation in the pulmonary veins (Carver and Mackinnon, 1994; Porth, 1994; O'Donnell, 1996).

Dyspnoea and increased respiratory rate ensue to meet the oxygen demands of the body and to counteract the developing hypoxia (Potter and Perry, 1995). As the pulse increases, the myocardium also requires more oxygen to cope with this workload (Porth, 1994). The increased respiratory rate is also indicative of hypoxia (Carver and Mackinnon, 1994).

When assessing vital signs for abnormality, it is important to remember that normality varies from individual to individual. On admission, all of the patient's vital signs must additionally be evaluated against physiological compensatory mechanisms.

Central cyanosis, evident from John's lips, is indicative of arterial desaturation of oxygen due to impaired pulmonary gaseous exchange (Porth, 1994). Pulmonary oedema may induce such cyanosis. Cardiac output is decreased because of failing compensatory mechanisms, and so blood is being oxygenated at a slower rate. Central cyanosis is a late sign of hypoxia (Potter and Perry, 1995) and a clinical sign of cardiogenic shock (Carpenito, 1995). The central cyanosis indicates that hypoxia has not developed recently, and that cardiogenic shock is entering the progressive stage (Barrows, 1996). Immediate treatment to reoxygenate the blood and counter cardiogenic shock is indicated, in order to avoid multiple, potentially fatal, complications (ie. multi-organ failure) (Barrows, 1996).

Central, crushing chest pain is common in patients with AMI, and is usually related to myocardial ischaemia, occurring secondary to coronary artery occlusion (Monahan *et al*, 1994). The pain arises as a result of unmet metabolic needs of the myocardial cells, caused by diminished or occluded coronary blood flow (Porth, 1994). The crushing, sub-sternal pain is a symptom of severe myocardial ischaemia, and arises from sympathetic interconnections between nerve fibres (Bullock and Rosendahl, 1992) or arteriospasm caused by acidosis.

A rise in temperature may be associated with several clinical conditions, most commonly infection. It is crucial to evaluate the slight rise in temperature in relation to all other vital sign measurements and the description of pain.

Anxiety may contribute to many signs and symptoms, and is common among patients with AMI (Cornock, 1996). Anxiety is associated with fear of death, complex environment and uncertain aetiology and prognosis in the immediate post-admission period (Brunner and Suddarth, 1989).

As John is the sole breadwinner in the family, he is naturally anxious about providing for his family. Anxiety may be exacerbated by the fact that he is unlikely to return to work as a labourer, as heavy physical activity at work and compromised pulmonary function are associated with AMI and myocardial strain (Barefoot *et al*, 1995; Roper *et al*, 1996). His wife may have to start looking for work, and the likelihood of this potential role reversal may further contribute to John's anxiety, making it an issue for his care (Roper *et al*, 1996). Also, labouring is associated with significant cardiovascular morbidity and mortality, increasing his risk of developing AMI complications (Lynch *et al*, 1995).

John smokes over 25 cigarettes a day and is under 45 years of age. Statistically, therefore, he is 33 times more likely to develop an AMI than a non-smoker of the same age (Negri *et al*, 1994). Being a smoker, he is also at greater risk of pulmonary complications (Fowler, 1996; Jousilahti *et al*, 1995), as pulmonary function is affected by hyperplasia of goblet cells and blockage of bronchioles and alveoli by mucous and tar (Porth, 1994). Together with pulmonary oedema, these added pulmonary complications severely reduce the gaseous exchange of oxygen and carbon dioxide. Furthermore, coronary vessel dilation is required to optimise oxygen perfusion to the myocardium, and nicotine is a vasoconstrictor (Carver and Mackinnon, 1994).

John is not overweight, so the link between excessive weight and cardiac problems is not relevant to him. However, his hobby is mountaineering, which has been shown to place a strain on the cardiovascular and respiratory systems and may have predisposed him to cardiac problems (Savourey *et al*, 1994). Strenuous activity at high altitude increases myocardial workload owing to the decreased availability of oxygen (oxygen saturation falls at higher altitudes) (Hoffman and Manzetti, 1996); exercise is, however, beneficial to the cardiovascular system.

Nursing diagnosis

Following this initial nursing assessment, the nurse should conclude that the oxygen supply to John's heart is compromised, and put forward a preliminary diagnosis of cardiogenic shock (progressive stage, compensatory mechanisms failing).

The nurse must then take immediate action to optimise recovery and prevent the development of further complications.

Goals for the first four hours of care

Priority 1: Management of cardiogenic shock

The central cyanosis observed during assessment indicates that John has hypoxia, a life-threatening condition (Carver and Mackinnon, 1994; Potter and Perry, 1995). Reoxygenation of tissues, to regain and maintain homeostasis and reperfuse the oxygen-starved myocardium, is top priority, in conjunction with thrombolytic therapy (Field, 1997). Cells become ischaemic after 20 minutes of oxygen deprivation and are less likely to recover (O'Donnell, 1996).

Mortality rates in post-AMI patients with ischaemia are 7.7% higher than in those without ischaemia, emphasising the need to counter cardiogenic shock and hypoxia through reoxygenation of blood and tissues (Carver and Mackinnon, 1994; Monahan *et al*, 1994). Supplemental oxygen administration also counters acidosis, helping to increase BP (Barrows, 1996). Administration of oxygen via nasal speculae (2–4l/min) is preferable to administration via a face-mask, as the face-mask is not tolerated as well and may further increase anxiety (Tremper-Mitchell, 1996).

The administration of inotropic drugs, such as dobutamine, will improve left ventricular function and cardiac contractility, countering cardiogenic shock by enhancing cardiac contraction and thus improving myocardial tissue oxygenation (Barrows, 1996).

Urinary output should also be monitored, as a urinary output of less than 0.5ml/kg/h may indicate that the patient is entering the progressive stage of cardiogenic shock (Barrows, 1996). Bed-rest should be advised to reduce myocardial workload. At this stage, unless the cardiogenic shock is treated, other interventions may prove futile.

Priority 2: Relief of pain

Pain relief is regarded as high priority in the acute management of AMI (Quinn, 1996). O'Connor (1995) found that nurses underestimate patients' pain in 46% of myocardial infarctions. Pain has physiological effects on the body, such as increased BP, heart rate and stroke volume (Rowe, 1995). These complications further compromise the myocardium by placing it under strain to meet the increased demands (Rowe, 1995).

Analgesia reduces the complications of pain, thereby improving the oxygen supply to the myocardium, causing vasodilatation and decreasing the workload of the heart, as well as reducing anxiety (Carver and Mackinnon, 1994; Monahan *et al*, 1994). Such benefits are clearly important in early management, as more oxygen is made available to the myocardium and myocardial oxygen demand is reduced (Friedman, 1995). Pain relief is also humane, and must be carried out concomitantly with the other priorities.

Diamorphine is the analgesic of choice for patients experiencing AMI, as it is rapidly effective and also reduces pulmonary oedema through venous dilatation, thus relieving pulmonary congestion (Trounce, 1994). Both of these actions are beneficial to John's condition. Slow intravenous injection of 5mg diamorphine, at 1 mg/min, is the route of choice for rapid therapeutic effect (*British National Formulary* [BNF], 1998). It is also the least traumatic route at a time when anxiety levels are high. Diamorphine also induces a state of euphoria, which will benefit John both physiologically and psychologically at this time (Trounce, 1994).

Priority 3: Limiting infarct size through reperfusion of the myocardium

Reperfusion of the myocardium is widely documented as a major priority in AMI management (medical and nursing), especially within the first few hours after the AMI, as the success of such treatment is time-related (Quinn and Thompson, 1995). Myocardial salvage is possible if thrombolytic therapy is initiated within 60 minutes of infarction (Resuscitation Council [UK], 1996).

The use of thrombolytic reperfusion therapy (eg. with streptokinase or tissue plasminogen activator [t-PA]) to increase myocardial oxygen supply has been widely reported to significantly reduce myocardial necrosis, and hence infarct size (O'Donnell, 1996; Field, 1997). Increasing myocardial oxygen supply through clot dissolution and coronary vasodilatation limits infarct size and improves left ventricular function, relieving symptoms and reducing the incidence of complications (Watters, 1997). John was immediately started on streptokinase 1.5 mega-units in 0.9% saline intravenously over 60 minutes.

Thrombolytic therapy has been shown to reduce mortality rates in AMI patients by up to 22% (Friedman, 1995), especially when administered within the first 1–6 hours of onset of pain (Quinn and Thompson, 1995). However, patients must be assessed for contraindications to such therapy (Griego and House-Fancher, 1996). Infarct size may also be limited by inducing coronary vasodilation with agents such as glyceryl trinitrate (BNF, 1998).

Priority 4: Cardiac monitoring for electrocardiogram (ECG) changes

Ten to twenty per cent of patients experience ventricular arrhythmias, the most common complication of AMI, within the first six hours (O'Donnell, 1996). Arrhythmias are strongly associated with mortality (Scognamiglio *et al*, 1994). There is a risk of sudden death from ventricular fibrillation (VF), which affects up to 60% of patients in the first hour (Carver and Mackinnon, 1994; Quinn and Thompson, 1995).

To ensure that complications are identified and treated immediately, heart rate and rhythm must be monitored continuously to detect changes (Riegel *et al*, 1995; Rowe, 1995). Repeat ECG should also be undertaken for patients reporting chest pain, to assess potential extension of the infarct (Quinn and Thompson, 1995).

Thus, continuous monitoring for life-threatening dysrhythmias such as VF and ventricular tachycardia is crucial; it is also important to look out for premature ventricular contractions (PVCs) which may indicate that reperfusion is taking place (O'Donnell, 1996).

Lignocaine hydrochloride infusion may be instituted at this stage if PVCs have been observed on the cardiac monitor.

Priority 5: Management of anxiety

Early anxiety management is well documented as a priority in the management of AMI (Carver and Mackinnon, 1994). Shiell and Shiell (1991) found that symptoms such as sweating, palpitations and chest pain may be anxiety induced, rather than symptoms of cardiac complications, verifying the need to eliminate anxiety to prevent it masking complications (Carver and Mackinnon, 1994).

Some researchers highlight the importance of treating psychological factors early on to ensure optimum recovery (Cornock, 1996). Also, seeing family members who are anxious or upset about the patient's condition may heighten patient anxiety. Research suggests that family members should be provided with information to meet their needs so as to reduce family anxiety (Quinn *et al*, 1996).

Untreated anxiety can raise metabolic rates and oxygen demand, further compromising the myocardium (Friedman, 1995; Potter and Perry, 1995). Thus, making anxiety management a priority in early treatment attends to both the psychological and physiological needs of the patient. Because of its intricate association with pain, anxiety management is assigned a high priority in the early management of AMI.

Concluding comments

This case study approach has demonstrated that knowledgeable and skilful nurses can carry out a comprehensive assessment of the health status of a critically ill person. It is important to remember that, although the objectives are prioritised, to some extent all the identified objectives are being attended to simultaneously, and therefore there is considerable overlap of interventions.

By using his/her extensive knowledge of pathophysiological processes and being aware of recent research literature, the nurse can prioritise appropriate goals for holistic care. Such a holistic approach has been shown to reduce early patient mortality in patients who have suffered an AMI (Lee *et al*, 1995), thus offering greater potential for saving lives (Quinn, 1996).

Key points

* Care of the patient with acute myocardial infarction is focused on dynamic interventions to induce early repair of myocardial tissue.
* Through a comprehensive analysis of clinical features, complications and underlying pathophysiology can be established.
* An understanding of the underlying pathophysiology of clinical features can aid in prioritising objectives with a view to providing optimum care and promoting early recovery.
* It is important to remember while the objectives are prioritised that, to some extent, all the identified objectives are being attended to simultaneously and therefore there is considerable overlap of interventions.

References

Abraham T, Wyper MA (1995) The patient with cardiovascular problems. In: Long BC, Phipps WJ, Cassmeyer VL, eds. *Adult Nursing: A Nursing Process Approach*. CV Mosby, London: 376–431

Barefoot JC, Larsen S, von der Lieth L *et al* (1995) Hostility, incidence of acute myocardial infarction, and mortality in a sample of older Danish men and women. *Am J Epidemiol* **142**(5): 477–84

Barrows JJ (1996) Shock. In: Lewis SM, Collier IC, Heitkemper MM, eds. *Medical–Surgical Nursing: Assessment and Management of Clinical Problems.* 4th edn. Mosby, St Louis: 117–41

BNF (1998) *British National Formulary* September 1998. British Medical Association and Royal Pharmaceutical Society of Great Britain, London

Brunner LS, Suddarth DS, eds (1989) *The Lippincott Manual of Medical–Surgical Nursing.* 2nd edn. Harper & Row, London: 214–363

Bullock BL, Rosendahl PP (1992) *Pathophysiology — Adaptations and Alterations in Function.* 3rd edn. JB Lippincott Co, Philadelphia

Carver K, Mackinnon C (1994) The cardiovascular system. In: Alexander MF, Fawcett JN, Runciman PJ, eds. *Nursing Practice: Hospital And Home — The Adult.* Churchill Livingstone, Edinburgh: 9–58

Carpenito LJ (1995) *Nursing Diagnosis — Application to Clinical Practice.* 6th edn. JB Lippincott Co, Philadelphia

Cornock M (1996) Cardiac distress. *Nurs Times* **92**(19): 44–6

Field D (1997) Cardiovascular assessment. *Nurs Times* **93**(35): 45–7

Fowler JP (1996) How to respond rapidly when chest pain strikes. *Nursing 96* **26**(5): 42–3

Friedman BM (1995) Early interventions in the management of acute myocardial uncomplicated infarction. *West J Med* **162**(1): 19–27

Griego L, House-Fancher MA (1996) Coronary artery disease. In: Lewis SM, Collier IC, Heitkemper MM, eds. *Medical–Surgical Nursing: Assessment and Management of Clinical Problems.* 4th edn. Mosby, St Louis: 884–931

Hoffman LA, Manzetti JD (1996) Respiratory system. In: Lewis SM, Collier IC, Heitkemper MM, eds. *Medical–Surgical Nursing: Assessment and Management of Clinical Problems.* 4th edn. Mosby, St Louis: 561–82

Jousilahti P, Toumilehto J, Vartiainen E *et al* (1995) Importance of risk factor clustering in coronary heart disease mortality and incidence in Eastern Finland. *J Cardiovasc Risk* **2**(1): 63–70

Lee KL, Woodlief H, Topol EJ *et al* (1995) Predictors of 30-day mortality in the era of reperfusion for acute myocardial infarction. Results from an International trial of 41021 patients. *Circulation* **91**(6): 1659–68

Lynch J, Kaplan GA, Salonen R *et al* (1995) Socio-economic status and carotid atherosclerosis. *Circulation* **92**(7): 1786–92

Monahan FD, Drake T, Neighbors M (1994) *Nursing Care Of Adults.* WB Saunders Co, Philadelphia

Negri E, La Vecchia C, Nobli A *et al* (1994) Cigarette smoking and acute myocardial infarction. A case control study from the GISSI-2 trial. *Eur J Epidemiol* **10**(4): 361–6

O'Connor L (1995) Pain assessment by patients and nurses, and nurses' notes on it, in early acute myocardial infarction. *Int Crit Care Nurs* **11**(4): 183–91

O'Donnell L (1996) Complications of Ml — beyond the acute stage. *Am J Nurs* **96**(9): 25–30

Porth CM (1994) *Pathophysiology — Concepts of Altered Health States.* 4th edn. JB Lippincott Co, Philadelphia

Potter PA, Perry AG (1995) *Basic Nursing — Theory and Practice.* 3rd edn. Mosby, St Louis

Quinn T (1996) Myocardial infarction. *Nurs Times* **92**(7): 9–12 (Professional development, part 3)

Quinn T, Thompson DR (1995) Administration of thrombolytic therapy to patients with acute myocardial infarction. *Acc Emerg Nurs* **3**(4): 208–14

Quinn S, Redmond K, Begley C (1996) The needs of relatives visiting adult critical care units as perceived by relatives and nurses. Part 1. *Int Crit Care Nurs* **12**: 168–72

Resuscitation Council (UK) (1996) *Advanced Life Support Manual*. 2nd edn. Resuscitation Council (UK), London

Riegel B, Thomason T, Carlson B (1995) Coronary precautions — fact or fiction. *Nursing 95* **25**(10): 52–3

Roper N, Logan WW, Tierney A (1996) *The Elements of Nursing — A Model for Nursing Based on a Model of Living*. 4th edn. Churchill Livingstone, Edinburgh

Rowe K (1995) Nursing a person who had suffered a myocardial infarction. *Br J Nurs* **4**(3): 148–54

Savourey G, Garcia N, Besnard Y *et al* (1994) Physiological changes induced by pre-adaptation to high altitude. *Eur J Appl Physiol* **69**(3): 221–7

Shiell J, Shiell A (1991) The prevalence of psychiatric morbidity on a coronary care ward. *J Adv Nurs* **16**(8): 1071–7

Scognamiglio R, Fasoli G, Nistri S *et al* (1994) Left ventricular function and prognosis after myocardial infarction: rationale for therapeutic strategies. *Cardiovasc Drug Ther* **8**(suppl 2): 310–25

Tremper-Mitchell J (1996) Lower respiratory problems. In: Lewis SM, Collier IC, Heitkemper MM, eds. *Medical–Surgical Nursing: Assessment and Management of Clinical Problems*. 4th edn. Mosby, St Louis: 621–81

Trounce JR (1994) *Clinical Pharmacology for Nurses*. Churchill Livingstone, Edinburgh

Tsunoda D (1996) Clinical snapshot: acute myocardial infarction. *Am J Nurs* **96**(5): 38–9

Walsh M (1990) *Accident & Emergency Nursing: A New Approach*. 2nd edn. Heinemann, London

Watters P (1997) RCN nursing update: Heart health: treatment. *Nurs Stand* **12**(3): 1–17

10

Fast track: early thrombolysis

Denise Flisher

The reduction of cardiac muscle damage post myocardial infarction depends on how fast intravenous thrombolytic therapy can be administered. This chapter looks at how the appropriately trained nurse can facilitate this early treatment.

For the past 20 years the delay in admission to hospital and effective treatment of patients presenting with an acute myocardial infarction (AMI) has been well documented (Smyllie *et al*, 1972; Morris, 1993). Early intravenous thrombolytic therapy reduces the mortality rate, especially when administered within six hours of the onset of the patient's symptoms. This has been proved in large clinical studies (GISSI, 1986; ISIS-2, 1988). There are two areas of concern:

1. Delay from onset of symptoms to admission to hospital.
2. Delay from hospital admission to the administration of thrombolytic drugs.

A British study involving 2373 patients from six district hospitals found that the mean delay from symptoms to admission was 60–90 minutes (Birkhead, 1992).

A similar study undertaken in the USA and involving 55000 patients, a much larger group, found that the mean delay from onset of symptoms to admission was 5.1 hours; from casualty to admission to coronary care was 1.7 hours; and from admission to coronary care to the administration of intravenous thrombolytics was 80 minutes (Morris, 1993). Results are not comparable between the two studies, but it should be noted that the American study involved a much larger sample of patients.

At Bedford Hospital, an audit carried out over a two-year period and involving 562 patients with AMI found that the mean delay from onset of symptoms to admission was 6.5 hours; from casualty to admission to coronary care was 1.2 hours; and from admission to coronary care to the administration of intravenous thrombolytics was 91 minutes.

It is difficult to address the delay from symptoms to admission as this involves patient education, which is virtually impossible without mass media coverage. At our hospital, the coronary care unit had a display dedicated to 'Don't hang on to your pain' on its open day. During the course of the day we spoke to 242 people about the fact that delay in coming to hospital causes more heart damage — but is this enough? It will take more than one hospital's efforts to improve the public's awareness.

Delay between admission and administration of the thrombolytic drug has been addressed at this hospital and has so far proven a great success.

History

Previously, most of our patients with chest pain were admitted directly to the coronary care unit via a GP. This caused confusion because the diagnosis was invariably non-cardiac, despite being 'chest pain'. The unit would therefore run out of beds when one was needed for a person sustaining AMI. In order to create more bed space on the coronary care unit, and to decide on a differential diagnosis for the chest pains, a 'bed state manager team' was first contacted by the GP. As a result, all patients with a primary symptom of chest pain were admitted directly to the casualty department.

Although this action stemmed the flow of non-cardiac patients being admitted to the coronary care unit, it created another problem in casualty. The casualty department was seeing sometimes up to 12 patients per day with a provisional diagnosis of AMI, which increased their workload considerably. The audit showed that the mean time from admission to casualty to transfer to the coronary care unit was in excess of 90 minutes. This delay, which was far too long and needed to be shortened by at least half, was usually caused by the casualty department being too busy or the casualty officer/on-call senior house officer wanting to wait for a chest X-ray to be taken.

A group of staff from both the casualty department and the coronary care unit, including the bed state management team, the cardiologist, audit officer and accident and emergency clinical director arranged a series of meetings in order to discuss a way of solving the problem. A system had to be devised whereby the patient was admitted to the coronary care unit and the thrombolytics given within a set time. A report produced by the North West Thames Coronary Heart Disease Focus Group indicated that thrombolysis within 30 minutes of arrival at hospital is a realistic target for patients with typical electrocardiograph (ECG) changes. It was a difficult goal to set, but was achievable with careful planning.

Action

All GPs now telephone the bed state manager to notify him/her of a pending chest pain admission. She then bleeps a designated member of the coronary care unit to let him/her know that the patient is on the way. As soon as the patient arrives in casualty, the coronary care nurse is bleeped again and he/she goes immediately to the department to record an ECG and obtain a brief medical history. This process is known as 'Fast track' (*Figure 10.1, Table 10.1*).

The designated coronary care nurse is trained in coronary care, ie. has obtained an appropriate English National Board Certificate 124, and passed an Advanced Cardiac Life Support course (ACLS) within the last three years. I also have to be satisfied that the nurse in question can diagnose an ECG with 'classic' hyper-acute changes and establish that there are no contraindications to thrombolytic therapy (*Table 10.2*). This is done through a series of teaching and testing over a period of at least one year.

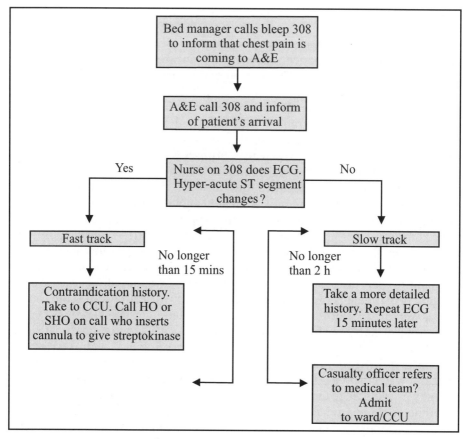

Figure 10.1: Fast track administration of intravenous streptokinase

If the ECG indicates a myocardial infarction without contraindications, the nurse bleeps the on-call senior house officer who meets the nurse and patient on transfer to the coronary care unit. On arrival, the senior house officer confirms the diagnosis and contraindication history, inserts a cannula if one is not already in situ, and the patient receives the prescribed thrombolytic therapy. If the SHO is delayed, the casualty officer will confirm the diagnosis and prescribe thrombolytics. The nurse contacts CCU to ask them to prepare the thrombolytic infusion to prevent further delay in 'door to needle time'. This has reduced the time between admission and administration of thrombolytics to 27 minutes and, in some cases, less.

If, however, the ECG shows ischaemic changes or the diagnosis is uncertain, the patient is admitted via a 'Slow track' system (*Table 10.1*) whereby he/she is seen in casualty by the casualty officer and referred to the on-call medical team. The patient may well end up in a coronary care bed or in a general ward, but obviously not as quickly as via Fast track admission. The ECG on these patients is repeated at 15-minute intervals in case it progresses to an infarction pattern, which would therefore change the admission category to Fast track. It must be stressed that the Fast track system has been developed for a nurse who is trained appropriately in coronary care for classic hyper-acute ECG changes only. Any doubts are referred directly to the on-call senior house officer.

Table 10.1: Indications for allocating to Fast or Slow track	
Fast track	Definite myocardial infarction (MI) with classic ST segment changes
Slow track	Patients presenting with a diagnosis of ?MI but with no ST changes
	Good history but no ST changes (allows time to carry out 15-minute ECGs)
	Angina diagnosis which could develop into an MI

Note: Slow track does not mean 'slow' patient care, but that streptokinase will not be administered as rapidly as on the Fast track system. The patient should not be in the accident and emergency department for longer than two hours

Table 10.2: Contraindications to streptokinase
Known allergy to streptokinase (had before in last year)
Recent streptococcal infection
Previous stroke (within last year)
Active peptic ulceration
Recent surgery (within 6 days)
Possible aortic dissection (call doctor)
Pregnancy
Anticoagulation therapy
Recent insertion of central or arterial line
Diastolic blood pressure above 110 mmHg
Diabetic retinopathy (call doctor)
Few of these contraindications are absolute. Take consultant advice

Produced as a guide which is laminated, reduced to pocket size and carried by each nurse working in the coronary care unit

Conclusion

Between August and November 1994 a total of 3564 patients were admitted to Bedford Hospital's casualty department with a provisional diagnosis of AMI. All patients were seen by a coronary care nurse within five minutes of arrival in casualty and 346 were Fast tracked to receive thrombolytic therapy. Each of those who went on the Fast track system had ECG changes and a significant cardiac enzyme rise indicative of an infarction before discharge from casualty.

Three hundred and sixteen patients with a primary diagnosis of unstable angina were Slow tracked, which meant that they were admitted to the coronary care unit at a slower rate. Eighteen of these patients developed a cardiac enzyme rise but no ECG changes and were therefore told that they did have a small AMI. The remainder of the 298 patients in the angina group were either treated with the appropriate medication or referred for angiography. This left 2902 patients with an initial diagnosis of chest pain, but with no obvious cause, who were either admitted to a general ward or discharged home.

Although this is only a small study, it shows that many of the patients admitted to the coronary care unit in this hospital with chest pain do not need to be in this area. More importantly, our previous door-to-needle time of 1.2 hours has been reduced to 27 minutes. It also shows that the CCU nurse is called to casualty for many non-cardiac cases. However, it is now easier to differentiate between the classic cardiac cases and those who have developed chest pain after pulling a muscle. The important issue is that the 'door to needle time' has decreased dramatically. This can only be an improvement in patient care.

Since the publication of this article the door-to-needle time has been reduced to less than 15 minutes. A new system has been set up whereby the thrombolysis is administered in the accident and emergency department by the coronary care nurse. This is used in conjunction with strict protocols and if the patient does not fulfil the criteria but still needs thrombolysis we resort back to the original Fast Track system. The new system is called 'Accelerated Fast Track' but with both systems in place the door-to-needle times will always be less than 30 minutes.

Key points

* There is a delay in the admission to hospital and the treatment of patients having sustained a myocardial infarction.
* The door-to-needle time should be no longer than 30 minutes.
* Fast track enables the thrombolytic therapy to be administered more quickly than does a conventional admission.
* Fast track nurses should be trained appropriately to diagnose classic hyper-acute electrocardiographic changes.

References

Birkhead J (1992) Time delays in provision of thrombolytic treatment in six district hospitals. *Br Med J* **305**: 445–8

GISSI (Gruppo Italiano per lo studio della Streptochinasi nell'infarto miocardico) (1986) Effectiveness of IV thrombolytic treatment in acute myocardial infarction. *Lancet* **i**: 397–401

ISIS-2 (International Study of Infarction Survival 2) (1988) A multicentre, randomised trial of IV streptokinase and aspirin in acute myocardial infarction. *Lancet* **ii**: 349–60

Morris DC (1993) Early treatment of acute myocardial infarction: the myths, mystery and magic. *Heart J* **2**: 308–12

Smyllie HC, Taylor MP, Cunninghame-Green RE (1972) Acute myocardial infarction in Doncaster — delays in admission and survival. *Br Med J* **i**: 34–6

11

Role of the nurse in thrombolytic therapy — expanding the clinical horizons

John W Albarran and Heather Kapeluch

The use of thrombolytic agents is currently a major aspect of the care of patients with acute myocardial infarction (AMI). This chapter explores the nurse's role in the care of patients receiving this form of therapy, and the implications for the future.

In recent years the management of patients with AMI and the length of their hospital stay has changed dramatically. This may be partly due to the advent of thrombolytic agents. Thrombolytic or clot dissolving agents are administered to patients with an AMI when thrombus formation may lead to partial or complete coronary artery occlusion. At this stage, thrombolysis can be most effective. The mechanism producing clot dissolution involves the conversion of inactive plasminogen (an endogenous protein) to plasmin, which then dissolves the fibrin mesh (*Figure 11.1*). The goal of thrombolysis is a reopened coronary artery and a reperfused myocardial muscle (Chamberlain, 1989).

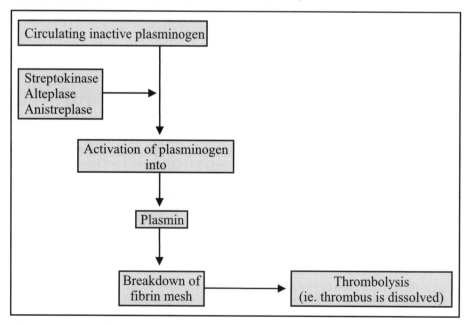

Figure 11.1: Mechanism of clot dissolution

Thrombolytic drugs

Currently in the UK the most common thrombolytic agents are streptokinase, alteplase, anistreplase and reteplase.

Streptokinase

Streptokinase is a non-enzymic protein derived from certain types of strepto-cocci. When administered intravenously it binds to circulating plasminogen to form an activator complex which converts plasminogen to plasmin and thus produces systemic thrombolysis (*Figure 11.1*; Kleven, 1988). Streptokinase is an antigen and may stimulate adverse reactions ranging from mild rashes to full anaphylaxis (Kleven, 1988; Kline, 1990). It produces systemic thrombolysis and has a half-life of 16 minutes. This may limit its use in patients requiring immediate invasive monitoring or other treatments. Also, repeated doses may be less effective, increasing the risk of complications and the level of antibody titres (Kleven, 1988).

Alteplase

In contrast to streptokinase, tissue plasminogen activator (t-PA) is a naturally occurring substance. When coronary occlusion occurs, the level of t-PA secretion is insufficient to bring about immediate clot dissolution. However, t-PA has now been produced by genetic engineering (alteplase; recombinant t-PA). Alteplase causes less allergic reactions than streptokinase (Kleven, 1988; Kline, 1990) and has a half-life of three to five minutes, which makes invasive intervention such as cardiac surgery or temporary pacemaker insertion less hazardous. Because it does not stimulate antibody formation it may be the drug of choice for patients who have previously had streptokinase.

With regards to administration, the GUSTO study (Global Utilisation of Streptokinase and Tissue plasminogen activator for Occluded arteries, 1993) reported that an accelerated regimen of intravenous t-PA and heparin (90 minutes in total), provided rapid reperfusion and a significantly improved survival rate when compared to streptokinase. There was, however, a higher rate of disabling strokes in the t-PA group in relation to the streptokinase group.

Anistreplase

Anistreplase (anisoylated plasminogen-streptokinase activator complex; APSAC) is a derivative and modified version of streptokinase that produces thrombolysis at the site of the clot but remains inactive in the systemic circulation. It is therefore more clot-specific. Anistreplase has a half-life up to 1.5 hours and may produce more lasting dissolution of thrombus. However, it predisposes the patient to more bleeding complications, without overcoming the allergic reactions associated with streptokinase (Chamberlain, 1989).

Reteplase

Reteplase is a new thrombolytic which can be administered as a double bolus, 10 mu given 30 minutes apart, and is as safe and clinically effective as streptokinase (International Joint Efficacy Comparison of Thrombolytics, INJECT, 1995; Weaver, 1996). Reteplase is a mutant form of t-PA with structural molecular differences that are produced by Escherichia Coli cells. In particular it has a half-life three times that of alteplase, allowing for the maintenance of therapeutic plasma concentrations and intravenous bolus administration. The benefit of an uncomplicated regime when compared to other thrombolytic drugs (*Table 11.3*) permits rapid initiation of therapy, which may potentially translate to a long-term reduction in morbidity and mortality. Additionally, the incidence of haemorrhagic complications, or other adverse events, is not increased and it also seems to have an advantage over streptokinase and related agents in that antibody formation is very low.

Additional therapy

Intravenous or subcutaneous heparin may be prescribed following thrombolytic therapy, not only to minimise coronary artery occlusion but also because the thrombolytic agents have such short half-lives (Daily, 1991). More recent analyses indicate that adding heparin to streptokinase may be associated with further bleeding risks without evidence of benefit. It is recommended however that alteplase is followed by intravenous heparin as this combination results in better patency of coronary arteries (Yusuf *et al*, 1996; The Task Force on the Management of Acute Myocardial Infarction of the European Society of Cardiology, 1996). GISSI-2 (1990) and ISIS-3 (1992) demonstrated that the addition of subcutaneous heparin does not influence in-hospital mortalities when combined with thrombolytic therapy and aspirin. However, these two major trials have reported that the addition of aspirin to thrombolytics results in significantly lower patient mortality rates (GISSI-2, 1990; ISIS-3, 1992). The immediate effect of aspirin is to reduce platelet aggregation, minimising progression to clot formation and possible coronary artery reocclusion.

Results

In the 1980s a number of multinational studies were undertaken; these have been reviewed elsewhere (Wilcox, 1992). The results suggest that thrombolytic agents reduce in-hospital mortality from AMI by 20–25%. This improvement is more dramatic when the treatment is given within two hours following the onset of chest pain; the benefits appear to decline with time, but some advantage may still be evident at 12 hours (Boersma *et al*, 1996). It has therefore been suggested that increasing public awareness on the importance of self-referral, following the onset of cardiac symptoms, is vital for ensuring that those at greatest risk of AMI receive treatment as early as possible (Weston *et al*, 1994; Boersma *et al*, 1996).

Studies have shown that risk factors are few but include hypotension, allergies, bleeding, cerebrovascular accidents and death (GISSI-2, 1990; ISIS-3, 1992). ISIS-3 and, more recently, Weaver (1996) reported that no particular agent was superior in terms of decreasing mortality rates, although there are more haemorrhagic strokes after alteplase and anistreplase than with streptokinase. Similarly, lower levels of hypotension and allergic reactions are recorded following alteplase.

The choice of agent may in part be dictated by market forces since streptokinase therapy costs approximately £80, whereas alteplase costs ten times as much and anistreplase somewhere in between. Additionally, apart from reperfusing myocardial muscle, the benefits of thrombolysis include shorter hospital stay and a reduction in nursing care hours (Sadaniantz *et al*, 1994).

Patient assessment

Thrombolytic therapy is considered when the patient fulfils certain criteria (*Table 11.1*). Careful patient assessment is a major priority, as time is very pertinent. As the nurse is often the first point of contact with the patient, he/she is in a unique position to utilise his/her clinical expertise and help medical staff to identify patients suitable for thrombolysis (Sait, 1988; Caunt,

Table 11.1: Inclusion criteria
ST elevation; 1mm in II, III and AVF; 1 mm in I and AVL; or 2mm in VI–V6
Clinical presentation, ie. severity, site, duration of chest pain, and the presence of other risk factors
Onset of chest pain less than 24 hours
Not contraindicated (see *Table 11.2*)

1992; Culbertson, 1992). Clearly, however, the decision to prescribe thrombolysis rests with the doctor but, with the introduction of well-designed clinical protocols, this trend is changing (Grijseels *et al*, 1995; Caunt, 1996).

One of the key aspects of assessment is a thorough evaluation of the patient's pain history (Sait, 1988; Daily, 1991). In particular, the onset, site, severity and duration of the pain are examined in detail to establish whether it is of myocardial origin. All patients presenting with chest pain must also have a 12-lead ECG to elucidate whether AMI has occurred. Elevation of the ST segment is evidence of such damage, although ECG changes are not always present and may develop at a later stage. The ability of the nurse to interpret ECG changes accurately is crucial to the patient's well-being (Daily, 1991; Lepley-Frey, 1991; Caunt, 1992). Other relevant aspects of assessment are blood pressure, heart rate and rhythm. An accurate assessment of the patient's total needs for care will enable the nurse to prioritise and implement appropriate actions. The assessment may also reveal those patients in whom thrombolytic therapy would be unsuitable because of an increased risk of bleeding (*Table 11.2*). In the past, those aged 75 years or more have been excluded from thrombolytic therapy because they were thought to be at high risk of bleeding complications and death (Kline, 1990). However, one study has suggested that the use of streptokinase in this age group is safe and significantly free of adverse effects (Kafetz and Luder, 1992).

Table 11.2: Exclusion criteria	
Absolute contraindications	Recent intracranial/spinal surgery (within two months)
	Uncontrolled severe hypertension
	Known blood dyscrasia, ie. haemophilia
	Active internal bleeding
	History of haemorrhagic cerebrovascular accident (within six months)
	Intracranial neoplasm, cerebral aneurysm, arteriovenous malformation
	Diabetic haemorrhagic retinopathy — treated by laser within one week
	Aortic dissection
	Liver disease
Relative contraindications	Surgery, biopsy, trauma within last ten days
	Cardiopulmonary resuscitation longer than 20 minutes
	Acute pericarditis, subacute bacterial endocarditis
	Cerebrovascular accident
	Patient taking anticoagulants
	History of gastrointestinal or genitourinary bleeding
	Pregnancy

Culbertson (1992) and Daily (1991) suggest that a flow chart may be a useful nursing tool to obtain patient details rapidly, provide a record of patient care and help to prioritise nursing resources. Culbertson (1992) added that a flow chart may have other advantages, eg. it may guarantee quality of care, provide a record of the patient's progress and be easily audited.

Administration of thrombolysis

Once it is established that a patient is eligible for thrombolysis the nurse must be involved in all stages of care, eg. giving simple explanations of the treatment and the ward environment as well as providing physical and psychosocial support for the patient and his/her family.

At present all thrombolytic drugs are administered intravenously. *Table 11.3* illustrates the dosages and methods of administration. With this form of therapy, baseline observations and continuous cardiac monitoring should be key nursing priorities, as this information can provide an objective measure of changes in the patient's condition (Ramsden, 1988). Because of the possibility of adverse effects, resuscitation equipment must be available (Moseley, 1992).

Table 11.3: Methods of administering thrombolytic therapy		
Agent	**Dose**	**Administration**
Streptokinase	1.5 mu	60 minutes
Alteplase	100 mg total (10 mg bolus, 50 mg for 1 hour, 40 mg for 2 hours)	3 hours
Anistreplase	30 units bolus	2–5 minutes
Reteplase	10 mm bolus	30 minutes apart

Drugs for managing anaphylaxis or sudden bleeding, eg. adrenaline, steroids, colloids and tranexamic acid, should be readily accessible and familiar to the nurse. Although the risk of intracranial bleeding remains low (0.5 to 1.4%; ISIS-3, 1992) many authors advocate that nurses should record and monitor the patient's neurological state (Sait, 1988; Daly, 1991). While treatment is in progress the nurse must record the pulse and blood pressure every 15 minutes (Rodriguez and Reed, 1987; Sait, 1988) because of the potential risks of hypotension bleeding and anaphylaxis. Once the treatment is completed, observations may be monitored hourly or according to unit or hospital policy.

During the first 48 hours of thrombolytic therapy the nurse must pay scrupulous attention to less obvious signs of bleeding as well as instigating strategies that will minimise trauma. For example, Daily (1991) suggested that urinary catheterisation should be avoided or delayed until the thrombolytic agent is considered to be inactive. Similarly, intramuscular injections, either before, during or up to six hours after therapy should be deferred. It is also recommended that patients avoid vigorous dental care, as well as wet shaving, during the first 24 hours (Rodriguez and Reed, 1987). In particular, the venepuncture site should be inspected on a regular basis, as this is the commonest bleeding site (Daily, 1991). The nurse should look for signs of redness, bruising or haematoma formation in this area. If any of these or any other detrimental changes develop then the infusion must be stopped.

The patient's urine should be tested daily for haematuria (Rodriguez and Reed, 1987). Rigors may also occur, and the patient should be advised that any unusual sensations during the treatment should be reported immediately.

The nurse must watch for evidence of coronary artery reocclusion (Ramsden, 1988), particularly as the incidence of this occurring is between 10–30% (Martin and Kennedy, 1994; Grines, 1996). If the patient's chest pain recurs and is unrelieved by nitrates, or if there is a rise in the ST-segment, cardiovascular instability, nausia or clamminess, then it is likely that the infarct-related coronary artery is reoccluding. Ensuring that the patient is optimally anti-coagulated requires clotting times to be kept at 1.5 times normal therapeutic values. This may be achieved by titrating the prescribed heparin (Ramsden, 1988).

Pain relief is a major nursing concern. Administration of opiates and the measurement of pain with visual analogue scales can enable the nurse to gauge whether the patient's pain is successfully controlled (Jowett and Thompson, 1989). To maximise pain relief and enhance myocardial function, nitrates or beta-blockers may be administered in conjunction with thrombolytic drugs (Daily, 1991).

Reperfusion

In terms of successful reperfusion there are four indicators that should be monitored, and the nurse is in the prime position to do this (Rodriguez and Reed, 1987; Daily, 1991; Moseley, 1992). First, the patient may report a sudden relief from chest pain. This may mean that coronary artery reperfusion is occurring and blood is reaching areas distant from the stenosed site. However, the pain relief may be due to opiates and the nurse needs to take this into account.

The second indicator is the appearance of reperfusion arrhythmias. One nursing study (Lepley-Frey, 1991) found that 80% of a sample of 41 subjects experienced reperfusion arrhythmias following the administration of alteplase. Of the sample, 36% had two or more disturbances, the most common being sinus bradycardia followed by an idioventricular rhythm. Reperfusion arrhythmias are associated with all thrombolytic drugs and their frequency tends to diminish over time, often without intervention. This phenomenon has been attributed to the wash-out of accumulated metabolites and other substances, which circulate around the heart once re-canalisation begins (Lepley-Frey,1991). Indeed, Lepley-Frey (1991) suggested that the absence of arrhythmias may be a sign that thrombolytic therapy has failed to reopen the blocked coronary artery.

A third and more sensitive indicator is the return of the raised ST-segment to the normal resting baseline. Experienced nurses may be able to observe this by continuously monitoring the trace from the ECG lead that affords the best quality interpretation. It is common practice to record a full 12-lead ECG one to four hours after thrombolysis to provide another measure of the effectiveness of the treatment.

The final indicator is the pattern of enzyme rise associated with AMI. Usually the serum creatinine phosphokinase level peaks at 24 hours following myocardial injury. However, if a thrombolytic agent is administered, reperfusion of the myocardium leads to a higher level peaking at 12 hours and subsiding sooner. Again, these changes are explained by the rush of blood through the underperfused myocardium. A more accurate way of assessing the degree of vessel patency achieved by thrombolysis is coronary angiography. This is a selective procedure that requires specialist services, is invasive and carries other risks.

Role of the nurse

Current opinion suggests that nurses caring for patients undergoing thrombolysis have specific responsibilities. Caunt (1992) and Ramsden (1988), for example, viewed the role of the nurse as pivotal both during and after treatment. It is the nurse who is closest to the patient and is first able to recognise signs of reinfarction. Therefore, the nurse's action influences the patient outcome.

Furthermore, the proximity of the nurse to the patient enables the identification of subtle changes (Benner, 1984). The expert nurse develops and maintains a unique diagnostic monitoring function in caring for the critically ill patients and, through this, becomes the patient's first line of defence (Benner, 1984), particularly when drugs have a margin for adverse effects and prompt detection is crucial.

Thrombolysis is beginning to have a wider application (Murray, 1992) and debate is also emerging as to the most suitable place for it in relation to AMI. The studies of Birkenhead (1992) and Parry *et al* (1993), have suggested that delays in the administration of thrombolysis were shorter when treatment was initiated in accident and emergency departments. The policy implications for nurses may include the development of a thrombolysis triage nurse (Birkenhead, 1992), in either casualty or in the coronary care unit where accident and emergency services are unavailable.

However, Caunt (1992) and experience suggest that nurses have already been playing some role in the primary screening of potential patients. A form of triage has often been practised by nursing staff when patients are admitted, but this seems to have been done on an informal basis.

One may reasonably speculate that a more formal triage role may need to be established in the future as the reduction in junior doctors' hours is realised. There may be added advantages for nurses in terms of autonomy and satisfaction, and for the consumers of healthcare in the better use of resources. There may also be an opportunity for nurses to take on a more proactive role in determining standards, in relation to auditing, and in developing multidisciplinary practice. A recent audit exemplified the contribution of nursing and showed that nurses enhanced the number of eligible patients prescribed thrombolysis by reminding junior doctors of this option (Hendra and Marshall, 1992).

Mounting evidence from other studies suggests that the expertise of coronary nurses enables them to safely assess and rapidly streamline patients with suspected MI and thus have an impact on reducing delay to treatment. For example, Quinn (1995) studied a small group of nurses and doctors regarding their 'intention to treat' a sample of patients admitted to CCU. The respondents were asked to state whether they considered thrombolysis was indicated and, if so, which agent they would recommend. There were no differences in nurses' and house officers' stated intentions in respect of thrombolytic therapy. A further 46 patients were assessed solely by coronary nurses on their management intentions which were then compared to the actual treatment prescribed. The findings suggest that nurses' management intentions were identical to those of the prescribing physicians. Quinn (1995) thus proposed that nurse-led thrombolysis should be instigated as such a role has the potential to reduce the delays to this vital treatment.

Another similar investigation has demonstrated the skill of experienced cardiac nurses in discriminating eligible patients for thrombolytic therapy on the basis of ECG findings and background clinical history (Storey and Rowley, 1997). This is of significance to patient outcomes, as accurate evaluation of 12-lead ECG can decrease delay in decision-making. In this study cardiac trained nurses' decisions to thrombolyse, according to the presence of ECG criteria, were comparable to those obtained by senior physicians. The research concluded that cardiac trained nurses have a valuable role in identifying patients who may be candidates for thrombolysis. It would thus appear that nurses are confident and competent in extracting relevant data to influence their judgements on patients with AMI. The studies of Quinn (1995), Storey and Rowley (1997) also seem to acknowledge the previously invisible triage role of nurses, as well as validating the level of expertise and decision-making skills. It may equally be reasoned that the use of well-established clinical and ECG criteria may enhance patient selectivity for thrombolysis.

The pro-activity of nurses in this area of practice has recently become widespread. For example, in response to increasing treatment times from admission to thrombolysis of more than one hour, Caunt (1996) undertook a small pilot study to assess the impact of a fast-track system of care. This involved three experienced cardiac nurses who were responsible for the initial assessment of patients (either in CCU or accident and emergency) and liaising with medical staff. In addition, part of their remit was to initiate immediate thrombolysis and other treatments jointly with a house officer according to strict protocols. Following implementation, an audit six months later revealed that of the patients who required thrombolysis for AMI, 42% had been assessed by these three nurses even though 24-hour cover was not available. Of the 21 patients who received thrombolytic therapy by these practitioners, the median time of administration from admission to hospital was <30 minutes. In contrast with 16 patients who were managed by a house officer, when there was no nurse available, the median time to thrombolysis was 43 minutes, with only seven receiving their treatment within 30 minutes. These specially trained nurses were also able to influence the management of patients because they were able to cannulate and request specific blood tests that were vital to decision-making. According to Caunt (1996), the benefits for the patients are early pain control, together with rapid assessment and the instigation of treatment. Arguably, nurses are also in a position to discriminate patients whose chest pain is non-cardiac in origin and to refer them appropriately.

In a similar venture, Flischer (1995) introduced a fast-track system to identify candidates who required thrombolysis and bring down the delays to treatment, as well as transfers to CCU, which were in excess of 90 minutes. Experienced nurses in possession of the coronary ENB course were recruited and further trained in ECG interpretation. In this project, once the designated nurse on duty has been notified of an admission, the individual is responsible for assessing the patient in the accident and emergency department and evaluating the ECG before contacting the senior house officer. This approach to fast-tracking has reduced the time between admission and treatment to 30 minutes or less as well as the level of duplication of information. Through this process nurses, together with medical staff, have also been able to screen those patients suitable for admission to coronary care from those being sent to other clinical environments, thus utilising clinical resources more effectively. Alderman (1996) has also described how the deployment of cardiac trained nurses to the accident and emergency unit, reduces the time taken to send patients for thrombolytic treatment. According to Weston *et al* (1994), causes of delay to treatment include duplication of assessments by different healthcare professionals and restrictive practices of limiting thrombolytic use to CCUs. From the above projects it is evident that nurses are actively engaged in identifying the challenges and overcoming obstacles through innovation and creativity. In this way, nurses are also developing cost effective and high quality services for patients with AMI. In addition, through these distinct strategies, nurses are assisting with the achievement of national targets; namely, that patients with obvious MI receive their treatment within 90 minutes of seeking medical assistance (Weston *et al*, 1994).

The impact of the nurse's role in thrombolysis is not solely confined to the institutional setting. In one prospective study to assess the safety and long term benefits of two thrombolytics initiated outside of the hospital environment, it was apparent that significant gain times to treatment and improved long term outcomes were feasible (Grijeels *et al*, 1995). However, the role of ambulance nurses in assessing and initiating thrombolysis in the pre-hospital phase, was seen as being of unique importance to the success of this study. The investigators also comment that while equipping specially trained nurses with additional skills may be costly, the results are offset by improvements in patients' acute clinical status.

The clinical horizons of the nursing role in the context of thrombolytic therapy are progressing and evolving, in many instances the contribution of practitioners being central to a patient's health status. Integrating core nursing values to the care of patients ensures that, as well as meeting reperfusion priorities, other concerns are addressed. The patient's experience thus reflects a holistic approach rather than one of being processed, a potential that could occur with fast-tracking.

Conclusion

Thrombolytic drugs reduce the mortality and severity of myocardial damage in patients following AMI and are reasonably safe. Optimum coronary reperfusion appears to be achieved if therapy is commenced soon after the onset of pain, and the addition of aspirin augments the benefits of thrombolysis.

In caring for this group of patients, nurses need to have an intimate therapeutic relationship, be highly trained and skilled, and have the authority to carry out treatment and make therapeutic decisions based on their own clinical observations. The key aspect of the nurse's role in relation to thrombolytic therapy must be the patient's safety and the prevention of complications. The nurse must be aware of the potential adverse reactions and of the relevant nursing interventions (*Table 11.4*).

Table 11.4: Problems with thrombolysis

Potential problems		Nursing actions/interventions
Hypotention as a result of therapy (ie. systolic pressure <90 mmHG)	1.	Stop infusion. (Vital signs must be monitored every 5–15 minutes during infusion. The patient must be warned that he/she may feel faint at the beginning of treatment.)
	2.	The patient must be placed supine and medical staff informed.
	3.	Blood products or inotropes may be administered if hypotension is profound. (If nitrates are in progress, also discontinue.)
Bleeding	1.	Stop infusion if there is any bleeding.
	2.	Monitor puncture site(s) for signs of haematoma.
	3.	If bleeding occurs, apply pressure until blood loss ceases.
	4.	Observe for signs of low back pain (ie. aneurysm), cardiac tamponade and changes in neurological state. (The recording of neurological and vital signs is crucial in the acute phase and up to 24 hours after therapy.)
	5.	To minimise bleeding, ensure that all iv access is established before therapy.
	6.	During treatment avoid any intramuscular injections, skin puncture or trauma; immobilise the limb with the infusion; and plug the cannula rather than removing it for a period of 24 hours. (For other nursing care refer to text.)
	7.	In severe cases of haemorrhage, antidotes such as tranexamic acid or blood products (ie. frozen plasma and platelets) may be administered.
Allergic reactions	1.	Patients must be instructed to report any itching, flushed sensation, nausea, rigors or shortness of breath.
	2.	Skin should be frequently assessed for evidence of a rash.
	3.	Mild reactions may be managed by antihistamines, corticosteroids, antiemetics and comfort measures.
	4.	Anaphylactic shock requires immediate response with intubation and adrenaline.
Reperfusion arrhythmias (most commonly accelerated idio-ventricular rhythm, bradycardia, ventricular ectopics and tachycardia)	1.	Continuous cardiac monitoring. A 12-lead ECG from the patient must be obtained before treatment.
	2.	The effects of reperfusion arrhythmias must be monitored through the vital signs. If the arrhythmia is brief and self-reverting, no treatment may be necessary.
	3.	If dysrhythmia compromises the cardiovascular state, alert medical staff and stop infusion. Further treatment may be needed, ie. antiarrhythmics.
	4.	The patient must be reassured that these rhythm disturbances are not unusual and may indicate that treatment is successful.
Reocclusion	1.	Maintain thrombolytic and anticoagulant therapy as prescribed. (Clotting parameters must be kept at one and a half times to twice the normal range.)
	2.	The nurse must monitor and evaluate: (a) symptoms or recurrent chest pain to exclude angina (other signs such as nausea and vomiting will be relevant) and (b) changes in ECG pattern, eg. new ST segment elevation (a 122-lead ECG must be obtained and compared with baseline).
	3.	Inform medical staff.
	4.	Give analgesia and supportive nursing care.
	5.	If reocclusion is confirmed, a further thrombolytic agent may be needed.

Table 11.4 contin.		
Anxiety or knowledge deficit	1.	Clear and simple explanations of all aspects of care must be given. This may need to be done on more than one occasion.
	2.	Information giving must be meaningful to the patient and supported by diagrams and written material as appropriate.
	3.	Family and relevant others must be involved with patient care.
	4.	Consistency of information must be maintained by all members of the team.

Nursing goals should also address the patient's unique set of problems, which may include relief of chest pain or information needs. The nurse must be concerned with the physical, psychosocial, spiritual and educational dimensions of nursing care. Without doubt, these high-tech drugs have expanded and extended the role of nurses, and practitioners must therefore define the unique contribution that nurses can make to patient care.

The literature on thrombolysis has largely been dominated by medical trials, with little evidence of research into the nurse's role in this context and how it varies in individual units. Similarly, the consequences of treating patients in casualty departments, in terms of patient supervision by nursing staff, and the knock-on effect on other patients waiting for treatment, are unknown.

However, there is an accumulating body of material which is accentuating the distinctiveness of the nurse's role in the early assessment and diagnosis of candidates for thrombolysis, and equally proactively responding to the existing clinical problems in delays to treatment. Such contributions emphasise the ongoing commitment and motivation of nurses to improve the delivery and quality of healthcare services.

Clearly, there are a number of resource implications. As more patients are treated with thrombolysis, the length of hospital stays becomes shortened further, and it is possible that continuity of care will be jeopardised because of the requirements for rehabilitation not being met. Thus, there appears to be a legitimate and desirable need to advance nursing research in these areas. According to Benner (1984),

> *Many drugs can only be used safely if their effects are observed and if their possible incompatibilities, contraindications, and adverse reactions are caught early.*

One may reason that without the input of expert nurses this cannot be achieved.

References

Alderman C (1996) Heart to heart. *Nurs Standard* **10**(34): 22–3

Benner P (1984) *From Novice to Expert*. Addison Wesley Publishing Company Inc, Massachusetts

Birkenhead JS (1992) Time delays in provision of thrombolytic treatment in six district hospitals. *Br Med J* **305**: 445–8

Boersma E, Maas A, Deckers J *et al* (1996) Early thrombolytic treatment in acute myocardial infarction: reappraisal of golden hour. *Lancet* **348**: 771–75

Caunt JE (1992) The changing role of coronary care nurses. *Intensive Care Nurs* **8**(2): 82–93

Caunt JE (1996) The advanced nurse practitioner in CCU. *Care of the Critically Ill* **12**(4): 136–9

Chamberlain D (1989) Thrombolysis in the treatment of acute myocardial infarction. *Care of the Critically Ill* **5**(5): 178–81

Culbertson P (1992) Thrombolytic agents: cardiac flow record. *J Emerg Nurs* **18**(2): 141–5

Daily EK (1991) Clinical management of patients receiving thrombolytic therapy. *Heart Lung* **20**(5): 552–65

Flisher D (1995) Fast-track: the early thrombolysis. *Br J Nurs* **4**(10): 562–5

GISSI-2 (1990) A factorial randomised trial of alteplase *vs* streptokinase and heparin *vs* no heparin among 12490 patients with acute myocardial infarction. *Lancet* **336**: 65–71

Grijseels EW, Bouten MJ, Lenderink T *et al* (1995) Pre-hospital thrombolytic therapy with either alteplase or streptokinase: practical implications, complications and long term results in 529 patients. *Eur Heart J* **16**: 1833–8

Grines CL (1996) Primary angioplasty — the strategy of choice. *New Engl J Med* **335**(17): 1313–15

Hendra TJ, Marshall AJ (1992) Increased prescription of thrombolytic treatment to elderly patients with suspected acute myocardial infarction associated with audit. *Br Med J* **304**: 423–5

INJECT (1995) randomised, double-blind comparison of reteplase double-bolus administration with streptokinase in acute myocardial infarction (INJECT): trial to investigate equivalence. *Lancet* **346**: 329–36

ISIS-3 (1992) A randomised comparison of streptokinase *vs* tissue plasminogen activator *vs* anistreplase and of aspirin plus heparin *vs* heparin alone among 41299 cases of suspected acute myocardial infarction. *Lancet* **339**: 1–16

Jowett NI, Thompson DR (1989) *Comprehensive Coronary Care*. Scutari Press, London

Kafetz K, Luder R (1992) Safe use of streptokinase in myocardial infarction in patients aged 75 and over. *Postgrad Med J* **68**: 746–9

Kline ME (1990) Clinical controversies surrounding thrombolytic therapy in acute myocardial infarction. *Heart Lung* **19**(6): 596–601

Kleven M (1988) Comparison of thrombolytic agents: mechanism of action, efficacy and safety. *Heart Lung* **17**(6): 750–5

Lepley-Frey D (1991) Dysrhythmias and blood pressure changes associated with thrombolysis. *Heart Lung* **20**(4): 335–41

Martin GV, Kennedy JW (1994) Choice of thrombolytic agent. In: Julian D, Braunwald E (eds) *Management of Acute Myocardial Infarction*. WB Saunders and Company Ltd, London: chap 3

Moseley MJ (1992) Thrombolytic therapy: a case study. *Crit Care Nurse* **12**(3): 62–8

Murray S (1992) Caring for patients undergoing treatment for vascular occlusion. *Br J Nurs* **2**(1): 17–19

Parry G, Wrightson WN, Hood L *et al* (1993) Delay to thrombolysis in treatment of myocardial infarction. *J R Coll Physicians Lond* **27**(1): 19–23

Quinn T (1995) Can nurses safely assess suitability for thrombolytic therapy? A pilot study. *Intensive Crit Care Nurs* **11**: 126–9

Ramsden CS (1988) Treatment strategies after successful thrombolysis in acute myocardial infarction. *Heart Lung* **17**(6): 777–81

Rodriguez SW, Reed L (1987) Thrombolytic therapy for MI. *Am J Nurs* **87**: 631–40

Sadaniantz T, Sadaniantz A, Garber C (1994) Coronary care unit requirements of patients with acute myocardial infarction treated with or without thrombolytic therapy: a pilot study. *Heart Lung* **23**(4): 328–32

Sait YN (1988) Case history: successful thrombolytic therapy in a patient with acute myocardial infarction. *Heart Lung* **17**(6): 782–6

Storey R, Rowley JM (1997) Electrocardiogram interpretation as a basis for thrombolysis. *J Roy Coll Physicians Lond* **31**(5): 536–40

The GUSTO investigators (1993) An international randomized trial comparing four thrombolytic strategies for acute myocardial infarction. *New Engl J Med* **329**: 673–82

The Task Force on the Management of Acute Myocardial Infarction of the European Society of Cardiology (1996) Acute myocardial infarction: pre-hospital and in-hospital management. *Eur Heart J* **17**: 43–63

Weaver WD (1996) The role of thrombolytic drugs in the management of myocardial infarction: comparative clinical trials. *Eur Heart J* **17**(suppl F): 9–15

Weston CV, Penny WJ, Julian DG (1994) Guidelines for the early management of patients with myocardial infarction. *Br Med J* **308**: 767–71

Wilcox R (1992) Choice of agent: optimal efficiency versus side effects. In: *Thrombolysis: Current Issues and Future Direction*. Medicine Publishing Foundation, Oxford: 9–15

Yusuf S, Anand S, Avezum A *et al* (1996) Treatment for acute myocardial infarction: Overview of randomised clinical trials. *Eur Heart J* **17**(supple F): 16–19

12

Lower limb amputation

Samantha Jane Donohue

1. Indications and treatment

Lower limb amputation is performed predominantly to alleviate acute and chronic limb ischaemia caused by vascular disease, poorly controlled diabetes or, occasionally, infection. Atherosclerosis is the primary cause of chronic arterial ischaemia and the most common reason for amputation. The vascular nurse has an important role in reducing the need for amputation, by providing information on health promotion and illness prevention to patients with vascular insufficiency to halt progression to amputation. This, first section, examines the indications for lower limb amputation in detail, and briefly outlines other treatment options including revascularisation techniques.

Lower limb amputation has decreased in incidence during the latter half of this century. While this is partly due to increased knowledge of the treatment of infection, it is predominantly the result of developments in vascular surgery and revascularisation techniques (Helt, 1994). Vascular insufficiency paired with poorly controlled diabetes or infection still often necessitates amputation. *Figure 12.1* shows the treatment pathway of a patient with vascular disease. The role of the vascular nurse is to halt the patient's progression through this pathway — by providing information on health promotion and illness prevention — and thereby reduce the number of people needing lower limb amputation.

Amputations are performed for a multitude of pathologies. At the turn of the century the predominant reason for performing amputation was trauma to the lower limb (Ham and Cotton, 1991). However, as the number of war casualties diminished, the reasons for performing amputation altered. Current indications for amputation can be divided into five broad categories: vascular disease; trauma; congenital malformations; malignant disease; and infection.

In Britain, amputations are now performed predominantly on people with irreversible tissue ischaemia due to vascular disease, poorly controlled diabetes mellitus or, occasionally, infection (Ham and Cotton, 1991).

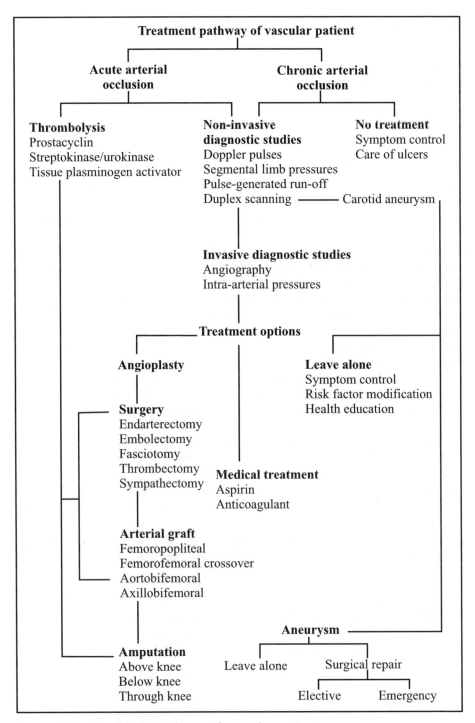

Figure 12.1: Treatment pathway of vascular patient

Vascular disease

Many amputees have previously had vascular reconstruction in the form of bypass surgery and may have had longstanding arterial and venous problems. Often, it is the coexistence of variables such as diabetes, rest pain, ischaemic ulceration and infection that indicate the need for amputation.

Chronic arterial ischaemia

Atherosclerosis: This is the primary cause of chronic arterial ischaemia. It accounts for more than half the deaths in the Western world (Ham and Cotton, 1991) and is the most common reason for amputation. It is a gradual and progressive narrowing of the arteries which eventually leads to total occlusion of the artery (Fahey and McCarthy, 1994). It can begin in the teenage years and spread rapidly; over 40% of middle-aged men have evidence of ischaemia due to atherosclerosis (Rose, 1992). The first clinical presentation may be sudden death, and even the non-fatal presentations (cerebrovascular event and myocardial infarction) may be irreversible. The prevalence of atherosclerosis appears to show a gender, social and geographical differential: it is more common in men, in manual and unskilled workers, and in south-west Scotland (Rose, 1992). This is related to differences in dietary intake of cholesterol and hereditary predisposition.

The pathogenesis of atherosclerosis is still debated (Ball and Mann, 1990), but it is generally believed to start with hyperlipidaemia which causes an alteration in the endothelial lining. The injury to the endothelium allows lipid-filled monocytes to move towards the smoother lining of the inner endothelium. This accumulation of cells, collagen and cholesterol forms a fibrous plaque. This may progress to form an atherosclerotic plaque, resulting in calcification of the vessel wall, and may also allow emboli to be carried 'downstream', often occluding a smaller vessel (Graham and Ford, 1994).

Cholesterol and triglycerides are essential components of the diet and cholesterol is an essential component of plasma membranes (Ball and Mann, 1990). Both circulate bound to specific apoproteins and the combination of lipid and protein is called lipoprotein. The lipoproteins contain varying densities of lipids and proteins: low-density lipoproteins (LDLs) have the highest concentrations of cholesterol, whereas high-density lipoproteins (HDLs) are predominantly protein (Higgins, 1997).

Ideally, serum cholesterol level should be less than 5 mmol/litre. Patients with hypercholesterolaemia paired with hypertension or smoking are at high risk of developing chronic occlusive disease (Rose, 1992).

Intermittent claudication: Patients presenting with intermittent claudication predominantly have chronic arterial occlusive disease. They experience muscular pain after walking a fixed distance. The pain most commonly occurs in the calf muscles and may extend to the buttocks, and is relieved by rest.

Exercise therapy is used to encourage the body to develop a collateral circulation to bypass the occlusion (Maune, 1994). Exercise programmes are an important treatment for people with chronic arterial occlusive disease, but advice should also be given on the detrimental effects of smoking, hypertension, hyperlipidaemia and poorly controlled diabetes, to avoid further deterioration of the peripheral circulation.

Rest pain: Rest pain indicates severe tissue and nerve ischaemia. It is characterised by a burning pain in the toes and feet. Local trauma may result in ulceration and tissue necrosis. The skin becomes dry and the limb discoloured. Patients with nocturnal rest pain often hang the affected limb out of bed to obtain relief (Fahey and White, 1994). The pain is often debilitating and indicates the need for amputation if bypass surgery is not possible.

Revascularisation and reconstructive surgery

Percutaneous transluminal angioplasty: PTA involves the insertion of a catheter into a stenotic or occluded artery, most commonly the common femoral artery. A deflated balloon is threaded through the catheter and inflated at the point of occlusion or stenosis, thus compressing the atheromatous material and widening the lumen of the artery. The procedure can be performed more than once and is often carried out during angiography, which is a precise method of depicting the location and extent of the arterial occlusion (Herbert, 1997).

Femoropopliteal bypass (Figure 12.2): The commonest site of an arterial occlusion is the lower point of the superficial femoral artery, just above the knee (Fahey and McCarthy, 1994). If there is adequate flow in the arteries below the knee, a femoropopliteal bypass may be performed. In this procedure, the bypass is formed from the patient's own saphenous vein, which is removed and reversed to make the venous valves ineffective. One end is then anastomosed to the femoral artery (above the common femoral artery) and the other to the popliteal artery. Occasionally the saphenous vein cannot be used, because it is varicosed or too small or because it has already been used. In this case, a Goretex or PTFE (polytetrafluoroethylene) graft is used.

Aortofemoral bypass and axillofemoral bypass: In aortofemoral bypass (*Figure 12.3*), graft made from plastic, such as Dacron or Teflon, is inserted. The graft is known as a bifurcated or trouser graft and is interposed between the abdominal aorta and the femoral arteries. This type of surgery is performed when there is extensive occlusive disease.

If surgery involving the aorta is not desirable, because of previous surgery or the presence of severe cardiorespiratory disease, then an axillobifermoral bypass (*Figure 12.4*) may be performed (Fahey and McCarthy, 1994). In this procedure a graft is tunnelled from the right axillary artery subcutaneously to the femoral arteries.

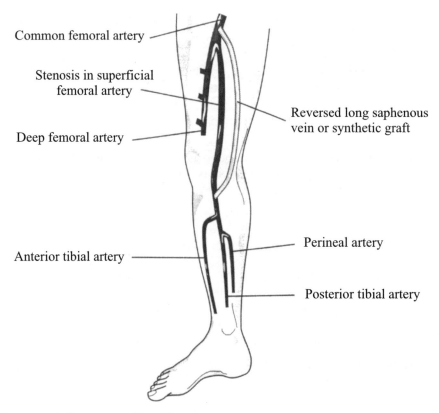

Common femoral artery

Stenosis in superficial
femoral artery

Deep femoral artery

Reversed long saphenous
vein or synthetic graft

Anterior tibial artery

Perineal artery

Posterior tibial artery

Figure 12.2: Femoropopliteal bypass

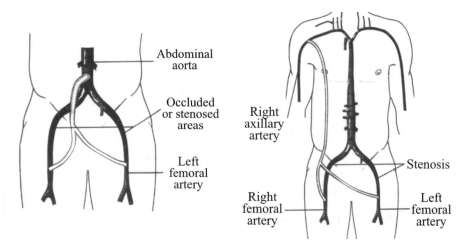

Abdominal
aorta

Occluded
or stenosed
areas

Left
femoral
artery

Right
axillary
artery

Stenosis

Right
femoral
artery

Left
femoral
artery

Figure 12.3: Aortobifemoral graft   **Figure 12.4: Axillobifemoral graft**

Acute arterial occlusion

Patients presenting with acute arterial occlusion classically exhibit certain symptoms: the limb is extremely painful, pale or mottled, and paralysed, and the pulse is not palpable or audible on Doppler ultrasound. The nurse has an important role in constantly assessing the state of the limb and in administering adequate analgesia to control the pain. The most essential diagnosis is determining whether the limb has a pulse as this will differentiate between an arterial and venous occlusion (McPherson and Wolfe, 1992). Acute obstruction of the vascular supply is a limb-threatening situation. It differs from chronic occlusive disease in that there is no time for a good collateral circulation to develop.

Acute arterial occlusion may be caused by an embolism, thrombosis or trauma, resulting in lower limb ischaemia. The most common cause of an arterial embolus is atrial fibrillation: the irregular atrial rhythm results in blood stasis, with the potential for thrombus formation. If an embolus is released into the circulation it may migrate and become lodged in a narrowing of the artery or at a bifurcation (Fahey and McCarthy, 1994). Approximately half of all emboli lodge at the common femoral bifurcation (Butler and Fahey, 1993).

Other cardiac causes of acute arterial occlusion are mitral stenosis (which produces a high left atrial pressure), myocardial infarction and endocarditis. Non-cardiac causes include atherosclerotic debris, aneurysm, and trauma to the artery caused by a crushing injury or fracture.

Treatment of an arterial embolus depends on how quickly the patient presents to the GP: irreversible ischaemia will necessitate amputation. Treatment consists of either dissolving the clot (thrombolysis) or removing it (embolectomy).

Thrombolysis: This involves infusion of a fibrinolytic agent, such as streptokinase or tissue plasminogen activator, locally into the stenosis through a catheter inserted into the occlusion. The procedure requires the patient to lay flat and still for up to 24 hours with a femoral arterial catheter in situ. Contraindications to this procedure include recent surgery duodenal ulceration and cerebrovascular haemorrhage.

Femoral embolectomy: In this procedure, a Fogarty catheter is used to extract the thrombus. The catheter is passed via the groin to a point distal to the occlusion; a balloon is then inflated and the embolus is removed.

Depending on the state of the ischaemic limb, fasciotomies to the anterior, lateral and posterior muscle compartments may be performed to avoid any inflammation and oedema causing tissue and nerve damage within the tight muscle compartments — often termed compartment syndrome (McPherson and Wolfe, 1992).

The nurse's role

All nurses working in a vascular surgery setting need to develop a working knowledge of the physiology and pathophysiology of the vascular and cardiovascular systems. When caring for patients with acute and chronic limb ischaemia it is vital for the nurse to be confident and competent in monitoring alterations in the limb using touch and visual observations, eg. the colour and warmth of the limb, and in detecting blood flow with a Doppler scanner.

Following revascularisation techniques, such as bypass surgery, hypotension and hypertension must be avoided in order to promote an optimum environment for the graft to function (Fahey and McCarthy, 1994). The patient is often extremely anxious at this time as successful revascularisation can mean the end of pain, ulcers and immobility. The nurse needs to be an empathic and skilled communicator, both in preparing the patient for the operation and in re-educating him/her with regard to lifestyle changes, such as smoking cessation and diet. This is dealt with in detail in the third section of this chapter.

Vascular disease and diabetes

Patients with diabetes mellitus are extremely susceptible to peripheral occlusive disease. Twenty years after their initial diabetic diagnosis, over 80% of diabetics have some form of vascular disease (Graham and Ford, 1994). In the USA, more than 45% of non-trauma amputations are performed on diabetics (Helt, 1994). Diabetic patients are more prone to lower limb lesions and ischaemia for a number of reasons.

Peripheral neuropathy: In 1993, the Diabetes Control and Complications Trial (DCCT Research Group, 1993) demonstrated a clear connection between poorly controlled diabetes and the onset of peripheral neuropathy and decreased peripheral circulation. Peripheral neuropathy is characterised by the loss of sensory and proprioceptive sensation in the peripheral tissues. Vulnerability to trauma to the feet is therefore increased, as is the likelihood of the injury going unnoticed. Peripheral neuropathy, together with the increased risk of infection due to hyperglycaemia and decreased tissue perfusion, makes the healing of lesions problematic.

Tissue perfusion: Diabetic patients are also vulnerable to peripheral tissue hypoxia as their circulating haemoglobin is prevented from delivering an adequate oxygen supply to the peripheral tissues owing to the accumulation of glucose on the red blood cell, ie. their glycosylated haemoglobin (HbA_{1c}) is raised.

Atherosclerosis: Diabetics tend to have a higher serum concentration of LDLs, and a lower concentration of HDLs which carry cholesterol to the liver to be removed. The aetiology of vascular disease is the same in diabetics and non-diabetics — only the prevalence is different.

Raynaud's disease

Raynaud's disease predominantly affects women and is characterised by bilateral attacks of ischaemia, usually affecting the fingers and toes. The skin becomes pale and the sufferer experiences burning and pain in the digits. The disease rarely extends beyond the metacarpophalangeal joint, and in severe cases can cause digital gangrene. Raynaud's syndrome differs in that affected individuals experience similar symptoms, but the onset is associated with other disease, such as systemic lupus erythematosus, sclerodoma and rheumatoid arthritis (Whitaker and Kelleher, 1994).

Arteritis

Arteritis is inflammation of an artery, often caused by an autoimmune response. One form of arteritis is Buerger's disease, or thromboangiitis obliterans. This is a rare disorder which is thought to be caused by heavy smoking; patients present with distal vessel occlusion which often necessitates amputation of the limb (Graham and Ford, 1994).

Venous disease

Ulceration, whether venous, arterial or mixed aetiology, can cause the sufferer immense discomfort and disability. Frequent dressing changes, uncontrolled pain, fetid odour and infection are all complaints aired by patients with venous and arterial ulcers. Venous ulcers differ from arterial ulcers in their speed of development and position on the leg. Arterial ulcers are more common on the lateral malleolus and foot whereas venous ulcers are more common on the medial malleolus (Nelson *et al*, 1996).

The use of the ankle-brachial pressure index can aid diagnosis of the ulcers; while many patients will present with ulcers of mixed aetiology, the extent of the arterial disease will dictate many of the treatment aims (Gilliland and Wolfe, 1992). Nelson *et al* (1996) noted that health professionals often underestimated the pain caused by ulceration. If the pain remains untreatable because of the mixed aetiology of the ulcers, amputation may be an option.

Trauma

Trauma is no longer the main cause of limb amputation in the Western world. However, amputation is still, occasionally, a life-saving procedure following industrial, farming and road traffic accidents (Ham and Cotton, 1991).

Any accident can involve extensive burns, tissue destruction, vascular impairment, bone non-union and neurological damage, and often the surgery must be performed immediately, thereby removing the opportunity for any psychological preparation. The development of rapid freezing procedures means that it may now be possible to implant limbs that have been severed; however, severe crushing injuries do tend to result in amputation.

Congenital malformations

Vitali *et al* (1986) estimated that one in every 1000 children are born in the West with a major deformity. Of these, 63% have defects in their upper limbs, 19% have defects in their lower limbs and 18% have bilateral defects. The cause of the defects is varied and the extent of the defects ranges from slight under- or overgrowth to complete failure of formation. Only children born with grossly deformed limbs are considered for amputation, and then it is with the future of a prosthesis in mind.

Malignant disease

A small percentage (approximately 3%; Herbert, 1997) of amputations are performed because of the presence of malignant disease, such as osteosarcoma. Osteosarcoma is a malignant growth of bone cells. The commonest sites of occurrence are the lower end of the femur, the upper end of the tibia and the upper end of the humerus. The tumour rarely occurs after the age of 20, and although radiotherapy is the primary treatment, amputation of the affected limb may be necessary (Macleod, 1986).

Infection

Hyerglycaemia causes changes in the body's glycoproteins, tissue hypoxia and nutritional changes and generally impairs the healing of infected lesions (Faris,1991). Diabetic patients are extremely prone to uncontrolled infection, including infection that is localised to a lesion, diffuse infection, such as cellulitis, and systemic infection. Ischaemic ulceration often leads to gangrene, and the primary task in such cases is to minimise damage by removing the necrotic, infected tissue and administering broad-spectrum antibiotics.

Uncontrolled infection, such as gas gangrene, is now less common; it was predominantly seen in warfare when wounds became contaminated with anaerobic organisms from the soil (Ham and Cotton, 1991). Gas gangrene requires immediate treatment; the patient exhibits the typical signs of infection and the wound gives off a fetid odour as well as producing a coppery discoloration of the skin. On X-ray, gas gangrene shows up as bubbles of air which may be felt when touching the subcutaneous tissues. Strict attention to hygiene is needed post-operatively with amputees, as faecal contamination of the stump will increase the risk of infection.

Prophylactic antibiotics, predominantly penicillin and metronidazole (Campbell, 1982), are usually advocated: cefuroxime may be used if the microorganism is resistant to penicillin or the patient is allergic to penicillin.

Key points

* Lower limb amputation is performed predominantly to alleviate acute and chronic limb ischaemia resulting from vascular disease, poorly controlled diabetes mellitus and infection.
* Atherosclerosis is the primary cause of chronic arterial ischaemia and the most common reason for amputation.
* The coexistence of limb ischaemia, rest pain, infection or poorly controlled diabetes in patients with vascular insufficiency all increase the likelihood of amputation becoming necessary.

❋ The vascular nurse has an important role in halting patients' progression to amputation, by providing information on health promotion and illness prevention.

References

Ball M, Mann J (1990) *Lipids and Heart Disease — A Practical Approach*. Oxford University Press, Oxford

Butler L, Fahey VA (1993) Acute arterial occlusion of the lower extremity. *J Vasc Nurs* **11**(1): 19–22

Campbell WE (1992) The ischaemic lower limb (2). *Hosp Update* May: 549–60

DCCT Research Group (1993) The effect of intensive treatment of diabetes on the development of progression of long-term complications in insulin-dependent diabetes mellitus. *N Engl J Med* **329**: 977–86

Fahey VA, McCarthy WJ (1994) Arterial reconstruction of the lower extremity. In: Fahey VA, ed *Vascular Nursing*. 2nd edn. WB Saunders, Philadelphia: 291–324

Fahey VA, White SA (1994) Physical assessment of the vascular system. In: Fahey VA, ed *Vascular Nursing*. 2nd edn. WB Saunders, Philadelphia: 53–72

Faris I (1991) *The Management of the Diabetic Foot*. Churchill Livingstone, Edinburgh

Gilliland EL, Wolfe JHN (1992) Leg ulcers. In: Wolfe JHN, ed *ABC of Vascular Diseases*. BMJ, London: 55–8

Graham LM, Ford MB (1994) Arterial disease. In: Fahey VA, ed *Vascular Nursing*. 2nd edn. WB Saunders, Philadelphia: 3–20

Ham R, Cotton L (1991) *Limb Amputation*. Chapman and Hall, London

Helt J (1994) Amputation in the vascular patient. In: Fahey VA, ed *Vascular Nursing*. 2nd edn. WB Saunders, Philadelphia: 509–35

Herbert LM (1997) *Caring for the Vascular Patient*. Churchill Livingstone, New York

Higgins C (1997) Measurement of cholesterol and triglycerides. *Nurs Times* **93**(15): 54–5

Macleod J (1986) *Davidson's Principles and Practice of Medicine*. 14th edn. Churchill Livingstone, New York

Maune J (1994) Therapeutic walking program: an alternative to a formal vascular rehabilitation program. *J Vasc Nurs* **12**(3): 80–4

McPherson GAD, Wolfe JHN (1992) Acute ischaemia of the leg. In: Wolfe JHN, ed *ABC of Vascular Diseases*. BMJ, London: 15–18

Nelson A, Ruckley V, Dale J *et al* (1996) Management of leg ulcers. *Nurs Times* **92**(20): 58–66

Rose G (1992) Epidemiology of atherosclerosis. In: Wolfe JHN, ed *ABC of Vascular Diseases*. BMJ, London 1–4

Whitaker L, Kelleher A (1994) Raynaud's syndrome: diagnosis and treatment. *J Vasc Nurs* **12**(1): 10–3

Vitali M, Robinson KP, Andrews BG *et al* (1986) *Amputations and Prostheses*. 2nd edn. Ballière Tindall, London

2. Once the decision to amputate has been made

This section examines the factors that need to be addressed once the decision to amputate has been made. It stresses the importance of preparing the patient and his/her family both psychologically and physiologically for the operation. The techniques and rationale for selecting the optimum level of amputation are then discussed. Finally, the specific levels of lower limb amputation are outlined.

Lower limb amputation is performed predominantly to relieve acute and chronic arterial ischaemia, although there are a number of other indications for this form of surgery. The indications for amputation, and the other treatment options available before the amputation stage is reached, are discussed in the first section of this chapter (*Indications and treatment*). Once it has been decided that the only possible surgery is amputation, there are a number of factors to consider. Of prime importance is that the patient and his/her family feel psychologically and physiologically prepared for the operation and understand the necessity for amputation and its implications for the future. The nurse's role is central to the patient's care and will be explored later in the chapter (*The role of the nurse*).

It is essential that amputation is not considered to be the result of 'failure' of medical therapy; instead, it should be seen as the most effective means of relieving the pain and suffering that a patient may have been living with for years.

Some patients see amputation as a positive step towards achieving some kind of quality of life for the first time in years, whereas others take a different view. Recently, a man with a long history of non-healing, painful ulcers said that the amputation would allow him to go to the cinema for the first time in years without worrying about the pain or the smell of the ulcers.

In contrast, another man who had spent the last 20 years progressing along the treatment pathway (outlined in *Figure 12.5*) stated that he viewed the amputation of his leg as the last stage before his death and that he had spent the last 20 years dreading the moment that he would consent to have his leg amputated.

The next decision to be made is the optimum level of amputation.

Selecting the level of amputation

As Mr Naylor, a Consultant Vascular Surgeon at Leicester Royal Infirmary, stated, 'Level selection is based on achieving the optimal chances of rehabilitation'.

He is insistent that the rehabilitation problems of many amputees are derived from the attitude of some professionals that amputation is a purely destructive not constructive procedure (Naylor, 1995). Amputations should not be performed by relatively junior medical staff, but by a skilled vascular surgeon. If the level of the amputation is not selected correctly, or the stump is not formed sufficiently, then any prosthesis fitting is extremely problematic.

The primary object of amputation is to remove sufficient diseased, infected and gangrenous tissue to permit the stump to heal but... retain adequate limb length for prosthesis.

(Ham and Cotton, 1991)

A variety of techniques are used to predict the optimum level of amputation. These are outlined in *Table 12.1*. However, Helt (1994) believes that,

To date, none of these tests have proved to be consistently more reliable than clinical judgement in predicting wound healing at a given level.

The most successful method appears to combine functional tests with simply examining the limb for ulceration and skin friability, assessing the general state of the patient and the possibility of a prosthesis, and ascertaining the patient's wishes.

Preservation of the knee joint is advantageous in rehabilitation, but as a patient once commented, 'I've always suffered from arthritis in that knee — what do I want to keep the bloody thing for'.

Table 12.1: Techniques used to predict the optimum level of amputation	
Angiography	Provides a static, anatomical image of the arterial tree to determine the patency of the vessels and evidence of collateral vessels
	Angioplasty to the iliac vessels may be required to ensure optimum flow to the stump
Segmental arterial pressures (ankle/brachial pressure index; ABPI)	Method of assessing the extent of occlusive disease. It involves calculation of the ratio of systolic blood pressure at the ankle, calf or thigh to brachial systolic pressure. The pressure of the lower limb should be equal to or slightly greater than the brachial systolic pressure (Whitson, 1996). Ideal ABPI = 1.0+
Laser Doppler flowmetry	Provides a quantitative measure of microcirculatory perfusion
Skin perfusion pressure	An invasive procedure that measures the pressure needed to halt blood flow to the skin
Infra-red thermography	Assesses blood flow to the skin by portraying temperature gradients

The different levels of lower limb amputation are shown on *Figure 12.5*.

Amputation of the foot

Autoamputation has been documented in the writings of the ancient Greeks (Helt, 1994). The gangrenous part of the limb demarcates and, once mummified, falls off. Autoamputation of digits is still promoted so long as there is no secondary infection present.

The main amputations of the foot are the ray, transmetatarsal and Syme's amputations (*Figure 12.6*).

Ray amputation

The surgeon cuts directly down to the bone proximal to the necrotic tissue. Any dead tissue, tendons and fascia are removed and no flap dissection is used.

Transmetatarsal amputation

The incision is made across the metatarsal joint, removing all of the digits. After an initial period, weight-bearing on the amputated foot can be achieved.

Syme's amputation

This involves a disarticulation through the ankle joint, normally at the lower end of the tibia. It is predominantly used in trauma surgery or in the presence of chronic infection, and the amputee will need a prosthesis for balance if weight-bearing (Ham and Cotton, 1991).

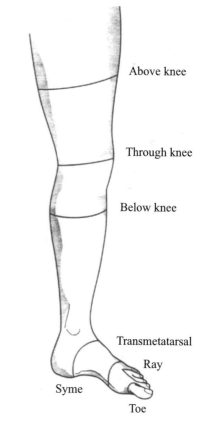

Above knee

Through knee

Below knee

Transmetatarsal

Ray

Syme

Toe

Figure 12.5: Levels of lower limb amputation

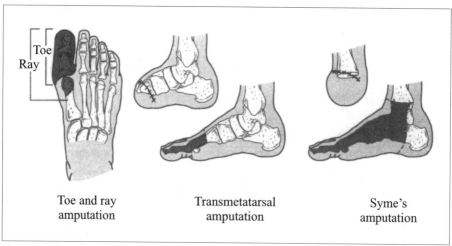

Toe
Ray

Toe and ray amputation

Transmetatarsal amputation

Syme's amputation

Figure 12.6: Main amputations of the foot

Below-knee amputation

The below-knee amputation (BKA) is traditionally favoured as preservation of the knee joint gives the amputee the best chance of being fitted with a fully functional prosthesis. The effectiveness of a long posterior flap in the BKA was popularised in the 1970s by Burgess (1968), who also highlighted the problems with this method, namely that a poorly designed flap may result in a deformed stump, and pressure and ulceration often cause difficulties with the prosthesis.

Robinson advocated the skew flap method, which is now predominantly used. By positioning the join of the flap obliquely, the tibial crest is covered by gastrocnemius muscle and the blood supply to the flap is maximised (Robinson *et al*, 1982).

Ideally, the BKA stump measures 14 cm from the tibial plateau; if this distance is less than 8 cm there will be a problem fitting a prosthesis (Naylor, 1995). Some surgeons divide the tibia into thirds, leaving the upper third, whereas others amputate at the largest diameter of the calf.

All surgery will be predominantly dictated by the extent of tissue damage and infection and also the rationale for surgery.

Through-knee amputation

A through-knee amputation (TKA) or knee disarticulation is a rapid and relatively bloodless amputation, as no bone needs to be cut. The TKA tends to be used when expectations of postoperative mobility are limited. Preservation of the patella allows the fitting of a prosthesis and also aids balance in a wheelchair.

Gritti stokes amputation

This amputation involves transection of the femur above the condyles and then attaching the femur to the end of the patella. The theory is that this will allow weight bearing, but as the fracture takes a long time to unite, and the femur often retracts up at the distal end, the operation is now rarely used.

Above-knee amputation

Many people with long-term peripheral vascular disease have few viable arteries below the knee joint. Often an above-knee (transfemoral) amputation is the only viable option.

The aim is to divide the thigh into thirds: a third is removed, leaving 25–30 cm from the greater trochanter. This should be sufficient to enable some kind of prosthesis to be fitted. The stump has anterior and posterior flaps that are equal in length, and the femur is sculptured and smoothed before the muscles are sutured together. The arteries and veins are ligated separately to allow the maximum number of collateral vessels to survive. A Redivac drain is usually inserted to prevent haematoma formation. Intensive physiotherapy is essential to avoid hip flexion.

Hip disarticulation

This amputation is generally only performed as a life-saving operation. The scar is anterior to avoid faecal contamination and it is essential that the patient is catheterised and receives intravenous antibiotics both pre- and postoperatively.

Mobility using a prosthesis is a possibility, but every effort must be made by healthcare team members to avoid contracture of the hip, infection and the wound breaking down.

Conclusion

There are many treatment options available before the amputation stage is reached. Many amputees have undergone previous vascular procedures and have considered amputation before admission. Those who present with an acute limb ischaemia may need an amputation without having time to prepare themselves physically, mentally or socially. Whatever the cause or route that leads to amputation, patients will need support from all members of the healthcare team to assist them through this traumatic period.

Key points

* It is essential that the patient and family feel psychologically and physiologically prepared for the amputation.
* Amputation should not be viewed as medical failure or a destructive procedure, but as a constructive procedure.
* Selection of the optimum level of amputation is a balance between the need to remove dead and infected tissue and the best chances of rehabilitation.
* All surgery will be dictated predominantly by the extent of tissue damage and infection, and by the rationale for surgery.
* Whatever the cause or route to amputation, the patient will need support from all members of the healthcare team to assist him/her through this traumatic time.

References

Burgess EM (1968) The below knee amputation. *Bull Prosthetic Res:* 19–25

Ham R, Cotton L (1991) *Limb Amputation.* Chapman and Hall, London

Helt J (1994) Amputation in the vascular patient. In: Fahey VA, ed *Vascular Nursing.* 2nd edn. WB Saunders, Philadelphia: 509–35

Naylor AR (1995) *Amputation: when and where.* Unpublished lecture, Leicester Royal Infirmary

Robinson KP, Hoile R, Coddington T (1982) Skew flap myoplastic below knee amputation: a preliminary report. *Br J Surg* **69**: 554–7

Whitson R (1996) Principles of Doppler. *Nurs Times* **92**(20): 66–70

3: The role of the nurse

This third section on lower limb amputation examines the role of the nurse in the pre- and postoperative care of patients undergoing amputation. The nurse has an integral role, not only in providing care, but also in liaising with other members of the multidisciplinary team in order to ensure that the person undergoing the amputation feels prepared for both the operation and discharge home. Amputation may greatly distort an individual's vision of him/herself as a person, a partner and a parent; ways in which this distortion can be minimised are explored.

Limb amputation is ideally a planned procedure. The preoperative period allows the nurse to carry out a full assessment of the physiological, psychological and social preparation required by the patient. The postoperative period is a time when the multidisciplinary team work together to fulfil these needs. The healthcare professionals are interdependent; effective communication between the team members is essential to the well-being of the amputee.

The multidisciplinary team outlined in *Figure 12.7* illustrates the network of support available to the amputee. This is not a definitive list and other health professionals such as the diabetic specialist nurse, community physiotherapist and occupational therapist may also have an input.

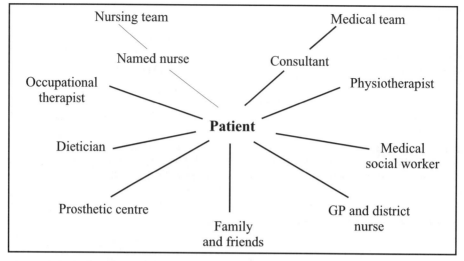

Figure 12.7: The clinical services and support available to the amputee

Preoperative role of the nurse

Physiological preparation

Patients awaiting amputation predominantly have acute arterial occlusion, long-standing chronic arterial occlusion and/or systemic infection. They are likely to be viewed as physiologically unprepared for an operation because of generalised cardiovascular disease, poor nutritional status and often uncontrolled diabetes mellitus.

Cardiovascular and respiratory stability: The anaesthetist and medical team will perform a full cardiovascular and respiratory assessment preoperatively. Hypertension, atrial fibrillation, chronic obstructive pulmonary disease, coronary heart disease and renal failure are common complications in patients awaiting amputation. Regular and accurate observations of blood pressure, pulse, fluid and electrolyte balance, respiratory rate and oxygen saturation by the nurse are required to ascertain whether any of the complications can be minimised preoperatively.

Infection: The level of the amputation will be affected by the extent of infected tissue (Helt, 1994). Infection may be localised to a lesion or be diffuse (eg. cellulitis) or systemic. The nurse can monitor the progression of infection by observing the limb regularly and documenting any changes in appearance, warmth, sensation and movement, as well as monitoring for pyrexia and hyperglycaemia. Ischaemic gangrene may rapidly develop into a life-threatening condition, with the circulating toxins causing septicaemia. Preoperative intravenous antibiotics may be necessary to control infection before surgery.

It is not unusual for a patient awaiting amputation to become acutely confused as a result of infection. This is an indication that immediate surgery is required.

Diabetic control: Preoperatively, diabetic patients undergoing vascular surgery are likely to have endocrine instability owing to the presence of pain and infection. They also tend to have a poor nutritional intake as their appetite has been suppressed by their physical condition (Holmes, 1996). The nurse has an essential role in assessing the patient's present and recent diabetic control. Uncontrolled blood glucose levels that cannot be corrected by the patient's normal regimen of insulin or oral hypoglycaemic drugs may necessitate a titrated intravenous infusion of insulin and glucose to achieve diabetic control preoperatively. The optimum blood glucose level before surgery is between four and ten mmol/litre (Marshall, 1996); however, surgery will occasionally have to be undertaken before control is achieved. The nurse should make the medical and anaesthetic staff aware of the patient's blood glucose level before he/she is taken to theatre so that they can closely monitor the levels perioperatively.

Many anaesthetists recommend that a diabetic patient is given preference on the theatre list. Fasting time should be determined from research-based practice. Chapman (1996) found that nurses are generally unaware of recent research on prescribed fasting times. Over 50% of anaesthetists in Chapman's study acknowledged that clear fluids given two to three hours before surgery did not significantly alter residual gastric volume or acidity, yet patients continue to be subjected to prolonged fasting times (Chapman, 1996).

Patients with non-insulin-dependent diabetes mellitus (NIDDMs) are often advised not to take their sulphonylurea (oral hypoglycaemic medication) on the day of the operation, regardless of where they are on the operating list, as drugs such as chlorpropamide are long acting and may cause a postoperative hypoglycaemic episode. Many patients with NIDDMs still possess sufficient endogenous insulin to carry them through the perioperative period. It is important to explain that if they do require insulin postoperatively to control their plasma glucose levels, this does not mean that they will always be dependent on insulin.

Diabetics may also have a preoperative assessment of retinopathy as anticoagulation can increase the risk of haemorrhage in patients with active proliferative retinopathy. It may be useful to contact the patient's diabetic centre to obtain the most recent retinopathy screening results.

Pain control: Many patients awaiting amputation will be experiencing uncontrolled pain. They may be prescribed opiates, such as morphine slow-release tablets and dipipanone, in an attempt to control the pain. Without adequate pain control, patients will find it extremely difficult to prepare themselves in other ways for the operation. However, because of the severity of the pain, adequate control is often difficult to achieve. The differential in pain perception by the patient and the nurse is widely documented (Seers, 1987; Field, 1996). The sensitivity of the ischaemic limb cannot be overemphasised — even the weight of a sheet can cause unbearable discomfort. Bed cradles are useful in alleviating pressure from the affected limb, and keeping the limb warm will promote reflex vasodilatation.

Verbal and non-verbal signals of pain should be used to ascertain the severity of the pain. There are many pain assessment tools now available (Schofield,

1995). In the John Radcliffe Hospital the majority of surgical wards now use a tool that encourages the patient to describe the pain and nausea experienced as well as incorporating a sedation score.

Diamond and Coniam (1991) found a correlation between the use of prophylactic preoperative pain relief and decreased post-amputation pain: 'Pain seems to be more common when the limb has been more painful prior to loss'. Bach *et al* (1988) found that an epidural block given before surgery to reduce the pain correlated with a reduction in the number of people complaining of phantom pain following amputation.

Problems of immobility: Pressure sores, chest infection, deep vein thrombosis, constipation and sensory deprivation can pose significant problems both preoperatively and post-amputation (Rubin, 1988). An ischaemic limb may render a person more immobile before the amputation than afterwards.

The patient's risk of developing pressure sores can be assessed using scores such as the Waterlow score (Waterlow, 1988).

The nurse is responsible for assessing the need for a pressure-relieving mattress and selecting a suitable mattress. Certain alternating-pressure mattresses should not be used for an amputee, because of the method in which the cells alternate. Huntleigh, for example, recommend that their Nimbus 1 is not used for an amputee as the sensor pad is central to the torso and the disproportioned weight of the amputee could lead to inappropriate cell pressure. (The Nimbus 1 is no longer in production and the Nimbus 2 and 3 are perfectly suitable for amputees.)

Passive limb and upper body exercises should be encouraged before the operation. The ward physiotherapist will assess current mobility and begin to discuss the exercise regimen that the patient shall commence following the amputation.

Nutritional intake: Ischaemia and ulceration can cause pain, infection and often an odour, all of which may adversely affect nutritional intake; this may result in malnutrition which, in turn, will affect healing and delay recovery.

Nurses have a key responsibility in pre-empting malnutrition (UKCC, 1997) and can work closely with a dietician, the patient and family in an effort to replete a patient's energy stores before surgery. The dietician may talk to the patient to find out which foods he/she prefers, and can provide a high protein diet and recommend suitable supplement drinks.

Psychological preparation

The psychological preparation of the patient and family should be viewed as a priority by the nurse. The first step is to introduce them to their nursing team, the ward and their named nurse. It is the named nurse's responsibility to assess how much psychological preparation is needed and what form it should take. The therapeutic effect of reducing postoperative anxiety by giving preoperative information has been documented by Swindale (1989). Although Swindale was studying anxiety levels following minor surgery, many patients have commented to me that they feel more able to cope with the surgery if they understand what to expect, rather than fearing the 'unknown'.

Each patient will have different psychological needs and these needs will be dynamic and constantly changing. Some patients will appear confident in their decision, anxious only for their partners and/or family, whereas others will see the amputation as the loss of their autonomy and capabilities as a person, and view their future existence only in terms of being an amputee.

Any person who faces radical surgery will also experience an alteration in the way they see their own body. Body image is neither a motionless nor a simplistic concept: the external environment can alter the way we see ourselves and we often utilise various coping strategies, both consciously and unconsciously, to cope with this alteration (Salter, 1988). Price (1990) developed a body-image care model where the body reality (how the body really exists), the body ideal (how we would prefer our body to look) and the body presentation (how we present our body to the outside world) are three equal components. A satisfactory body image is dependent on the equilibrium of these three components. Our social networks, our environment and our ability to utilise additional coping mechanisms help to promote a positive response to circumstances when the equilibrium is threatened.

For example, our ideal body and the reality of our body may be different and so we utilise coping mechanisms to find a mean body presentation that we are comfortable with. The environment has dictated a body ideal and we have been able to respond to that ideal by achieving an acceptable compromise.

However, when a person's internal environment dictates an alteration in the body presentation that is unwanted or unacceptable to that person, then the body image is seen as altered. Sometimes a person can utilise the external environment to manipulate internal changes, eg. if the individual dislikes the signs of ageing, he/she may use make-up, plastic surgery and fashion to manipulate the body reality. However, physiological changes, such as a limb amputation, cannot be manipulated and the body-image equilibrium is disrupted.

Environment constantly interacts with the individual and determines, in part, adaptation level.

(Roy, 1976)

The attribution of causes of an altered body image plays an important part in the individual's recovery, and the nature and intensity of the person's grief is seen to largely depend on to whom, or what, the individual attributes the cause of the physiological changes (Abramson and Martin, 1990). For example, a woman with NIDDM was recently admitted to the vascular unit requiring a below-knee amputation. She had originally developed a small lesion on her toe after wearing ill-fitting anti-embolism stockings while recovering from a minor operation. The lesion deteriorated, became infected and failed to heal. She was understandably bitter, especially as she had previously visited a podiatrist regularly and taken great care of her feet. In contrast, a man who had a below-knee amputation attributed the causes of his peripheral vascular disease to his refusal to give up smoking. He stated that nothing would ever stop him smoking and acknowledged his responsibility in causing the amputation.

Preoperatively, an assessment of the patient's present body image and self-esteem by the nurse is important. It should also be remembered that patients facing an amputation may already have an altered body image due to uncontrolled pain or non-healing ulcers, but they should still be assisted in the preparation for the loss of a limb. In addition, a person who has already had one limb amputated will experience a further alteration in body image if the remaining limb is amputated. They may feel that society will reject them as a bilateral amputee because of their increased dependence on others, and this fear needs to be addressed.

In predicting an individual's ability to cope with the forthcoming operation, an assessment of their support systems by the nurse is useful. For example, if a person fears the responses of others to his/her altered body state, an empathetic response by the person's close family and friends will be important. If those significant others are included in preoperative discussions concerning the surgery, they are more likely to provide that empathic response and assist in the redevelopment of a satisfactory body image (Price, 1990).

The presence of other amputees on the ward can often be useful in demonstrating coping strategies. Some people have the confidence to talk to other patients and share their fears and experiences. Others may rely on their nurse to suggest the possibility of discussing experiences with other amputees rather than instigate it themselves. Obviously, every person's ability to cope with situations differs and this individuality in needs will help to structure the nursing input.

Social preparation

Preoperatively, a full assessment of the individual's daily life needs to be undertaken if a successful discharge is to be the final goal. The discharge plan needs to commence on admission. Unfortunately, most people who have undergone lower limb amputation because of peripheral vascular disease have bilateral disease and an extremely poor life expectancy. Nearly 30% of these people will have their remaining limb amputated within two years and over 50% will die within five years of their first amputation (Ham *et al*, 1985). A poorly planned discharge could be wasting valuable moments in the lives of these people and is unacceptable.

In the vascular unit in Oxford the nursing assessment is structured around Roy's model of nursing. Roy (1976) sees the person as an adaptive system that is fluid in its ability to respond to external or internal stimuli. Adaptive behaviours can be assessed by interviewing the person, and tentative judgements can be made as to the effectiveness of the person's behaviours. Using the model the social assessment can provide a base on which to make those tentative judgments: by building up a picture of the person's family, social network and adaptations to the illness so far, we can develop an individualised and effective discharge plan (*Figure 12.8*).

Individualised discharge plan				
Patient label **Bill Watson** **cr no: 246318B**	**Discharge planning information**			
	Nursing team Blue	**Primary/named nurse** Sam Donohue		
	Ward 6A	**Admission date** 27.2.97		
Social situation				
	• Bill was widowed in 1992 • Bill lives alone in a ground floor, warden controlled flat that is wheelchair accessible • District nurse visits twice daily to re-dress ulcers, GP and DN aware of admission • No other social services received			
List key discharge needs:	**Referrals**	**Name**	**Date**	**Reason**
• Self-management of diabetes • Stump wound healing • Confident in wheelchair • Inform DN and GP and warden • TTO's	**Physio**	Gerry	on admission	Pre-amputation advice and post-op care
	or	Vera	"	Wheelchair, stump board, home assessment
	Social worker	Sheila	"	Advice for benefits
	Community nurse	Paul	5/3/97	Discharge from community hospital-check blood glucose
	Community hospital	Bicester	5/3/97	Convalescence — one week
	Dietician	Jane	"	Diabetic, loss of weight
A self-medication programme needed prior to discharge? No	**Podiatrist**	Steve	"	Advice and foot assessment

Figure 12.8: Individualised discharge plan

Communication with the occupational therapist and physiotherapist to ascertain how they feel the person will cope following the amputation is integral to the discharge plan. Many homes need alterations to allow wheelchair access and if the person lives alone or his/her home is not able to be accessed by a wheelchair, then the social work team will need to be involved; they will also be able to give financial advice concerning social security benefits and allowances that may be available.

Postoperative role of the nurse

Physiological needs

During the initial postoperative period, the attention given to the amputee is similar to that given to any other patient. Hypo- or hypervolaemia, disturbed cardiac, renal and respiratory function, pressure area care and pain control are all normal postoperative concerns.

Haemodynamic stability: The amount of blood lost during the operation differs according to the level of the amputation. A through-knee amputation is a relatively bloodless amputation, whereas a below- or above-knee amputation will have more effect on haemodynamic stability. Blood pressure, pulse and urinary output should be monitored regularly, with the parameters similar to those in any other postoperative condition. Intravenous hydration will continue until the patient is tolerating fluid and diet adequately.

Below- and above-knee amputees tend to return from theatre with a suction drain, such as a Redivac drain, in situ, to avoid haematoma formation in the stump. The drain is not normally sutured in place; this allows its removal without disturbing the bandages that are helping to form the stump.

Diabetic control: All patients will show a metabolic response to surgery. Hepatic glycogenolysis and gluconeogenesis are stimulated as a result of the rise in circulatory levels of hormones, such as adrenocorticotrophic hormone, catecholamines (adrenaline and noradrenaline), glucagon and growth hormones (Marshall, 1996).

Non-diabetic individuals possess the ability to suppress the catabolism of fats and proteins into glucose by releasing insulin from the beta cells in the pancreas and therefore keep their blood glucose level within the normal limits, ie. 4–7 mmol/litre.

Insulin-dependent diabetics (IDDMs) do not have this ability to naturally halt these catabolic processes, and if they are not given the required amount of insulin they are potentially at risk of becoming ketoacidotic. People with NIDDM possess adequate insulin levels to halt lipolysis, but still need to have their blood glucose levels monitored closely. If the reading appears abnormally high or low, a venous sample should be sent for analysis.

Once the patient can tolerate an adequate diet, his/her normal regimen of insulin or oral hypoglycaemic tablets should be reinstated. The nurse should continue to monitor the blood glucose levels closely, as once the trauma of surgery is over and any infected/necrotic tissue has been removed, the mean blood glucose level may drop and the patient may become hypoglycaemic.

The wound: The bandages surrounding the stump help to form the stump and reduce oedema. For this reason, many vascular units have a policy of leaving the bandages intact for up to five days unless there is significant rationale for their removal, ie. haemorrhage, odour or staining. The flap of the stump is normally stitched using a continuous suture that can be removed after ten days. Some surgeons prefer to use clips; however, their use has been correlated with a higher incidence of wound pain (Galvani, 1997).

Transmetatarsal amputations tend to have individual sutures along the wound. Plaster of Paris is sometimes used to help form the stump and avoid flexion contracture; this is removed approximately five days later. Hypovolaemia and malnutrition can prevent the wound from healing and may necessitate revision of the stump to a higher level. This is yet another indication of the importance of the nurse's role in assessing and addressing any nutritional and fluid imbalance.

Mobility: The amputee will normally begin an exercise programme the day after surgery. Prevention of joint contracture, as well as the other complications associated with immobility, is essential and so the physiotherapist will teach the amputee how to develop strength in the amputated limb, the remaining limb and the upper body (Andrews, 1996). If the amputee is not physically able to begin gentle exercise, then the physiotherapist will spend time teaching him/her how to optimise respiratory function. Early mobilisation will help to improve the person's confidence about future independence (Andrews, 1996). The first time the amputee gets out of bed will be traumatic, unless adequate explanations and reassurance have been given.

Many amputees are nursed on an alternating-pressure mattress to avoid the development of pressure sores. However, these often make independent movement from bed to wheelchair difficult. This can be eased by deflating the mattress, thus enabling the person to move across the mattress with minimum energy expenditure. Transmetatarsal and Syme's amputations will require the amputee to be non-weight-bearing for up to five days. The amputee can move from bed to chair, but will only be able to use the heel to aid mobilisation. Ideally, a wheelchair should have been delivered preoperatively. The position of the wheels will differ according to the level of amputation; all amputees who have had a below-, through- and above-knee amputation need to have a stump board fitted to the wheelchair to support the stump at all times.

Pain control: As well as correlating with poor postoperative pain relief and respiratory and cardiovascular complications (Hollinworth, 1994), inadequate pain control will restrict an amputee's postoperative mobilisation.

The pain experienced initially will differ from the ischaemic pain experienced before amputation. Immediately following the amputation the pain is of an acute, traumatic nature instigated by tissue damage, neurological disturbance and anxiety — often termed stump pain.

Stump pain can often be successfully relieved by the use of opiates, non-steroidal anti-inflammatory agents and local anaesthetics. However, a poorly fitting prosthesis, neuroma formation on the stump and joint pain may cause the stump pain to continue for up to six months after the operation (Davis, 1993b).

The type of pain that many amputees experience but are not prepared for is phantom limb pain. This is literally pain experienced in the limb that has been amputated and is often described as a crushing, tearing pain. The episodes of pain may differ in intensity and frequency and may cease after a short period or persist indefinitely (Diamond and Coniam, 1991). Phantom limb pain has been described as one of the worst clinical pain syndromes (Melzack and Wall, 1995) and its true cause is poorly understood. The phenomenon of phantom limb pain should not be underemphasised. Krebs *et al* (1984) found that 60% of amputees were still experiencing phantom limb pain seven years after amputation. Pain that continues six months after surgery is generally extremely difficult to treat (Davis, 1993b).

Phantom limb sensation differs from phantom limb pain in that it may not be a painful sensation that is experienced. The absent body part may be felt to be touching, tickling, itching or twisting. Initially, the illusory limb may appear identical to the amputated limb, and then gradually shrink or become distorted and grotesque (Chapman, 1986). Jensen and Rasmussen (1995) have divided the clinical characteristics of phantom pain into three categories: simple sensations, eg. touch, itching and heat; more complex sensations, eg. the limb's length, posture and size; and limb movement, eg. spontaneous or willed movements.

Amputees are often shocked and upset by the sensations and pain experienced. One man said that his wife only realised the extent of the problem when she sat on his bed to have a cuddle and he shouted at her to get off the bed. She had sat down where his amputated leg would have been and he felt the crushing pain coinciding with her sitting down.

There are a variety of treatments available for phantom limb pain and sensation. The current treatment choices tend to combine tricyclic antidepressants, such as carbamazepine, and anticonvulsant drugs, such as sodium valproate, with non-invasive stimulatory techniques such as transcutaneous electrical nerve stimulation (TENS). In TENS, electrodes are placed over the stump and/or remaining nerves in order to stimulate the release of A-beta fibres which are thought to halt the pain impulse passing up the spinal cord to the cerebral cortex (Davis, 1993a).

Hypnosis has been shown to be effective in a study of 37 patients who had undergone either arm or limb amputations and were experiencing phantom limb pain (Cedercreutz and Uusitalo, 1967, cited in Hildegard, 1986). Following hypnosis, 20 were asymptomatic and more than 10 felt that their condition had improved. Up to eight years later, 8 people were still symptom free and 10 still felt that their symptoms had improved.

The preparation of amputees for phantom limb pain and sensation tends to be an ad hoc process. Predominantly, because of poor understanding of its cause and fear that forewarning people about phantom pain may cause the person to experience it (Wilson, 1994), many people are not alerted to the phenomenon preoperatively.

The nurse's postoperative assessment of pain is essential in order to distinguish between stump pain, phantom limb pain and phantom limb sensation. Pain assessment charts can supply the nurse with comprehensive information concerning the type, location and intensity of the pain, as well as information concerning the pain experience, ie. blood pressure, pulse and respiratory rate.

However, as highlighted by Mackintosh (1994), pain questionnaires and charts rely heavily on the individual's ability to verbalise the pain that is being experienced. Culture, gender and age all affect expression of pain (Seers, 1987). Some cultures advocate wailing when in pain, whereas others are notoriously stoical. The pain experienced following an amputation may scare and confuse people.

The sensations may be attributed to a loss of sanity and constant explanations and reassurance by all members of the healthcare team involved in the patient's care is essential. One woman who had had an above-knee amputation became increasingly withdrawn, despite being physiologically stable. After much discussion, she stated that she felt she 'had gone mad' as she was having constant pain in her toes and desperately wanted to massage them, but was fearful of the other patients seeing her and laughing. She feared the loss of her sanity. By the day that she was due to return home she was able to laugh about the sensations and pain experienced as she understood their significance.

All health professionals involved in nursing people undergoing limb amputation should educate themselves about the various pain responses to the surgery in order to help control the pain and support those experiencing it.

Psychological needs

Postoperatively, the psychological needs of the amputee can often depend on the preparation they receive before the operation. Initially, the amputee may show an awareness of losing the limb, and the role of the nurse, with both the patient and family, is to encourage them to express their true feelings (Helt, 1994).

> *Body-image sustenance and development is achieved best within a supportive social support framework. Social support networks... provide the milieu in which a normal body is first formed and an altered body image is reintegrated into society.*

(Price, 1990)

The altered body part should be referred to by its proper name, not 'your bad leg', and privacy to investigate the limb and to express feelings about it should be allowed. The patient may wish to conceal the limb with bedding or clothing until he/she feels able to cope with viewing the limb. When the person is ready, he/she will begin to acknowledge the changes that have occurred and will start to become more inquisitive as to the future. Integration with other amputees and engaging in activities where others are present is an important step.

The nurse needs to be truthful and non-judgemental yet help to facilitate rehabilitation goals by guiding the person through recovery. A person who has undergone such a major alteration in body image is not going to possess a fully constructed body image by the time of discharge. However, a trusting, truthful relationship that involves realistic appraisal and ongoing evaluation of progress is essential.

Social needs

Ideally, the discharge process should have commenced before surgery and the nurse should have already liaised with the physiotherapy, occupational therapy and social services departments. The occupational therapist may decide to perform a washing and dressing assessment, as well as a home visit, to aid his/her assessment of the amputee's needs on discharge.

Family and carers may approach the nurse with questions concerning discharge home and the future. Documenting discussions, information given and unaddressed needs will allow the nursing team to achieve continuity in their care. Information, such as the address of the Limbless Association (BLESMA, Frankland More House, 185–187 High Road, Chadwell Heath, Romford RM6 6NA. Tel No: 0181 590 1124) and the local prosthetic service should be given before discharge.

Discharge advice: Depending on the cause of the amputation, the discharge process should include information on looking after the remaining limb. Advice should be given concerning foot care, care of the stump and how to limit the risk of developing or exacerbating peripheral vascular disease.

Diabetics should be referred to a podiatrist because of their increased risk of peripheral lacerations, and relatives/carers should also be given information on how to care for the stump and the remaining limb. Some amputees will continue to smoke despite knowing the risks of doing so. Many of them state that it is their only pleasure left and remind us of the fact that when they fought in the Second World War they were given cigarettes as part of their pay.

Conclusion

The nurse has an integral role in optimising the care of a person undergoing lower limb amputation. From admission to discharge the needs of the amputee are constantly changing, therefore the ability of the nurse to continuously assess these needs and formulate plans of care to meet these needs is paramount. The nurse has a central role in liaising with other members of the multidisciplinary team, in co-ordinating communication, and in evaluating care, as he/she has the most regular contact with the patient.

The primary role of the nurse is to assist and support the person and family through a dramatic, life-changing experience in a positive way, which will hopefully allow them to return home with the strength needed to face the future.

Key points

* The nurse plays a central role in assessing and addressing the patient's physiological, psychological and social needs, both before amputation and postoperatively.

* As life expectancy of people undergoing lower limb amputation, because of vascular disease and poorly controlled diabetes, is extremely poor, their discharge home should not be delayed by poor planning; a discharge plan therefore needs to be commenced on admission.

* Amputation may be viewed as the release from years of pain and disablement due to ulcers and infection.

* People facing amputation will react differently and should be nursed as individuals who have individual needs.

References

Abramson LY, Martin DJ (1990) Depression and the causal inference process. In: Gross RD, ed. *Key Studies in Psychology*. Hodder and Stoughton, London

Andrews KL (1996) Rehabilitation in limb deficiency: the geriatric amputee. *Arch Phys Med Rehabil* **77**: 14–17

Bach S, Moreng MF, Tjellden NU (1988) Phantom limb pain in amputees during the 12 months following amputation, after pre-operative lumbar epidural blockade. *Pain* **33**: 297–301

Chapman R (1986) Pain, perception and illusion. In: Sternbach RA, ed. *The Psychology of Pain*. 2nd edn. Raven Press, New York: 153–79

Chapman A (1996) Current theory and practice: a study of pre-operative fasting. *Nurs Stand* **10**(18): 33–36

Davis P (1993a) Opening up the gate control theory. *Nurs Stand* **7**(45): 25–7

Davis RW (1993b) Phantom sensation, phantom pain, and stump pain. *Arch Phys Med Rehabil* **74**: 79–86

Diamond AW, Coniam SW (1991) *The Management of Chronic Pain*. Open University Press, Oxford

Field L (1996) Are nurses still underestimating patient's pain postoperatively? *Br J Nurs* **5**(13): 778–84

Galvani J (1997) Not yet cut and dried. *Nurs Times* **93**(16): 87–9

Ham RO, Thornberry DJ, Regan JF *et al* (1985) Rehabilitation of the vascular amputee — one method evaluated. *Physiother Practice* **1**: 6–13

Helt J (1994) Amputation in the vascular patient. In: Fahey VA, ed. *Vascular Nursing*. WB Saunders: Philadelphia: 509–32

Hildegard ER (1986) Hypnosis and pain. In: Sternbach RA, ed. *The Psychology of Pain.* 2nd edn. Raven Press, New York: 197–221

Hollinworth H (1994) No gain? *Nurs Times* **90**(1): 24–7

Holmes S (1996) The incidence of malnutrition in hospitals. *Nurs Times* **92**(12): 43–7

Jensen TS, Rasmussen P (1995) Phantom pain and other phenomena after amputation. In: Melzack R, Wall PD. *Textbook of Pain*. 3rd edn. Churchill Livingstone, London: 651–66

Krebs B, Jenson TS, Kroner K *et al* (1984) Phantom limb phenomenon in amputees seven years after limb amputation. *Pain* (Suppl) **2**: 585

Mackintosh C (1994) Do nurses provide adequate pain relief? *Br J Nurs* **3**(7): 342–7

Marshall SM (1996) The peri-operative management of diabetes. *Care Crit Ill* **12**(2): 64–7

Melzack R, Wall PD (1995) *The Textbook of Pain*. 3rd edn. Churchill Livingstone, London

Price B (1990) A model for body-image care. *J Adv Nurs* **15**: 85–93

Roy C (1976) *Introduction to Nursing: An Adaptation Model*. Englewood Cliff, New Jersey

Rubin M (1988) The physiology of bedrest. *Am J Nurs* **1**: 50–5

Salter M (1988) *Altered Body Image: The Nurse's Role*. John Wiley and Sons, Chichester

Scholfield P (1995) Using assessment tools to help patients in pain. *Prof Nurse* **10**(11): 703–6

Seers K (1987) Perceptions of pain. *Nurs Times* **33**(48): 37–9

Swindale J (1989) The nurse's role in giving preoperative information to reduce anxiety in patients admitted to hospital for elective minor surgery. *J Adv Nurs* **14**: 899–905

UKCC (1997) Nurses are responsible for feeding patients. *Register* **20**: 5

Waterlow J (1988) Calculating the risk. *Nurs Times* **83**(39): 58–60

Wilson PG (1994) Phantom pain. In: Tollison CD, ed *Handbook of Pain Management*. 2nd edn. Williams and Wilkins, Baltimore: 497–502

13

Primary nursing care of people who have had a stroke

Sue Palmer

This chapter describes the care of two people who have had a stroke. It explores how their primary nurse and her colleagues learned to identify communication needs, and examines the development of strategies to help meet those needs.

Communication was described by Houghlan-Adkins (1991) as a, '... universal, dynamic process by which means human beings exchange ideas, impart feelings and express needs'.

In a model of interpersonal interaction Hargie (1993) emphasised the fact that effective communication is a two-way process involving both participants on an equal basis (*Figure 13.1*). He also described the factors that influence the ability of those involved to achieve an effective interaction. These include:

1. Personal factors, such as appearance and physical and mental well-being.
2. Situational factors, which include the environment, past experience and the role played by each participant.
3. Issues such as motivation and the goals set by each person (either consciously or subconsciously).

Disruption to each or any of these factors by either party can be a barrier to effective communication (Hargie, 1993).

The aim of this chapter is to highlight these barriers by analysing the difficulties in communication experienced by two people who have had a stroke. In addition, the strategies employed to overcome or to alleviate the results of such barriers are examined. The term strategy has been carefully chosen and is used intentionally. Bury (1991) defined strategy as follows,

> *The term strategy, in contrast to 'coping', directs attention to the actions people take, or what people do in the face of illness, rather than the attitudes people develop.*

Nurses have a key role in the facilitation of these strategies.

The issue of effective communication is of paramount importance for anyone who has had a stroke. Buckwalter *et al* (1989) stated that effective communication underlies all aspects of care for people who have had a stroke. They described it as being an essential part of any rehabilitation process and quoted research undertaken by the Institute of Medicine (1986) in the USA. This suggested that as people who cannot effectively communicate find difficulty in maintaining control over their lives, the resulting loss of control is often

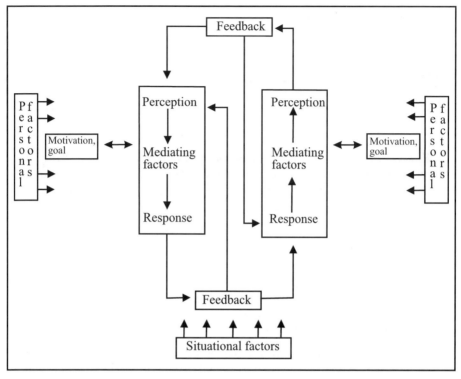

Figure 13.1: Extended model of interpersonal interaction (from Hargie, 1993)

augmented by loss of the use of a limb, sight or memory. The inability to express anger, opinions and needs leads to further frustration and helplessness. There is evidence to suggest that quality of life after a stroke is not only affected by functional capacity but also by emotional, behavioural and cognitive ability (Sissons, 1995); this adds weight to the need for effective communication in order to influence these factors, which in turn has an impact on quality of life.

People who have had a stroke may experience communication difficulties in a variety of ways. For example, a cerebrovascular accident in the left (dominant) hemisphere is likely to cause aphasia or dysphasia. The range of deficit can vary widely from mild symptoms to severe disruption of expression and/or comprehension (Houghlan-Adkins, 1991).

The two people described in this chapter present two different types of difficulty with interpersonal interaction which result from having a stroke. These difficulties are summarised in *Table 13.1*.

Table 13.1: Difficulties with interpersonal interaction experienced by John and Jane		
	John	**Jane**
Personal factors	Impaired memory led to no perception of physical or mental well-being. He had no awareness of why he should be in hospital	Reduced ability to concentrate
Situational factors	No recall of past experiences. No concept of uniform meaning doctor or nurse. No structure to the day (although he slept all night)	Impairment of social roles due to lack of social skills, eg. patience, talking in turn. Reduced concept of hospital environment, eg. talked loudly in the middle of the night
Motivation and goals	Memory loss meant goals were all short-term, eg. need for a cigarette or for the toilet	Self-centred motivation in conversations. Not able to prioritise, eg. her safety was secondary to question or comment
Perception	Severely disrupted as memory of only 30 seconds	Self-perception disrupted, eg. body image. Lack of memory/ concentration on what was said to her
Response	Repetitive response, often regardless of what had just been said	Fluctuating ability to comment appropriately because of altered perceptions
Feedback	Difficulty giving or receiving feedback as he could not remember what was happening to him	Feedback difficult to interpret due to disrupted responses and understanding. Some comments not relevant to activities

Care study 1

Assessment

Memory has been described and analysed since the days of Plato. Pioneering work was undertaken by Korsakoff in 1889 which is referred to and quoted 100 years later (Ellis and Young, 1988) when memory is described as an 'elusive construct' (Dye, 1989). However, memory is still not clearly or completely understood. There appear to be three main elements; registration, retention and retrieval (Ellis and Young, 1988). It has proved difficult to test which of these elements are affected by brain injury such as a stroke.

> **Case study 1**
>
> John was 76 years old. When he was found wandering
> in the street hear his home and brought to hospital he
> could remember his name and most events up until
> 1960. He remembered his daughter and son-in-law but
> not his grandchildren and he did not remember that his
> wife had died four years previously. A brain scan
> showed a localised area of ischaemia causing severe
> memory loss but no other apparent deficits.

John's difficulties with communication were twofold:

• From his point of view, he could not remember anything from one moment to the next, so he was impaired emotionally and socially. With reference to the factors identified by Hargie (1993) as influencing communication, John had severe memory loss which had an impact on personal and situational factors. For example, he was not able to recount previous experience and so did not recognise uniforms as correlating with roles. In addition, his motivation and goal-setting abilities were severely impaired and his perception, responses and feedback were disrupted as a result of the memory loss. This demonstrates the range and depth of the barriers to communication that John faced.

Church (1985) described the importance of being able to remember recent information, ie. it allows a person to 'function normally' and 'remain oriented'. Added to this, Bleathman and Morton (1996) describe the 'devastating' effect of loss of memory on sense of self and identity. As a result of his memory loss John was unable to build relationships with nurses and other patients and needed reassurance that he was 'in the right place' and could remain there. Anxiety in itself is recognised as being a barrier to communication (Hargie, 1993).

• From the nurses' point of view, frustration was the major barrier to effective communication with John. The fact that there was no opportunity to build rapport or a relationship with him added to this problem. The nurses' goal was to make some progress in reducing John's anxiety and to increase his ability to recognise familiar people or places. This process was slow and unrewarding and after three months on the ward John would still show surprise if a nurse approached him and used his name.

Frustration was not a consistent problem for John. He would become more anxious as the day wore on, but essentially he maintained a cheerful and humorous outlook on life. The nurses observed that this behaviour made it easier for them to care for John than if he were constantly frustrated or irritable and complaining. His personality therefore prevented him from becoming an unpopular patient; Stockwell (1972) stated that the ability of people to 'laugh and joke' with the nurses made them more popular.

According to Stockwell, the least popular patients on a ward fall into two groups, and John had the potential to fit into either group. The first category include people who demonstrate by their behaviour that they do not want to be in that ward, or who constantly complain or demand attention. The second group were those people whom nurses perceive as not having a need to be in hospital — or in that particular ward — **and** whose personalities do not outweigh this judgement.

John required much attention and spent a long time on the ward while waiting to find accommodation, as he was unable to return to his own home. Strategies for overcoming the obstacles to communication needed to fulfil two functions:

1. To focus on and alleviate the anxiety and fear felt by John.
2. To minimise the frustration felt by staff.

Alleviating John's anxiety

A major component of John's anxiety was his expressed desire to go home. He was also worried that his family did not know where he was. John had never left his wife alone for long periods as she had been in poor health, and he did not remember that she had died. This foundation for anxiety emerged through talking with Maggie, his daughter. Maggie told the nurses she had initially felt that gently reminding John that his wife had died was an appropriate way of helping him to remember her death. However, it had caused John to become distressed because each time she told him was as painful as the first.

Bleathen and Morton (1996) suggest a solution within which the goal of achieving an understanding of reality is seen as less important than communicating to ease distress and restore self-worth. It involves concepts from validation therapy, acknowledging anxieties and losses without trying to force 'new insights' (Feil, 1992). In this case, both Maggie and the nurses caring for John found it very uncomfortable to repeatedly tell him that his wife had died. They adopted a strategy of encouraging him to remember where she was and that she was not in any danger. After a period of time John began to ask for his sisters or for Maggie and he did not refer to his wife so much.

Initially John was unable to remember that his family came regularly to visit him and would express anxiety that they did not know where he was. This meant that he was constantly asking to speak to his daughter or to be taken to his sister's house. Telephoning his daughter did not solve the problem because he would soon forget that he had spoken with her. Church (1985) reported that reality orientation is a useful tool for helping people feel less threatened by their environment. Reality orientation was instituted in this case in the form of a visitors' book. John's sisters would write a message and the date and sign their name each time they visited and Maggie and her family did the same.

The visitors' book became a very useful aid to communication because it was a constant reminder for John of when his family had visited. It also provided written evidence that they knew where he was and cared about him. John seemed to find this helpful and it reassured him and alleviated his anxiety temporarily. He also had photographs and tapes of his favourite Irish music.

According to Church (1985), people with poor short-term memory are more dependent upon their environment. John remained in the same bed area during his time on the ward. He could occasionally identify which of three beds was his and he could usually find his way to the toilet from his bed. Part of his care plan involved guiding him back to his bed area if he was anxious or distressed, in the hope that he would find comfort in his most familiar environment.

Minimising nurses' frustration

The measures described above were all facilitated by the way in which nursing was organised on the ward, namely primary nursing. Fairlie (1992) recognised this as a promising strategy for strengthening communication between patients and nurses. However, Menzies (1970) noted that nurses sometimes distance themselves from their patients because of stressful or frustrating situations, thus fulfilling a need to protect themselves. Therefore, while primary nursing fosters clear communication channels on the one hand, it can increase feelings of frustration or stress on the other.

The potential for feelings of impatience or frustration to become a problem was alleviated by open discussion and acknowledgement of such feelings at daily handover times if it was felt necessary. Strategies were discussed or reviewed, feelings were shared and resolutions were sought. At the beginning of each shift, all nurses received a priority handover. This identified the most important strategies for each patient during that shift. The nurse caring for John would then receive more detailed information from the nurse who had been working with him for the previous shift.

Priorities for John were threefold:

1. The potential for him to smoke in an unsafe place, as he could not remember that there was a smoking area.
2. There was a potential for him to be lost as he could not recall his way around the ward.
3. There was a chance that he might leave the ward and become lost in the hospital.

The ward nurses could therefore share the responsibility for John's safety, although his allocated nurse was accountable. This system also ensured that all nurses were aware of the things that increased John's sense of comfort and security. For example, everyone knew where his matches were kept. This removed the need to ask him questions that he was unable to answer or to find his primary nurse when he wanted to light a cigarette.

All the above strategies were outlined in John's care plan along with his identified self-care deficits (Orem, 1991), goals and nursing interventions. His care was evaluated at each shift and a reassessment of his needs was carried out every two weeks by his primary nurse.

John became less anxious and some rapport was built up with staff. It remained difficult to tell whether he felt that his needs were met, despite his difficulty with communication, or whether any rapport was established for him.

Discharge

John moved to a residential part three home near to his sisters which had special provision for people with memory loss. He was accompanied to his new home by his daughter and his primary nurse. This enabled a verbal and written description of his needs to be discussed with the nurses caring for him in the new setting.

Case study 2

Assessment

According to Pimental (1986), there is still a great deal that is unknown about the effects of right-hemisphere brain injury. However, some issues have been identified in relation to communication. Often people who have suffered a right-sided stroke talk excessively but find it hard to get to the point. In addition, they may be unable to add expression or emotion to what they are saying and may have difficulty in recognising emotion in others. Alexander *et al* (1989) observed that people with right-hemisphere injury often also have limited insight into their condition or disabilities.

Jane had a number of difficulties with interactions, although she did not perceive these herself. From the nurses' perspective the main barrier was that the language deficit was not striking, unlike the aphasia or dysphasia experienced after left-hemisphere brain injury. Thus, it did not appear to be so devastating. In people who have had a right-sided stroke it is common for difficulties to go unnoticed, thereby creating a barrier to effective communication. After working with Jane over a number of weeks, her communication difficulties became apparent and could then be addressed.

Case study 2

Jane was 60 years old when she experienced a right-hemisphere (non-dominant) cerebrovascular accident resulting in a dense left-sided weakness and a deficit in her communication skills.

Jane's difficulties were focused upon three areas:

• She was easily distracted from what she was doing. This is a common symptom of right-brain injury (Houghlan-Adkins, 1991). Jane talked continuously and had little awareness of others in the room or insight into her own safety. For example, she would continue to talk while undertaking a potentially hazardous transfer from her bed to her chair and so be unable to concentrate fully on the manoeuvre. She would ask her fellow patients questions while they were talking to their visitors, or start a conversation with a nurse who was in mid-sentence with another patient. Pimental (1986) attributed this type of behaviour to impulsiveness, verbosity and inattention, which are all symptoms of organic right-hemisphere injury. The person exhibiting these symptoms should not be labelled as rude by nurses or other patients.

• Jane had little or no insight into the effect that her stroke was likely to have on her life. She was very optimistic and talked of plans to go abroad on holiday with her friend. She also spoke about going home for the night and picking up her cat.

• Jane would often look down or away while she was talking. Pimental (1986) highlighted the fact that reduced eye contact and less facial animation is a common feature following a right-sided stroke. This is significant for communication, as Hargie *et al* (1994) described the face as a rich source of information regarding the emotional state of the individual. These authors went on to discuss the importance of eye contact, which has an impact on interactions because it demonstrates that the listener is paying attention to what is being said.

Care plan

The strategies employed by the nursing staff to overcome barriers to communication were again facilitated by the use of primary nursing. This allowed continuing assessment of Jane's communication abilities and difficulties.

The issue of concentration was highlighted in Jane's care plan. Nursing interventions included directing Jane through tasks which she needed to accomplish by employing firmness in a kindly way. Continuous repetition was necessary as Jane would easily revert to her previous behaviour. Houghlan-Adkins (1991) advocated the reinforcement of socially correct behaviour in a firm but kind manner.

Jane's lack of insight was a barrier to effective communication for both Jane and the nurses caring for her. Jane would talk of plans and schemes which the nurses felt unable to dismiss as ridiculous, although they could not reinforce them. The nurses also felt uncomfortable at the idea of having to shatter all Jane's illusions by telling her the truth. This situation was made more complicated by the fact that it was not clear to what extent Jane would eventually recover. Therefore, Jane's care plan reflected a balance, in that nurses would not reinforce her unrealistic ideas (*Figure 13.2*) but, instead, would encourage her to think more thoroughly about what she was saying. For example, when she wanted to go home for the night it was helpful to ask how she would get into bed, to make her think through her suggestion. Pimental (1986) advocates letting the client know when statements do not make sense. This strategy seemed to help Jane to realise that some of her ideas were unrealistic or difficult to achieve, without leaving her with a sense of hopelessness.

To establish eye contact, the care plan emphasised the importance of approaching Jane from her left side. This is acknowledged to be good practice by Houghlan-Adkins (1991) and is a well-known strategy. One of the most important factors in managing Jane's care was that the nurse caring for her understood why she had less eye contact and reduced facial expression, and why she might interrupt or appear discourteous. This topic was introduced through discussion about the medical diagnosis and the pathological alterations influencing behaviour.

Discharge

Jane was on the ward for two months and was then transferred to a specialised rehabilitation ward near to where she lived. While on the ward she made considerable progress, both physically and in terms of realising her potential capabilities.

Self-care (patient problem)	Goal	Nursing action	Signature
Jane does not seem to understand the full impact of her stroke and the effect it will have on her life	Jane will say she knows what is happening and has an idea what the future will hold	1. Avoid reinforcing Jane's optimism 2. Keep reminding Jane of her capacities and that she will need help for quite a while yet	

Figure 13.2: An extract from Jane's care plan

Conclusion

Anyone with communication difficulties following a stroke may experience frustration, embarrassment, irritation, depression and aggression. This is further exacerbated if speech therapy is intermittent or discontinued as a result of slow progress (Buckwalter *et al*, 1989). It is clear that nurses and other members of the multidisciplinary team must work together to identify and develop strategies to deal with these difficulties.

With John and Jane the communication difficulties were not solved entirely. However, nurses were able to go some way towards alleviating the distress and discomfort which emerged as a direct result of inability to communicate. It was difficult to evaluate the degree of success in overcoming John's communication problems as the only measure was his level of anxiety, which was reflected in his agitation and activity. Jane's problems were alleviated to some degree. People who have experienced irreversible damage to their brain as a result of a stroke rarely regain their previous level of communication. However, it is possible to overcome some of the difficulties and so minimise some of the disadvantages and discomfort experienced by people with these handicaps. Stockwell (1972) found the people nurses enjoyed caring for were able to communicate readily with them.

Popularity may have assisted the communication process with John and Jane. However, the literature reveals that popularity is underpinned by strategies emerging from a thoughtful and critical approach to nursing care. This presents a particular challenge to the nurse caring for people who have communication handicaps resulting from a stroke.

Key points

* Effective communication underlies all aspects of care for people who have had a stroke.

* After a stroke the range of communication deficit can vary enormously from person to person.

* Effective communication is a complex process involving internal and external factors.

* Communication deficits from right-hemisphere brain injury are not always immediately obvious and can be overlooked.

* The patient's ability to communicate seems to have a direct correlation with his/her popularity on the ward.

Acknowledgements

Figure 13.1 is reproduced by kind permission of Croom Helm. Thanks are due to Angela Heslop and Anna Collins, without whom this chapter would have remained a handwritten essay.

References

Alexander MP, Benson DF, Stuss DT (1989) Frontal lobes and language. *Brain Lang* **37**: 656–91

Bleathman C, Morton I (1996) Validation Therapy: a review of its contribution to dementia care. *Br J Nurs* **5**(14): 866–8

Buckwalter K, Cusak D, Siddles E *et al* (1989) Increasing communication ability in aphasic/dysarthric patients. *West J Nurs Res* **11**(6): 736–47

Bury M (1991) The sociology of chronic illness. A review of research and prospects. *Sociology of Health and Illness* **13**(4): 451–68

Church MA (1985) Forgotten something? *Nurs Times* **81**(30): 22–4

Dye CA (1989) Memory and Ageing: a nursing responsibility. *Recent advances in nursing* **23**: 53–65

Ellis AW, Young AW (1988) *Human Cognitive Neuropsychology*. Lawrence Embaum Associates, Hove

Fairlie A (1992) Nurse-patient communication barriers. *Sen Nurse* **12**(3): 40–3

Feil N (1992) Validation therapy with late onset dementia populations. In: Jones GMM, Meisen B (eds) *Care Giving in Dementia*. Routledge, London

Hargie O (1993) *The Handbook of Communication Skills.* 1st edn. Croom Helm, London

Hargie O, Saunders C, Dickson D (1994) *Social Skills in Interpersonal Communication*. 2nd edn. Croom Helm, London

Houghlan-Adkins ER (1991) Nursing care of clients with impaired communication. *Rehabil Nurs* **16**(2): 74–6

Institute of Medicine (1986) *Improving Quality of Care in Nursing Homes.* Report No 10m–85–10. National Academic Press, Washington DC

Menzies I (1970) *The Functioning of Social Systems as a Defence Against Anxiety.* Tavistock Institute, London

Orem DE (1991) *Nursing Concepts of Practice.* 3rd edn. McGraw Hill, New York

Pimental PA (1986) Alterations in communication. *Nurs Clin North Am* **21**(2): 321–37

Sissons RA (1995) Cognitive status as a predictor of right hemisphere stroke outcomes. *J Neurosci Nurs* **27**(3): 1520–6

Stockwell F (1972) *The Unpopular Patient.* Royal College of Nursing, London

14

Diabetic control in the patient with acute myocardial infarction

Karyn Noy

Diabetes mellitus affects 2% of the population and up to 5% of people over 65 years of age (Thomas, 1993). Diabetic patients have more coronary artery disease and a higher mortality from acute myocardial infarction (AMI) than the rest of the population (Patmore and Jennings, 1996). They have similar-size infarcts to those without diabetes, but the total mortality post-MIs is higher (Karlson et al, 1993). This article examines the literature on AMI in diabetic patients to ascertain the most effective management of these patients and hence improve their prognosis.

Diabetes mellitus is a clinical syndrome characterised by hyperglycaemia due to a deficiency or diminished effectiveness of insulin (Perkins, 1992). Approximately a quarter of sufferers are insulin dependent (type 1) and the rest are non-insulin dependent and are controlled by diet alone or by diet and oral hypoglycaemic agents (type 2). It is thought that, in type 1 diabetes, there is an immunological cause for the destruction of insulin-secreting islet beta cells in the pancreas, resulting in an insulin deficiency requiring insulin treatment (Bodansky, 1989). There is also a genetic predisposition to the development of diabetes. The aetiology of type 2 diabetes involves impaired insulin secretion and decreased tissue responsiveness (insulin resistance). Obesity, increasing age and family history are additional contributory factors (Paton, 1989).

Premature atherosclerosis is the most common cause of complications and death in diabetes. The Framingham study (Abbott *et al*, 1988) found an increased frequency of myocardial infarction (MI) and angina in diabetics, particularly women. Diabetic patients are not only at greater risk of sustaining a MI, but also have almost double the mortality from MI compared with the non-diabetic population (Patmore and Jennings, 1996). The Minnesota Heart Survey (Sprafka *et al*, 1991) and GISSI-2 (1990) found that the relative mortality rate in hospital and at six months ranged from 1.5 to 2.5, depending on gender and the type of diabetes, with type 1 diabetics having the worst prognosis.

Karlson *et al* (1993) concluded from their research on 858 patients in Sweden that re-infarction and left ventricular failure (LVF) were more prevalent in the diabetic population, but that there was no evidence that diabetic patients had larger infarcts than non-diabetic patients. The Corpus Christi Heart project (Orlander *et al*, 1994) examined 1357 patients and found that the size of the infarct was not a predictor of the increased morbidity or mortality seen in the group with diabetes. The increased long-term mortality of diabetic individuals was considered to reflect more rapid progression of coronary heart disease and cardiac failure, which was related to the effect of diabetes on processes such as thrombogenesis and accelerated atherosclerosis. Coexisting hypertension — seen in 60–80% of individuals with type 2 diabetes (Orlander *et al*, 1994) — is thought to have a synergistic effect with diabetes, causing myocardial interstitial fibrosis. This results in diastolic dysfunction, which contributes to the excess cardiac failure.

Abbott *et al* (1988) examined the Framingham study with a view to comparing the impact of diabetes on survival following acute MI (AMI) in men and women. Among non-diabetic patients, the risk of fatal coronary heart disease was significantly lower in women than in men (relative risk 0.6). In the presence of diabetes, however, women had double the risk of recurrent MI compared with men. Women with diabetes developed cardiac failure four times more often (16%) than women without diabetes (3.8%), reflecting the fact that women with diabetes lack the coronary vascular disease protection normally enjoyed by the female sex, ie. the predisposing factors related to having diabetes outweigh the protective mechanisms of the female sex hormones.

The precise cause of this increased incidence of morbidity and mortality is not known. It may be explained by the greater degree of coronary atheroma (perhaps due to altered carbohydrate and fat metabolism) in these patients, or it could be a consequence of coexistent diabetic complications. Jowett and Thompson (1986) believe that autonomic neuropathy of the heart or diabetic microangiopathy of cardiac tissues (similar to that found in the retina and kidney) may also be implicated. Patmore and Jennings (1996) point out that diabetic patients have been found to have abnormalities of platelet function and haemostatic factors which would predispose them to coronary thrombosis. GISSI-2 (1990) reported that reperfusion after thrombolysis, assessed non-invasively, was achieved less frequently in diabetic patients; one can speculate that this reflects the thrombogenic tendency in diabetes.

As previously stated, diabetic patients have a much higher mortality and incidence of LVF following MI. The cause of the higher incidence of LVF in diabetic patients with AMI is still unclear. It may result from the presence of autonomic neuropathy, preceding hypertension, previous unrecognised MI or diabetic cardiomyopathy (due to microangiopathy). Metabolic alterations, such as increased circulating free fatty acids and decreased availability of intracellular glucose, may also reduce cardiac output by inhibiting anaerobic glycolysis (Fava *et al*, 1993). There is some evidence to suggest that raised systemic insulin levels (in both type 1 and type 2 diabetes) may be atherogenic (Pidcup, 1997). Hyperinsulinaemia may also raise arterial blood pressure by stimulating sympathetic nervous system activity, thereby promoting renal sodium reabsorption and inducing vascular smooth muscle hypertrophy. It may also cause atherogenic changes in blood lipids (Pidcup, 1997).

Many clinicians consider that the increased mortality and morbidity in diabetic patients is due, at least in part, to the silent ischaemia caused by autonomic neuropathy (Nesto *et al*, 1988; Orlander *et al*, 1994; Patmore and

Jennings, 1996). Fava *et al* (1993) found that the proportion of patients with delayed presentation or atypical/absent chest pain was similar in the diabetic and control groups; these results are similar to those of Smith *et al* (1983) and Callaham *et al* (1989). Airaksinen and Koistinen (1992), however, claim that the association of autonomic neuropathy with unrecognised MI or silent MI is unsubstantiated. They point out that the increase in silent coronary artery disease is quite similar to that in painful and overall coronary artery disease in the diabetic population. Another possible explanation for the poor prognosis of diabetic patients post-AMI may be the increased prevalence of previous coronary heart disease reported by these patients (Orlander *et al*, 1994).

Management

Patmore and Jennings (1996) recommend that all diabetic patients who sustain a MI should receive aspirin on exactly the same basis as non-diabetic patients. Aspirin may be even more important in diabetics, because of the hyperreactivity of the platelets, although there is no trial evidence to support this theory. The optimum daily dose of aspirin in diabetes has not been studied, but there is some evidence that the usual standard dose of 75–150 mg may be too low (Zuanetti *et al*, 1993).

Thrombolysis has been shown to be a vital part of the management of diabetics post-MI. When thrombolysis was first introduced there were concerns about the risk of retinal haemorrhage and visual loss in patients with proliferative retinopathy. However, this has not been the case in practice, and proliferative retinopathy is now considered only a relative contraindication to be weighed against the undoubted benefits of thrombolysis (Lynch *et al*, 1994).

Diabetic patients included in the large trials of thrombolysis such as GISSI-2 (1990) and ISIS-2 (1988) did not have a higher complication rate in terms of bleeding or stroke than non-diabetic patients (Zuanetti *et al*, 1993). Jenkins *et al* (1996) studied survival in diabetic patients up to one year following admission for AMI pre- (1987) and post- (1990) thrombolysis. The data suggest that thrombolysis may improve one-year survival in diabetic subjects (Jenkins *et al*, 1996). Lynch *et al* (1994), using a much larger sample size, found that the introduction of thrombolytic therapy was accompanied by a significant reduction in mortality and incidence of LVF among both diabetic and non-diabetic patients — a result that was compatible with those of the major thrombolytic trials. Unfortunately, Fava *et al* (1993) pointed out that because of a higher incidence of contraindictions fewer diabetic than non-diabetic patients received thrombolytic therapy. Bradbury and Cruickshank (1993) highlight the potential complications associated with thrombolytic therapy for all patients (including diabetics): spontaneous and iatrogenic bleeding; acute hypotension; allergic and anaphylactic reactions; febrile reactions; and reperfusion arrhythmias.

Oswald *et al* (1984) reported an overall prevalence of undiagnosed diabetes mellitus of 5.3%. They were concerned that, at that time, the contribution of undiagnosed diabetes mellitus to total mortality following AMI seemed to be underestimated. Recent research on the prognostic implications of hypergly-caemia post-MI has acknowledged the importance of accurate glycaemic control for all patients (Malmberg *et al*, 1995). MI stimulates an acute stress response with secretion of catecholamines, cortisol and glucagon and suppression of insulin secretion, resulting in a relatively insulin-resistant state (Patmore and Jennings, 1996). Insulin enhances the uptake of glucose, the major energy substrate of ischaemic myocardium, and reduces non-esterified fatty acid concentrations which, it has been suggested, increase infarct size (by increasing myocardial oxygen consumption), reduce myocardial contractility and are associated with post-MI arrhythmias (Gwilt *et al*, 1984).

Small studies carried out before the advent of thrombolysis failed to prove the efficacy of insulin in reducing infarct size (Gwilt *et al*, 1984), but did find a significant reduction in the incidence of cardiac arrhythmias (Clark *et al*, 1985) and mortality (Rackley *et al*, 1981). Gwilt *et al* (1984) showed insulin infusion to be safe post-MI, with no significant problems of hypoglycaemia or hypokalaemia. Malmberg *et al* (1995) found that rigorous control of plasma glucose by insulin infusion resulted in a one-year mortality that was 29% lower than that in the control group. They concluded that,

Insulin-glucose infusion followed by a multidose insulin regimen improved long-term prognosis in diabetic patients with acute myocardial infarction.

These authors are currently researching which part of the treatment is the most beneficial: infusion alone or infusion plus subcutaneous injections for three months. The stimulus for this study was the fact that physicians are reluctant to commence all diabetics on insulin therapy at home, owing to the cost implications. This poses an ethical dilemma for health professionals: should patients get the best therapy regardless of cost?

Gwilt *et al* (1984) and Lynch *et al* (1994) found that the admission blood glucose level is an independent predictor of mortality in diabetic patients presenting with AMI. A positive relationship between hospital mortality and admission glucose was found in both periods; however, the number of patients presenting with blood glucose levels greater than 20 mmol/litre has decreased with time. More research needs to be carried out to determine whether insulin infusions could benefit patients with lesser degrees of hyperglycaemia.

Diabetes management aims to achieve precise blood glucose control, usually within a range of 5–10 mmol/litre, with insulin therapy (Webster and Thompson, 1991). It is standard practice now to give insulin infusion to the majority of diabetic patients for the first 24–72 hours following AMI. The precise blood glucose level can be varied according to the needs of the patient, and can be simply, effectively and safely controlled. Webster and Thompson (1991) point out that giving insulin via an infusion pump can limit mobility and thought needs to be given to help the patient retain maximum independence; a battery-powered pump may be useful.

Metformin is useful as a first-line oral hypoglycaemic agent for the treatment of overweight patients with type 2 diabetes who remain hyperglycaemic after dietary manipulation, and as dual therapy in combination with a sulphonylurea (Hart and Walker, 1996). Severe heart failure can cause tissue hypoxia which increases lactate production; in addition, renal hypoperfusion results in reduced renal clearance of metformin, which can lead to metformin-associated lacticacidosis (MALA). For these reasons it is standard practice to stop metformin treatment in patients presenting with AMI or LVF. If it is not restarted, a deterioration in glycaemic control may result.

Metformin has been used in the UK for over 500000 patient years and there have been only three reported episodes of lacticacidosis associated with therapeutic doses of metformin (Ryder, 1984; Hutchinson and Catteral, 1987; Tymms and Leatherdale, 1988). Hart and Walker (1996) state that, in patients who present with AMI or LVF, there is no reason why metformin therapy should not be restarted once the acute event has resolved if the plasma creatinine concentration is normal.

Most physicians believe that patients should be discharged on the same medication they were taking when admitted, unless glycaemic control becomes problematic. Webster and Thompson (1991) believe that if the patient has already been injecting insulin, the dose required post-MI is likely to be 20–40% more than the usual daily total dose. MI is known to cause stress hyperglycaemia and abnormal glucose tolerance may persist for up to three months after the acute event (Patmore and Jennings, 1996). Subsequent diabetic management is decided on an individual basis. As recent research indicates (Malmberg *et al*, 1995), all diabetic patients who have had an AMI should be discharged home on subcutaneous insulin for a period of three months. This would involve liaison between hospital and community medical and nursing staff to ensure the patient is administering the required dosage of insulin to maintain the optimum blood glucose level of 5–10 mmol/l.

The use of beta-blockers post-MI has been shown to improve survival, although they should be avoided in patients with some respiratory disorders, eg. asthma. Traditionally there have been concerns about prescribing these agents to diabetic patients. In insulin-treated patients, beta-blockers may prolong hypoglycaemia by inhibiting glycogenolysis and impairing hypoglycaemia awareness. In non-insulin-treated patients, blockade of pancreatic $beta_2$-receptors could lead to a deterioration in diabetic control. Beta-blockers may also worsen symptoms in peripheral vascular disease, precipitate heart failure and have an undesirable effect on lipids, all of which are common problems in diabetic patients.

Beta-blockers are contraindicated in patients with LVF, of which there is a higher incidence in diabetic patients (Karlson *et al*, 1993). The Acute Infarction Ramipril Efficacy (AIRE) study (1993) showed that angiotensin-converting enzyme (ACE) inhibitors have had a considerable impact on the outcome following AMI in those with LVF. ACE-inhibitors can reduce microalbumin excretion and delay progression to nephropathy. They also have no adverse effects on lipid and carbohydrate metabolism and so are a common choice for treatment of hypertension in diabetes. Calcium channel blockers (eg. diltiazem) may also be used post-MI to decrease mortality and morbidity. The exception is when the patient has LVF as the deleterious effects of calcium channel blockers outweigh the possible benefits (Waters, 1997; Persson, 1995). This group of drugs has been shown to have beneficial effects on glucose homeostasis, lipid metabolism and renal function in diabetic patients (Caldwell, 1993).

Role of the CCU nurse

In the acute stages following an MI, the nurse's actions are aimed at achieving optimum recovery. A holistic approach to nursing care is essential at all times. This is achieved through research-based practice and co-ordinating the activities of the multidisciplinary team. The nurse should ensure that the patient receives the appropriate medical management as described above, eg. thrombolysis if appropriate, and that good glycaemic control is maintained. The nurse is also responsible for monitoring blood glucose levels, informing medical staff if there are problems and administering the insulin and oral hypoglycaemics.

A sliding scale insulin regimen should be prescribed according to the individual needs of the patient in much the same way as intravenous nitrates, ie. as maximum and minimum doses, with a phrase such as 'titrate according to blood sugar'.

Expanded role

Norris (1995) states that central to professional autonomy is power over diagnosis and doctors have been extremely reluctant to relinquish control over diagnosis to nursing colleagues. She points out that the reason doctors welcome nurses' role expansion is unclear,

> *Whether they recognise nurses' skills and expertise or simply wish to offload tasks that they no longer want to carry out — an extension and expansion of the role of the nurse as physician's assistant — is debatable.*

Norris (1995) points out that the breaking up of nursing work into discrete tasks (as in task allocation) ensures that no nurse has an integrated view of the nursing function. A holistic approach to nursing care, in which physical, mental and social factors are taken into account, will go some way to developing the nurse's autonomy. The coronary care unit (CCU) nurse looks after all aspects of the patient's well-being, including attending to his/her psychological, social and physical needs.

Frequently the work of nurses and doctors overlap, particularly in technical areas. CCU nurses often already carry the responsibility of being in the front line of assessing and monitoring a patient's condition, and responding quickly to change, as well as providing psychological support to patients and their families in times of great stress (Caunt, 1996).

The Scope of Professional Practice (UKCC, 1992a) removes the requirement that nurses undertaking an extended role are trained by a medical practitioner who then gives him/her a certificate following training (Mitchinson and Goodlad, 1996). Using the *Code of Professional Conduct* (UKCC, 1992b) as a guide and a safeguard, the nurse can negotiate the expanded role and make the appropriate judgements and decisions relevant to education and training. These protocols must be drawn up in agreement with the managers and employers in order to ensure their vicarious liability (Hunt and Wainwright, 1994). The scope of nursing practice is already well developed in most CCUs, with the establishment of protocols for defibrillation, first-line drugs, venepuncture and cannulation.

According to Darley (1996), the complexity of modern care is such that no single profession can reasonably assume accountability for all care. The professions should understand this and their regulatory bodies should put forward a mutually supportive framework for accountability.

Diabetes is recognised by the medical profession as an incurable and devastating illness (Bodansky, 1989). The patient, especially if newly diagnosed, may have many questions about the illness, its management and the future. Webster and Thompson (1991) point out that the main barriers to effective care include the constraints of limited knowledge, skills and time. CCU nurses may not be adequately prepared to provide patients with the support and information they need. The patient's typically short-stay on the CCU is unlikely to be long enough for the nurse to provide the support that is necessary, and in any case the first 48 hours are probably not the best time to give information as pain, anxiety, nausea and drugs are likely to limit retention.

Educating patients and relatives about diabetes should take place in conjunction with cardiac rehabilitation. Education must include advice on monitoring and interpreting blood glucose levels, and how to adjust diet and insulin accordingly; the effects of exercise, stress and illness on blood glucose must be explained. Attention also needs to be paid to other factors linked with micro- and macrovascular complications, such as obesity, smoking, hyper-lipidaemia and hypertension (Hale, 1992; Merrin, 1992). The role of the nurse is to provide sufficient information to enable the patient to make an informed decision about his/her lifestyle. Knowledge is only one factor contributing to compliance; the patient's perceptions and the personal and social circumstances within which he/she lives are also crucial in the decision-making process.

Caring for the diabetic patient post-MI is a complex and highly specialist aspect of the CCU nurse's role. The nurse requires a high level of understanding and an ability to relate theoretical knowledge to practice. It is the author's experience that many nurses understand very little about this subject area.

Conclusion

Diabetes mellitus increases the risk of heart disease and doubles the risk of dying following an AMI. The causes are complex, but the increased risk may briefly be explained by the greater degree of coronary atheroma and coexistent diabetic complications in these patients. Diabetic patients have a higher incidence of LVF post-MI and reinfarction. The prognosis for women with diabetes is as poor, if not worse, than that in men.

Management should be similar to that of non-diabetic patients, bearing in mind that rigorous control of blood glucose has been shown to improve the long-term outcome of these patients. Caring for diabetic patients post-MI is an essential component of the role of specialist CCU nurses. This involves diagnosing hyperglycaemia, initiating treatment (through informing the medical staff), administering the prescribed medication, monitoring its effect, providing psychological support for the patient and his/her family, and educating them about the disease.

Recommendations

- informal and formal teaching sessions about diabetes and heart disease should be introduced for nursing staff on CCUs
- a core care plan that will encourage the assessment, planning and implementation and evaluation of care suitable for diabetic patients on CCUs should be written
- educational literature and tapes for people from different groups should be acquired from the British Diabetic Association
- further research is needed in the long- and short-term management of diabetic patients following an AMI
- further investigation of the changing role of the CCU nurse in relation to diabetes management, with particular reference to education and prescription, is advisable
- the increased mortality of diabetic patients post-MI should encourage CCU nurses to monitor patients' progress carefully and watch for signs of LVF
- diabetic retinopathy should be considered only a relative contraindication to thrombolysis
- blood sugar levels should be carefully monitored at all times throughout the patient's stay in hospital (and once discharged), as he/she may remain abnormal for up to three months post-MI.

Key points

* Diabetic patients are at greater risk of sustaining an acute myocardial infarction (AMI), and also have almost double the mortality from AMI compared with non-diabetic patients.
* Thrombolysis is a vital part of the management of diabetic patients.

* Rigorous control of plasma glucose has been shown to improve the long-term outcome of diabetic patients.

* AMI is known to cause stress hyperglycaemia and abnormal glucose tolerance may persist for up to three months after the acute event.

* The coronary care nurse looks after all aspects of the patient's well-being, including attending to his/her psychological, social and physical needs.

References

Abbott R, Donahue R, Kannel W *et al* (1988) The impact of diabetes on survival following myocardial infarction in men *vs* women. *JAMA* **260**: 3456–60

Acute Infarction Ramipril Efficacy (AIRE) study (1993) Effect of Ramipril on mortality and morbidity of survivors of acute myocardial infarction with clinical evidence of heart failure. *Lancet* **342**: 821–8

Airaksinen K, Koistinen M (1992) Association between silent coronary artery disease, diabetes and autonomic neuropathy (fact or fallacy). *Diabetes Care* **15**(2): 288–92

Bradbury M, Cruickshank JP (1993) Use of thrombolytic therapy in acute myocardial infarction. *Br J Nurs* **2**(12): 619–24

Bodansky H (1989) The natural history of type 1 diabetes. *Pract Diabetes* **6**(1): 7–9

Caldwell BV (1993) Treating hypertension in the diabetic patient: therapeutic goals and the role of calcium channel blockers. *Clin Ther* **15**(4): 618–36

Callaham P, Froelicher V, Klein J *et al* (1989) Exercise induced silent ischaemia: age, diabetes mellitus, previous myocardial infarction and prognosis. *J Am Coll Cardiol* **14**: 1175–80

Caunt J (1996) The advanced nurse practitioner in CCU. *Care Crit Ill* **12**(4): 136–9

Clark R, English M, McNeil G *et al* (1985) Effect of intravenous infusion of insulin in diabetes with acute myocardial infarction. *Br Med J* **291**: 303–5

Darley, M (1996) Right for the job. *Nurs Times* **92**(30): 28–31

Fava S, Azzopardi J, Muscat H *et al* (1993) Factors that influence outcome in diabetic subjects with myocardial infarction. *Diabetes Care* **16**(12): 1615–8

GISSI-2 (1990) A factorial randomized trial of alteplase versus streptokinase and heparin versus no heparin among 12490 patients with AMI. *Lancet* **336**: 65–71

Gwilt D, Petri M, Lamb P *et al* (1984) Effect of intravenous insulin infusion on mortality among diabetic patients after myocardial infarction. *Br Heart J* **51**: 626–30

Hale P (1992) Setting the standards for diabetes care: hyperlipidaemia. *Pract Diabetes* **9**(3): 88–9

Hart S, Walker J (1996) Is metformin contraindicated in diabetic patients with chronic stable heart failure? *Pract Diabetes Int* **13**(1): 18–20

Hunt G, Wainwright P (1994) *Expanding the Role of the Nurse. The Scope of Professional Practice*. Blackwell Scientific Publications, Oxford

Hutchinson S Catteral J (1987) Metformin and lacticacidosis — a reminder. *Br J Clin Pract* **41**: 673

ISIS-2 (Second International Study of Infant Survival) collaborative group (1988) Randomized trial of intravenous streptokinase, oral aspirin, both or neither among 17187 cases of suspected acute myocardial infarction. *Lancet* **77**: 349–60

Jenkins D, Lamb P, Krentz A *et al* (1996) One year survival following acute myocardial infarction in diabetic patients. *Pract Diabetes Int* **13**(1): 6–8

Jowett N, Thompson D (1986) Diabetic heart disease. *Nurs Times/Nurs Mirror* **82**(44): 33–4

Karlson B, Herlitz A, Hjalmarson A (1993) Prognosis of acute myocardial infarction in diabetic and non-diabetic patients. *Diabet Med* **10**: 449–54

Lynch M, Gammage MD, Lamb P *et al* (1994) Acute myocardial infarction in diabetic patients in the thrombolytic era. *Diabet Med* **11**: 162–5

Malmberg K, Ryden L, Efendic S *et al* (1995) Randomized trial of insulin-glucose infusion followed by subcutaneous insulin treatment in diabetic patients with acute myocardial infarction (DIGAMI Study): effects on mortaility at one year. *J Am Coll Cardiol* **26**: 57–65

Merrin P (1992) Setting the standards for diabetes care: hypertension. *Pract Diabetes* **9**(3): 91–4

Mitchinson S, Goodlad S (1996) Changes in the roles and responsibilities of nurses. *Prof Nurse* **11**(11): 734–6

Nesto R, Phillips DJ, Kett K *et al* (1988) Angina and exertional myocardial ischaemia in diabetic and non-diabetic patients: assessment by exercise thallium scintigraphy. *Ann Intern Med* **108**: 170–5

Norris E (1995) Achieving professional autonomy for nursing. *Prof Nurse* **11**(1): 59–61

Orlander P, Goff D, Morrissey M *et al* (1994) The relation of diabetes to the severity of acute myocardial infarction and post-myocardial infarction survival in Mexican-Americans and non-hispanic whites. The Corpus Christi Heart Project. *Diabetes* **43**: 897–901

Oswald G, Corcoran S, Yudkin J (1984) Prevalence and risks of hyperglycaemia and undiagnosed diabetes in patients with acute myocardial infarction. *Lancet* **1**: 1264–7

Patmore J, Jennings P (1996) Myocardial infarction in the diabetic patient. *Care Crit Ill* **12**(6): 203–5

Paton RC (1989) The natural history of type 2 diabetes. *Pract Diabetes* **6**(1): 10–13

Perkins J (1992) How much should we tell them? (Patient education for people with diabetes). *Prof Nurse* **8**(2): 130–3

Persson S (1995) Update on the use of angiotensin converting enzyme inhibitors and calcium antagonists in post infarction patients. *J Hypertens* **13**(2): S57–63

Pidcup J (1997) Cardiovascular disease in diabetes mellitus. In: Pidcup J, Williams G, eds. *Textbook of Diabetes*. 2nd edn. Blackwell Science, Oxford: 1–22

Rackley C, Russell R, Rogers W *et al* (1981) Clinical experience with glucose-insulin-potassium therapy in acute myocardial infarction. *Am Heart J* **102**: 1038–49

Ryder R (1984) Lactic acidosis coma with multiple medication including metformin in a patient with normal renal function. *Br J Clin Pract* **38**: 229

Smith J, Buckels L, Carlson K *et al* (1983) Clinical characteristics and results of non-invasive tests in 60 patients after acute myocardial infarction. *Am J Med* **75**: 217–23

Sprafka J, Burke G, Folsom A *et al* (1991) Trends in prevalence of diabetes mellitus in patients with myocardial infarction and effect of diabetes on survival. The Minnesota Heart Survey. *Diabetes Care* **14**(7): 537–43

Thomas L (1993) An overview of current research into diabetes. *Prof Nurse* **9**(1): 15–8

Tymms T, Leatherdale B (1988) Lactic acidosis due to metformin therapy in a low risk patient. *Postgrad Med J* **64**: 230

UKCC (1992a) *The Scope of Professional Practice*. UKCC, London

UKCC (1992b) *The Code of Professional Conduct for the Nurse, Midwife and Health Visitor*. UKCC, London

Waters D (1997) Calcium channel blockers: an evidence-based review. *Can J Cardiol* **13**(8): 757–67

Webster RA, Thompson R (1991) The diabetic patient in the coronary care unit: a nursing perspective. *Pract Diabetes* **8**(1): 13–5

Zuanetti G, Latini R, Maggioni A *et al* (1993) Influence of diabetes on mortality in acute myocardial infarction: data from the GISSI-2 study. *J Am Coll Cardiol* **22**: 1788–94

Section 3: Essential psychological and rehabilitation elements in cardiovascular nursing

15

Transfer anxiety in patients with myocardial infarction

David A Jenkins and Helen Rogers

When patients are transferred from a coronary care unit to a general ward they often experience transfer anxiety. A structured pre-transfer teaching programme is suggested as a tool which may improve patient care.

Anxiety has been described as a multidimensional phenomenon which requires a person to draw upon the strength of his/her past experiences, expectations, social background and various conscious and subconscious coping mechanisms (Selye and Tache, 1985). Peplau (1964) considered that any threat to an individual's security produces anxiety.

Anxiety is one of the primary problems affecting patients who have suffered myocardial infarction (MI) (Hacket *et al*, 1968; Lowe, 1989; Thompson and Webster, 1989; Malan, 1992). Using the Hospital Anxiety and Depression Scale (HADS; Zigmund and Snaith, 1983), Shiell and Shiell (1991) found that 44% of the 50 patients admitted to a coronary care unit (CCU) experienced high levels of anxiety or depression. They concluded that some of the symptoms, such as sweating, palpitations and chest pain, might have been related to anxiety rather than to any direct sequelae of MI.

After an MI, patients are subjected to a barrage of experiences, many of which may create anxiety or be considered stressful. Research suggests that transfer from the CCU to the general ward is one such stressful experience (Klein *et al*, 1968; Schactman, 1987; Saarman, 1993). A patient's length of stay on a CCU depends upon his/her physical condition and the demand for beds for new admissions. Transfer from the CCU is inevitable and may occur within a few hours of completion of thrombolytic therapy. A patient's physiological status may have improved sufficiently for transfer, but his/her psychological adaptation may lag behind. Patients have been known to ask: 'Can't I stay here a little longer?'

Anxiety creates stress. Tortora and Anagnostakos (1993) defined stress as, 'any stimulus that creates an imbalance in the internal environment' and Selye (1978) described it as, 'the non-specific response of the body to any demand made upon it'.

The body's physiological response to stress is that of the 'flight or fight' mechanism, during which adrenaline is released from the adrenal medulla due to stimulation of the sympathetic nervous system. This causes an increase in the heart rate together with dilatation of the blood vessels to the heart, lungs, brain and major muscles. Blood vessels to the kidneys, skin and other organs, however, are constricted in the effort to conserve the blood supply to the vital organs and ensure immediate survival. Sweating increases, lowering the body temperature and eliminating waste products. The rate of respiration also increases and the airways dilate to allow improved oxygenation and elimination of carbon dioxide. As a result of these physiological changes, there is an increased demand for oxygen which may lead to ischaemic chest pain, arrhythmia or sudden death in a patient with MI who already has an irritated and damaged myocardium (Toth, 1980; *Figure 15.1*). A recent study by Moser and Dracup (1996) also demonstrated the relationship between high anxiety after acute MI and a subsequent increased high risk of cardiac complications. Their study emphasised the need for research on early psychosocial intervention in patients after acute MI.

Klein *et al* (1968) reported a high level of patient stress, with a high incidence of cardiac arrhythmias, during the transfer of patients from CCU to the general ward.

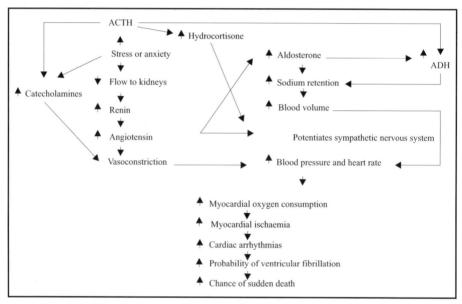

Figure 15.1: A modification of Folkow and Neil's (1971) hypertension stress model. From: Toth (1980). ACTH = adrenocorticotrophic hormone; ADH = anti-diuretic hormone

Transfer anxiety

Transfer anxiety has been defined as a separation anxiety (Freud, 1963; Saarman, 1993) involving loss of the close relationships developed between the patient, nurses and doctors. CCUs are often reported as being highly stressful environments for patients (Mackellaig, 1987; Pearce, 1988). Conversely, there is also strong evidence that patients consider the CCU to be a secure, familiar and safe environment (Minkley *et al*, 1979; Poe, 1982; Miracle, 1986; Saarman, 1993). When patients are transferred, they move forward into the unknown, into areas where they will become one of many and will lose the intensive observation of CCU staff (Poe, 1982).

Nurses are usually responsible for managing transfers. The complexities of transfer anxiety need therefore to be fully identified, and appreciated, in order to initiate preventive activities within patient care.

Components of transfer anxiety

Bowlby (1960) discussed three conditions which are specific components of transfer anxiety; primary anxiety, expectation of transfer, and fright on transfer.

Primary anxiety: Primary anxiety can be directly linked to the onset of patients' defence mechanisms, which may have both psychological and physiological components. Primary anxiety arises from the type and timing of transfer, and the disruption of interpersonal relationships. It occurs when patients do not have the opportunity to transfer gradually. Abrupt transfer, which could be due to emergency admissions of other patients, or inadequate transfer preparation, does not give the patient sufficient time to assimilate the positive characteristics of the transfer. Consequently, he/she may view the entire process as one of rejection. Klein (1968) found this to be a common feature.

Another problem associated with sudden transfer arises from the positioning of patients on the new wards. If there are patients who are critically or terminally ill nearby, then the transferred patients may view this as a contraindication of any improvement in their own condition (Klein *et al*, 1968). Owens (1978) high-lighted a positive aspect of the placement of transferred patients on general wards. He noted that anxious patients tended to discuss their feelings of anxiety when they were in a group of patients with similar circumstances and, by doing this, became less anxious themselves. Abrupt transfers can also exacerbate feelings of abandonment, loss and insecurity (Saarman, 1993). If there is no choice but to transfer at night, then a recognition of these potential problems should be identified and nursing actions adopted to minimise them.

Expectation of transfer: A possible condition which might lead to anxiety is the patient's expectation of transfer. Patients may be anxious and poorly prepared for transfer; they will probably be expecting care to continue in the same supportive manner as in the CCU. They may also consider themselves still to be critically ill and have difficulty in perceiving their condition in the same light as the staff who are looking after them (Klein *et al*, 1968) and who are prepared to transfer them.

Fright on transfer: Fright can cause patients to demonstrate two major behavioural responses (Bowlby, 1960): the escape behaviour and immobility. Escape behaviour may simply be demonstrated by patients asking verbally for transfer because they feel they have improved very quickly and therefore no longer need to be in the CCU. They may also communicate their desire to leave non-verbally, by climbing out of bed or removing cardiac monitor electrodes.

Immobility, or emotional freezing, can be seen in patients who do not move about in bed, or do not speak in anything other than monosyllabic terms.

Feelings of fright may also arise when patients do not know what to expect in a given situation. One method of giving patients a fairly accurate outline of what is expected of them is to present them with a set of written guidelines that show a planned gradual progression from dependence to independence. As each patient's condition improves, staff can reduce the treatment, observations and amount of supportive equipment. This gradual reduction in care serves to reassure patients of steady improvement (Saarman, 1993). It is infinitely better than a sudden discontinuation of supportive measures, which may cause suffering to patients from unwarranted fears that any deterioration in their condition may go undetected. The physical condition of patients is monitored closely and continuously during their stay in the CCU. Hacket *et al* (1968) discovered that the majority of patients were reassured by the presence of the monitoring system.

How to improve patient transfer

Pre-transfer teaching programme: If nurses in the CCU prepare patients for transfer by explaining what is happening and why, and by giving maximum support, then aspects of transfer anxiety can be reduced or even eliminated. In order to achieve this, it is suggested that the CCU nurse begins the planned preparation for transfer through a structured pre-transfer teaching programme at the earliest appropriate point after admission. Toth (1980) researched this problem and her findings indicate that such an approach is very effective in reducing patient anxiety.

It is recognised that Toth's programme is very behavioural in its orientation, with little scope for taking account of individual patient idiosyncrasies, and that a more open and less structured approach, such as that of Peplau (1964), could be offered. For any programme to work it has to be easily and effectively used by all nursing staff. If a less structured approach is used, a definitive identification of the various transfer anxieties may prove difficult. A structured pre-transfer teaching programme should help CCU nurses to identify the three components of transfer anxiety, as described in the flow-chart format in *Figure 15.2*.

The use of this chart could clearly formulate nursing actions, using patients' own resources to help to reduce those conditions which lead to transfer anxiety. Toth (1980) noted that patients on structured pre-transfer programmes had lower blood pressures and heart rates than a control group — although anxiety levels of the same groups showed no significant differences. Holland (1977) emphasised that any nursing intervention which reduces the risk of cardiac arrhythmias must include patient teaching from the moment of admission to the CCU.

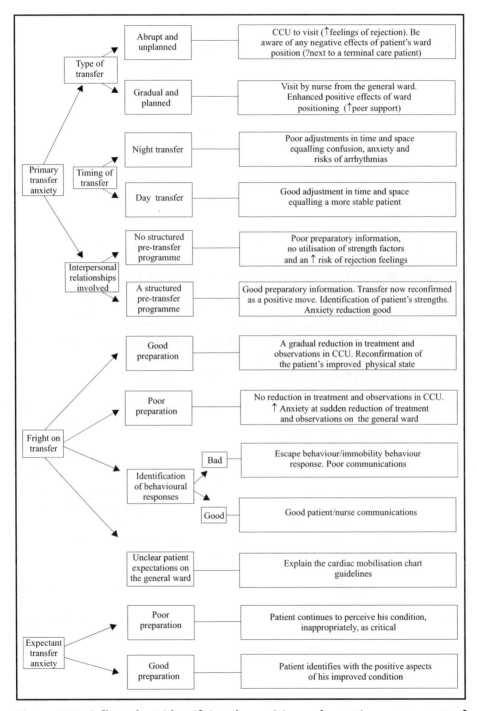

Figure 15.2: A flow chart identifying the positive and negative components of transfer anxiety

Psychological support: Naismith e*t al* (1979) highlighted the fact that fear, depression and anxiety were all common experiences for patients on transfer from the CCU, and that there was a lack of psychological support within CCUs. Good interpersonal skills in nurses have been shown to provide some pain relief, and to improve pulse and respiratory rates (Gerrard, 1978), indicating the importance of such skills.

To minimise the effects of transfer anxiety, patients need to be mentally prepared for transfer out of the CCU. Poe (1982) suggested that emphasising the need for transfer as a result of an improvement in the patient's condition, would enable patients to see the event in a positive light. In planning patient transfers, CCU nurses should identify ways in which individual patients maintain their own independence in order to gradually wean them away from psychological dependence on the CCU nurse.

Research into the effects of preparatory information on the emotional responses of patients by Lazarus (1968) indicated that such information was effective in reducing emotional distress and anxiety. Before transfer from the CCU, patients should be informed that it is not unusual for them to feel isolated, confused and insecure at times. Once patients can accept that these feelings are a possibility, they can be encouraged to use their own resources to cope with them (Popkess, 1981). In order to reduce fright it should also be possible to give patients physical evidence of improvement by discontinuing cardiac monitoring a couple of hours before the actual transfer (Minkley *et al*, 1979).

Patients can be given a great psychological boost by a visit from a nurse from the receiving ward before transfer, as well as a visit from the CCU nurse after patients have been transferred to the general ward (Miracle, 1986). This promotes continuity of care and reduces the effect of the transition into a strange environment (Klein *et al*, 1968).

Use of relatives: Nurses may receive a lot of help and support from patients' relatives at transfer time. Schwartz and Brenner (1979) considered that patient stress was significantly reduced if patients' relatives were present and involved in the transfer. Doerr and Jones (1979) explored the hypothesis that anxiety from family members could be transferred to patients. Thompson and Webster (1989) presented a study which advocated that counselling of male patients post-MI, together with their partners, would reduce anxiety for both.

Patients must understand that they have reached a state of improvement and stability when they no longer require intensive care or observation. The transfer should be presented in a positive manner and confirmed as something that patients and their families have been waiting for. In this way, the act of transfer is used as an opportunity for anxiety reduction.

Conclusion

Transfer anxiety is only one of the many stresses that patients may encounter following MI. Nevertheless, it is an important aspect of patient care which CCU nurses should address as they have considerable control over the organisation of transfers to general wards.

Although much has been written on this subject over the last 30 years or so, and it is acknowledged to be an important aspect of care, it has not been widely covered in British nursing journals. At this time, with the current pressure for beds in CCUs, it is appropriate that the matter is addressed.

There will be many occasions when a hard-pressed unit has to transfer a patient abruptly to a busy general ward. CCU nurses should be able to identify the components of transfer anxiety, using the flow chart in *Figure 15.2* . As CCU nurses become more conversant with the ways in which they can alleviate transfer anxiety, they will be in a position to reduce the incidence of transfer anxiety in patients before, during, or just after transfer to the general ward.

Key points

* With current pressure for bed allocation within CCUs, patient transfer anxiety needs to receive more attention.

* A structured pre-transfer teaching programme may assist nurses in recognising transfer anxiety.

* By using such a tool, care/advice may be offered by nurses which will enhance psychological support and reduce the problems relating to transfer anxiety.

References

Bowlby J (1960) Separation anxiety. *Int J Psychoanal* **41**(2/3): 89–113

Doerr BC, Jones JW (1979) Effects of family preparation on the state anxiety level of the coronary care unit patient. *Nurs Res* **28**(5): 315

Folkow B, Neil E (1971) *Circulation*. Oxford University Press, New York

Freud S (1963) *The Problem of Anxiety*. Norton, New York

Gerrard N (1978) Nurses' level of empathy and respect in simulated interactions with patients. *Int J Nurs Stud* **20**(2): 83–7

Hacket TP, Cassem NH, Wishnie HA (1968) The coronary care unit — an appraisal of its psychological hazards. *N Eng J Med* **279**: 1365–70

Holland JM (1977) *Cardiovascular Nursing: Prevention, Intervention and Rehabilitation*. Brown and Company, Boston: 106–21

Klein RF, Kliner VA, Zipes DP *et al* (1968) Transfer from a coronary care unit. *Arch Intern Med* **122**: 104–8

Lazarus H (1968) Emotions and adaptations: conceptual and empirical relations. *Nurs Res* **31**(4): 172–6

Lowe L (1989) Anxiety in a coronary care unit. *Nurs Times* **85**(45): 61–3

Mackellaig JM (1987) A study of the psychological effects of intensive care with particular emphasis on patients in isolation. *Intensive Care Nurs* **2**(4): 176–85

Malan SS (1992) Psychological adjustment following MI: current views and nursing implications. *J Cardiovas Nurs* **6**(4): 57–70

Minkley BB, Burrows D, Ehrat K *et al* (1979) Myocardial Infarction Stress of Transfer Inventory: development of a research tool. *Nurs Res* **28**(1): 4–10

Miracle V (1986) Transfer anxiety and the myocardial infarction patient. *Kentucky Nurse* **34**(1): 15–16

Moser DK, Dracup K (1996) Is anxiety early after myocardcial infarction associated with subsequent ischemic and arrhythmic events? *Psychosom Med* **58**: 396–410

Naismith LD, Robinson JF, Shaw GB *et al* (1979) Psychological rehabilitation after myocardial infarction. Papers and Originals. *Br Med J* **1**: 439–46

Owens JF (1978) Cardiac rehabilitation. A patient education programme. *Nurs Res* **27**(3): 148–50

Pearce J (1988) The power of touch. *Nurs Times* **84**(24): 27–9

Peplau H (1964) *A Working Definition of Anxiety. Some Critical Approaches to Psychiatric Nursing.* Macmillan, New York

Poe C (1982) Minimizing stress-of-transfer responses. *Dimens Crit Care Nurs* **1**(6): 364–74

Popkess SA (1981) Diagnosing your patient's strengths. *Nursing* **11**(7): 34–7

Saarman L (1993) Transfer out of critical care: freedom or fear. *Crit Care Nurs Q* **16**(1): 75–8

Schactman M (1987) Transfer stress in patients after myocardial infarction. *Focus Crit Care* **14**(2): 34–7

Schwartz LP, Brenner ZR (1979) Critical care unit transfer: reducing patient stress through nursing interventions. *Heart Lung* **8**(3): 540–6

Selye H (1978) *The Stress of Life.* 2nd edn. McGraw Hill, New York: 55

Selye H, Tache J (1985) On stress and coping mechanisms. *Issues Ment Health Nurs* **7**(14): 3–24

Shiell J, Shiell A (1991) The prevalence of psychiatric morbidity on a coronary care ward. *J Adv Nurs* **16**: 1071–7

Thompson DR, Webster RA (1989) Effect of counselling on anxiety and depression in coronary patients. *Intensive Care Nurs* **5**(2): 52–4

Tortora GJ, Anagnostakos NP (1993) *Principles of Anatomy and Physiology.* 7th edn. Harper International Edition, New York: 23

Toth JC, (1980) Effect of structured preparation for transfer on patient anxiety leaving coronary care unit. *Nurs Res* **26**(1): 28–34

Zigmund AS, Snaith RP (1983) Hospital anxiety and depression scale. *Acta Psychiatr Scand* **67**: 361–73

16

Sexual healing: caring for patients recovering from myocardial infarction

Lynne Marie Whitaker

Sexuality is rarely addressed when patients are recovering from myocardial infarction (MI). This chapter discusses both nurses' and patients' attitudes to sexuality, and examines ways to increase nurses' awareness so that they can offer sexual advice and apply a truly holistic approach when caring for patients following an MI.

Health education and rehabilitation play a large part in the role of the coronary care nurse. The ultimate aim is for patients to resume their normal daily activities of living and eventually return to work.

Many patients admitted to the coronary care unit (CCU) may have enjoyed a sexual relationship with their partner before admission. Therefore, if nurses regard the care they deliver as being holistic and aim to restore the coronary patient to his/her optimum level of functioning, the patient's sexuality and sexual function must be considered when planning care and during subsequent health education sessions (Thompson, 1980).

Myocardial infarction (MI) is a major life event, both for patients and their families, and often means that patients have to adapt their lifestyle following discharge. The resumption of sexual activity can be an area of concern for the patient and his/her partner.

Sexuality does not appear routinely on patient care plans and is rarely addressed when patients are recovering from MI. Is this because of embarrassment from both the patient and the nurse? Does the nurse look upon the patient as being too old? Does the patient regard sexual activity as being detrimental to his/her health? This chapter attempts to answer these questions and also offers suggestions for nurses caring for patients recovering from MI.

Attitudes

The patient

Many patients believe in the misconception that resuming sexual activity following discharge may be a danger to their perceived fragile health. Many are under the impression that sexual intercourse has a higher energy expenditure than playing football, and associate it with an increased workload on the heart, linking this with the possibility of further chest pain or reinfarction.

In many cases, heart disease is associated with the natural ageing process.

Patients suffering MI may feel that the condition is an untimely reminder of their ageing and consequently abstain from sexual activity after discharge. Those who view themselves as being old are reluctant to verbalise their sexual feelings as they fear that other people will see them as depraved (Griffiths, 1988).

People who have been seriously ill may regard themselves as being less sexually attractive (Jones, 1992). Papadopoulos *et al* (1983) found that one of women's main worries was that their partners would no longer find them attractive. Fear of an inability to perform to their usual sexual standard post-discharge may also affect patients who are considering resuming sexual activity. This may also be accompanied by concerns about reinfarction and that their spouse will seek another sexual partner.

The length of stay in hospital may influence patients' rehabilitation in general, and affect their resumption of sexual activity post-discharge. If the stay in hospital is longer than the average six to seven days, this may be associated with complications of infarct size and may precipitate emotional problems and depression (Jones, 1992).

Patients' partners will also have fears, most commonly the dread of their partner dying during sexual intercourse. McCann (1989) found that if they communicate these anxieties it may help to reinforce patients' concerns regarding their own health, and lead to sexual dysfunction. Papadopoulos *et al* (1983) found that couples who did not resume sexual activity post-discharge suffered a deterioration in their emotional relationship. This failure to communicate sexually may therefore lead to failure in communication in other areas of marriage.

The nurse

Often, nurses who are expected to carry out assessments on patients are newly qualified, young and still unconfident about their own sexuality (Savage, 1990). This leads to the nurse becoming embarrassed if the subject is broached by the patient and therefore he/she may give the patient vague advice such as 'take it easy'. This means that fears and misconceptions regarding sexual activity are not alleviated.

The nurse may also be guilty of sexual prejudice. It is well documented that single patients, the elderly, and homosexuals do not receive as much information as married heterosexual patients. Booth (1990) found that many nurses presumed that elderly patients did not have sexual needs, did not think that it really mattered at that age, and concluded that it was highly unlikely that they would be having sexual relations.

Sexuality is not covered as an in-depth subject in general nurse training. Thompson (1980) found that this lack of awareness and knowledge of sexuality and the normal physical effects of sexual intercourse may mean that the subject of sexuality is not approached at all when assessing the patient. Many nurses look upon sexuality, the activity of living, as pertaining to intercourse only and, because of this, may not discuss the subject of sexuality with patients who are sexually inactive.

McCann (1989) states that sexuality is an integral aspect of personality and self-esteem, and a significant part of health, whether a person is sexually active or not. Webb (1985) adds that sexuality includes the totality of being human. Sexuality is not only about intercourse, but also touch, self-image and self-esteem; while sexual needs are linked with emotional needs of love, closeness and caring.

Why give sexual guidance?

Nurses must be aware of the great need for sexual guidance following MI. The age of male patients in the CCU is reducing, and many patients may be in their early forties (Cohen, 1980). These are very productive years and therefore patients will be hoping to return to work and resume their everyday activities of living, including an active sex life.

Sexual guidance for female patients tends to be more infrequent than for male patients (Baggs, 1986). Most female patients admitted to CCU are post-menopausal (Wenger, 1985) and many nurses are of the opinion that female sexual dysfunction consists of failure to reach orgasm, failure of vaginal lubrication or vaginismus, and loss of libido, all of which are associated with the menopause (Jones, 1992).

It is well documented that compared to the male patient there is a reduction in the amount of counselling available to female patients (Baggs, 1986; Jones, 1992). Papadopoulos *et al* (1983) found that 51% of female patients feared resuming sexual activity, and only a quarter went back to premorbid levels post-discharge. As early as 1933, Kinsey *et al* (1948) observed that women become less inhibited and more interested in sex as they move through their forties, fifties and sixties. Does this not indicate then the importance of sexual guidance for both men and women, regardless of their age?

It has been recognised that one of the most important parts of rehabilitation for the patient following an MI is the reconstruction of a normal sex life as this may help him/her to feel 'whole' again (Jones, 1992). Personal relationships may suffer if sexual activity is not resumed post-discharge, as tension and frustration between the patient and his/her partner may be created. The partner rarely discusses his/her anxieties through fear of initiating chest pain or reinfarction, and the patient's fear of resuming sexual activity because of lack of encouragement may be more dangerous than the activity itself (Thompson, 1990; Piper, 1992).

Anyone recovering from a life-threatening illness needs to feel loved and cared for; the partner may want to show his/her love but be afraid of any intimacy. Patients should not be deprived of this relationship through lack of counselling. Nurses may not know how to approach this subject because they feel inadequately prepared. The more knowledge nurses have, the more favourable their attitudes will be, and they will feel more able to give the advice that is needed (Webb, 1985).

Main concerns

Once it has been identified that sexual guidance following an MI is a large area of cardiac rehabilitation that is not addressed by either medical or nursing staff, how can sexual healing be achieved and who should be the one to provide it?

Goodman (1989) found that many patients reported receiving no information about resuming sexual activity, although cardiac physicians felt that they had covered the subject. Counselling and sexual guidance must be based on trust. The primary nurse is the person most likely to establish a rapport with the patient and is in the prime position to alter false opinions and give corrective advice. Without counselling, patients can only rely on ignorance, misinformation, misconceptions and superstition to cope with their own fears regarding their illness and sexual inadequacy (Cohen, 1980).

Fear of death during coitus is a major concern both for the patients and their partners. It is important that all their anxieties are alleviated. Ueno (1963) found that only 0.6% of 5559 cases of sudden death were precipitated by sexual activity, and three quarters of these were associated with extramarital intercourse. Therefore, people who have illicit affairs in unfamiliar surroundings appear to be more at risk. This must be pointed out to the patient.

It must also be stressed that sexual activity within a long-term and mutually committed relationship is of great importance, and ordinary sexual activity within this relationship can and should be restarted as soon as moderate exercise is restarted (Thompson, 1990).

However, anal intercourse, which may be practised by both homosexual and heterosexual couples, can have the most impact on coronary health. Anal intercourse stimulates the vagus nerve, which slows the heart rate, the conduction of impulses, and the coronary blood flow (Bloch *et al*, 1975). This may result in diminished cardiac performance and induce chest pressure or pain.

This information is vital to patients who usually engage in anal intercourse as they may be at risk. It is important, therefore, to offer guidance on sexuality, with the emphasis on giving and receiving pleasure through holding and caressing, rather than concentrating on performance-driven sexual activity.

Many patients may abstain from sexual activity because of a decreased exercise tolerance, which precipitates angina pectoris. The association of sexual intercourse with high energy expenditure may prevent a couple from resuming their normal sexual activity. This misconception must be rectified, and sexual activity must be considered along with all other daily living activities.

The energy expenditure during intercourse with a familiar partner is equivalent to that of climbing stairs (Thompson, 1980) and less than arguing, driving to work, or watching exciting television (Hellerstein and Friedman, 1970). Patients who do experience angina pectoris either during or after intercourse may be advised to take a dose of glyceryl trinitrate as a prophylactic measure, although this may mean that they have to cope with a headache.

Almost all infarct patients become depressed. Concern regarding sexuality is one of the causes of depression. The nurse must try to help reinstate a positive attitude to self-esteem and body image. The patient's partner may also find it difficult to cope with the stress which may lead to depression and denial of the patient's illness. Since depression tends to precipitate a lack of interest in sexual activity, efforts should be made by staff to diminish this reaction during the acute stage (Thompson, 1980).

Effects of cardiac drugs

Many patients will be discharged from hospital on drugs which may considerably affect their sexual performance or libido, either directly, by altering hormone levels, or indirectly, as a result of drug-induced depression (*Table 16.1*). Because sexuality is frequently overlooked, many nurses may be unaware of the effects that some drugs have on sexual performance. This may lead to the misconception that a patient's sexual dysfunction is as a result of his/her MI rather than his/her medication.

If patients are given more information regarding the effects of drugs on sexual performance, it may help to prevent depression and change the patient's outlook of his/her own sexuality, as they realise that their sexual dysfunction may be reversed. Patients who are affected by medications may be advised to have intercourse in the morning when drug levels will be at their lowest. Sexual dysfunction caused by beta-blockers is dose related and therefore improves as doses are reduced.

Table 16.1: Cardiac drugs that may affect sexual performance	
Digoxin	Lowers testosterone levels and negatively influences libido
Thiazide diuretics	Decrease libido and are associated with impotence, which is also reported with spironolactone
Beta-blockers	Impotence is well documented with propranolol. Labetalol causes delayed ejaculation rather than impotence
Methyldopa	Causes impotence due to central catecholamine depletion and drug-induced depression

Cardiovascular effects of sexual activity

In order to offer sexual guidance to the patient, nurses must have a basic knowledge of the cardiovascular effects of sexual activity. There are four stages to the normal sexual response, in which changes in blood pressure and heart rate occur.

Stage 1: Excitement

Excitement is precipitated by psychogenic or peripheral stimuli, which increases sexual tension resulting in vasocongestion. This phase lasts from several minutes to hours.

Stage 2: Plateau

Plateau occurs with intensified sexual tension. The heart rate increases to about 180 beats per minute and blood pressure increases by 20–80 mmHg systolic and 20–40 mmHg diastolic. This phase lasts from 30 seconds to three minutes.

Stage 3: Orgasm

The heart rate increases to 180 beats per minute, blood pressure by 40–100 mmHg systolic, 20–50 mmHg diastolic, and hyperventilation occurs. Orgasm lasts for three to fifteen seconds. Energy expenditure during orgasm is around 5.5 metabolic equivalents (METs) (1 MET is the basal oxygen requirement of the inactive body which is 3.5 ml oxygen/kg/min), which is equivalent to climbing two flights of stairs (Thompson, 1990). However, little has been discovered about the energy expenditure in females who are multiorgasmic.

Stage 4: Resolution

This is where the body returns to its resting state. If orgasm occurs, resolution is rapid (10–15 minutes), but if orgasm does not occur, resolution may take two to six hours (Thompson, 1980). Many patients may experience palpitations or chest pain during the resolution stage. This may be due to the Valsalva manoeuvre which is initiated by breathholding before orgasm. This may cause a transient decrease in venous return, precipitating hypotension, reflex tachycardia and chest pain (Lefkowitz, 1975, cited in Thompson, 1980). If the nurse is aware of this, he/she can advise the patient to concentrate on breathing regularly during intercourse.

Guidelines for nurses

If nurses have an in-depth knowledge of sexuality and the cardiovascular effects of sexual activity, they are well prepared to give specific information and advice to the patient and partner. However, information given to the patient while in hospital may not be recalled.

Elliot and Smith (1985) found that stress factors reduced the individual's ability to retain and comprehend much-needed information, and Braulin *et al* (1982) found that frequent repetition of details given was necessary to ensure that the information was understood.

An in-depth study of sexuality must be included in the RGN syllabus, and individual students must be encouraged to look at their own attitudes and prejudices to sexuality and increase their own awareness. The nurse who feels embarrassed about discussing sexual activity with a patient may not be able to look towards colleagues for guidance, as they may also feel inadequate.

One-day workshops or in-service training are ways of improving the qualified nurse's knowledge of sexuality. Peer group support can be encouraged during group discussions, and protocol written to help guide nurses when discussing sexual activity with patients.

Nurses must also be aware that it is not just the married heterosexual male who may suffer an MI. Little is written regarding single, homosexual or female patients following an MI. However, if the nurse is aware of all the different sexual options, this may help to reduce prejudice, which could lead to the nurse ignoring the patient's cues or concerns.

If nurses' attitudes affect their ability to give sexual guidance, the patient must be referred to a colleague who can meet his/her needs for support and guidance. Thompson (1980) found that psychologically induced, permanent impotence may result if the patient does not receive sexual guidance.

There are many recommendations for those involved in dealing with the sexual problems of coronary patients. Nurses must be aware of these, and adapt this information for use in their own area.

Annon (1976) described the PLISSIT model, which is still recommended and useful when approaching the subject of sexual activity with post-coronary patients. The model provides four levels of approach: permission; limited information; specific suggestion; and intensive therapy (*Table 16.2*). It is important that advice and counselling take place in a comfortable, private environment and include, if possible, the patient and his/her partner. However, single patients must not be denied this information.

Table 16.2: The PLISSIT model	
Permission	To discuss and ask questions about sex. The counsellor may need to bring the subject up first if the patient is unwilling to do so
Limited information	Directly relevant to the patient's particular situation and sexual concern
Specific suggestion	Involves careful and detailed assessment of the problems, goals and expectations
Intensive therapy	Usually means referral to a sexual counsellor, clinical psychologist, or sexual dysfunction clinic
Source: Annon, 1976	

The patient may be advised to include a range of sexual activities such as holding, caressing and mutual masturbation, as these help to rebuild self-confidence before progressing to full intercourse. Advice must be given on what to avoid before sexual activity. These include: heavy meals; restrictive clothing; extreme temperatures; illicit affairs; unfamiliar surroundings; emotional outbursts; excessive alcohol; and fatigue. All of these put additional strain on the cardiac workload (Thompson, 1990).

The couple may also be advised to start with relaxed positions which facilitate easy breathing, such as female-superior or lateral positions. However, it must be stressed that there is little difference on cardiac workload between different coital positions or between intercourse and masturbation (Hellerstein and Friedman, 1970).

Following assessment of the patient, the care plan will be written which should include aspects of the patient's sexuality. Assessment may include previous patterns of sexual activity, any previous pain or sexual difficulties, and the patient's and partner's attitudes regarding resuming sexual activity. This pre-written protocol may then be adapted to the couple's needs, or the needs of the individual. The nurse may find that questionnaires for the patients to fill in may facilitate discussion of their fears or problems.

Conclusion

Sex and sexuality is life-affirming and enjoyable and can greatly assist in the rehabilitation of a person's mental and physical status following MI. It is extremely important that each patient is viewed as an individual, and no assumptions made as to his/her health education and rehabilitation needs (Jones, 1992).

Nurses must be aware that sexuality is an important aspect of patient care, and must overcome the apparent reluctance to incorporate this information into health promotion sessions. It is important that the patient and partner are informed of the effects of the illness on sexual functioning. The main aim of offering sexual guidance is to facilitate communication between the couple and restore sexual activity to pre-illness levels. The patient usually needs to restore his/her self-confidence and self-esteem, and time spent getting to know his/her partner again may help to achieve this.

The nurse must guide the patient towards regaining some sense of sexual normality following MI and help him/her to return to as near a normal life as possible. The heart is the symbol of love and caring and, as nurses, with education and awareness we can help patients and their partners resume their caring, and let the heart continue its extra special function of loving.

Key points

* Sexual activity is not discussed with the patient for a number of reasons, eg. general attitudes to sexuality, and embarrassment on behalf of the patient, partner or nurse.

* Nurses must face up to their own sexuality and prejudices, and realise the importance of sexuality in everyone's life.

* The nurse must not withhold valuable information from the patient because of feelings of inadequacy.
* Nurse education lacks the in-depth tuition needed on the subject of sexuality and moves must be made for the subject to be incorporated into training and education.
* Nurses must be supported by managers and colleagues, so they can give valuable education and support to the patient following myocardial infarction.
* Once educated, the nurse is in a prime position to alter any false opinions and can offer specific advice so that the patient can make an informed choice.

References

Annon J (1976) *The Behavioural Treatment of Sexual Problems: Brief Therapy.* Harper and Row, New York

Baggs J (1986) Nursing diagnosis: potential sexual dysfunction after MI. *Dimen Crit Care Nurs* **5**(3): 178–81

Bloch A, Maeder JP, Haissly JC (1975) Sexual problems after MI. *Am Heart J* **90**: 536–7

Booth B (1990) Does it really matter at that age? *Nurs Times* **86**(3): 50–2

Braulin JLD, Rook J, Sills GM (1982) Families in crisis; the impact of trauma. *Crit Care Q* **5**(3): 38–46

Cohen J (1980) Sexual counselling of the patient following MI. *Crit Care Nurs* **6**(6): 18–27

Elliot J, Smith DR (1985) Meeting family needs following severe head injury. *J Neurosurg Nurs* **17**: 111–13

Goodman RE (1989) Sex-counselling for the post coronary patient. *Br J Sex Med* **16**(1): 25–28

Griffiths E (1988) No sex please we're over 60! *Nurs Times* **84**(1): 340–50

Hellerstein HK, Friedman EH (1970) Sexual activity and the post coronary patient. *Arch Intern Med* **125**: 987–99

Jones C (1992) Sexual activity after MI. *Nurs Standard* **6**(48): 25–28

Kinsey AC, Pomeroy WB, Martin CE (1948) *Sexual Behaviour in the Human Male.* WB Saunders, Philadelphia

McCann ME (1989) Sexual healing after attack. *Am J Nurs* **89**: 1133–38

Papadopoulos C, Beaumont C, Shelley S *et al* (1983) MI and the sexual activity of the female patient. *Arch Intern Med* **143**: 1528–30

Piper KM (1992) When can I do 'it' again nurse? Sexual counselling after a heart attack. *Profess Nurs* **8**(3): 168–72

Savage J (1990) Sexuality and nursing care: setting the scene. *Nurs Standard* **4**(37): 24–25

Thompson D (1980) Sexual activity following acute MI in the male. *Nurs Times* **76**(45): 1965–67

Thompson D (1990) Intercourse after MI. *Nurs Standard* **4**(43): 32–33
Ueno M (1963) The so called coital death. *Japanese J Legal Med* **17**: 333–37
Webb C (1985) *Sexuality, Nursing and Health*. John Wiley, Chichester
Wenger NK (1985) Coronary disease in woman. *Ann Rev Med* **36**: 285

17

Cardiac rehabilitation: structure, effectiveness and the future

Karyn Noy

Despite advances in the investigation and treatment of angina and myocardial infarction, and increased knowledge of the factors associated with the development and progression of ischaemic heart disease, it remains the leading cause of death and morbidity in the majority of industrialised countries. Cardiac rehabilitation provides a means of modifying lifestyle and other risk factors in patients presenting with established, symptomatic coronary artery disease, thereby reducing the risk of further cardiac events. It has also been proven to be cost-efficient.

Ischaemic heart disease remains the most common cause of death in Western societies, and the highest rates in the world are found in parts of the British Isles (Horgan *et al*, 1992). In 1991, the government's consultative document for health in England, *The Health of the Nation*, set a target of a 30% reduction in deaths from heart disease in people under 65 years of age by the year 2000.

This is a massive task, as Fawcett (1993) pointed out, and health education plays a major part in attempts to achieve it. Cardiac rehabilitation programmes have been proven to reduce mortality and morbidity at minimal cost.

This chapter reviews the literature on cardiac rehabilitation to determine what exactly it is, and then describes its benefits and limitations to ascertain what improvements can be made to existing programmes.

What is cardiac rehabilitation?

Jowett and Thompson (1996) define cardiac rehabilitation as,

... the process by which patients with coronary heart disease are enabled to achieve their optimal physical, emotional, social, vocational and economic status.

This optimistic definition is based upon the World Health Organization's (WHO's) most recent definition of cardiac rehabilitation (WHO, 1993), which reads as follows,

The rehabilitation of cardiac patients is the sum of activities required to influence favourably the underlying cause of the disease, as well as the best possible physical, mental and social conditions, so that they may, by their own efforts, preserve or resume when lost, as normal a place as possible in the community.

Cardiac rehabilitation programmes have become an accepted method of follow-up after acute myocardial infarction (AMI) (Levin *et al*, 1991). The aim of the rehabilitation is to help patients achieve a physically active lifestyle, including return to work, and to reduce the risk factors for coronary artery disease such as smoking, hypertension and hyperlipidaemia.

Exercise, as a treatment for heart disease, is as old as our knowledge of the condition. In 1768, Heberden noted that his patients with angina pectoris were nearly cured by sawing wood for half an hour a day (Coats *et al*, 1990). However, this treatment was forgotten until early in the 20th century, when heart disease was recognised as a serious health problem. Up until the late 1960s, bed rest for up to six weeks was advised for patients following AMI. Much research has since been carried out to determine the physical benefits of mobility post-AMI and cardiac rehabilitation programmes throughout the Western world now include exercise.

Who should receive cardiac rehabilitation?

Rehabilitation is important for patients following AMI, coronary artery bypass grafting (CABG), cardiac transplantation, valve surgery, angioplasty or stent, physiological pacemaker implantation, repair of congenital heart defects and prosthetic valve surgery. It also benefits those who suffer from angina or heart failure (Horgan *et al*, 1992; Chua and Lipkin, 1993). Initially, most rehabilitation programmes were introduced for younger patients post-AMI, but the client group is changing as the procedures for treating heart disease are being developed.

Skelton *et al* (1994) reported an increase in the number of patients requiring cardiac rehabilitation following CABG. In their study in Edinburgh, less than one in ten patients referred to the service were post-myocardial infarction (post-MI). Almost 25% of men and 40% of the women admitted were over the age of 65 years. Studies have reported a poorer uptake of cardiac rehabilitation programmes by women compared with men (McGee and Horgan, 1992).

Traditionally, patients with heart failure have been considered unsuitable for rehabilitation programmes, but this attitude is now changing and it has been shown that exercise and advice on lifestyle modification can substantially relieve the symptoms of heart failure (Jones and West, 1995).

The disparate nature of the groups who would benefit from cardiac rehabilitation emphasises the importance of tailoring programmes to individual patient needs (Horgan *et al*, 1992).

Cardiac rehabilitation should be available to all suitable patients, but limited resources often necessitate prioritisation. There is a lack of conclusive research evidence as to which types of patient benefit most from cardiac rehabilitation, the ideal time at which to commence rehabilitation, and the effect of newer treatments such as thrombolysis and angioplasty on outcome following rehabilitation (Oberman, 1989). Nonetheless, it has been suggested that the patients who might benefit most from inclusion are those who have multiple cardiac risk factors, and/or a low exercise capacity, or are slow to adjust psychologically to a new lifestyle, or have had recent cardiac surgery (Chua and Lipkin, 1993).

Contraindications to exercise training include unstable angina pectoris, ventricular arrhythmias, uncontrolled hypertension and severe aortic stenosis (Chua and Lipkin, 1993). Age is not an absolute contraindication, although it imposes obvious constraints if associated with poor mobility or co-morbidity (Siddiqui, 1992).

The British Cardiac Society reports that only 74% of UK health authorities offer both inpatient and outpatient rehabilitation programmes (Davidson *et al*, 1995). Horgan *et al* (1992) believe that even when such programmes are available, the provision of cardiac rehabilitation varies greatly between hospitals, and there is little consistency in the level of funding, selection criteria or programme content. They suggest that every major district hospital that treats patients with heart disease should provide a rehabilitation service.

Structure and content of cardiac rehabilitation

Cardiac rehabilitation should begin at the time of diagnosis of coronary artery disease, or as soon as possible following admission with an acute event (WHO, 1993).

Cardiac rehabilitation programmes comprise three phases (Certo, 1985):

- Phase I: inpatient hospital phase beginning in the coronary care unit (CCU)
- Phase II: outpatient hospital-based phase for two to four months
- Phase III: maintenance phase from four months onwards.

It is important to realise that the ability to absorb and retain information in the acute phase of the illness is limited (Williams, 1993), and therefore points need to be repeated at various stages of the programme.

A major focus of cardiac rehabilitation is modification of lifestyle to reduce the known risk factors for coronary heart disease (Chua and Lipkin, 1993). WHO (1993) suggests that a comprehensive approach should be taken (*Table 17.1*) and that partners and other close family members should be involved in the rehabilitation process.

Newens *et al* (1995) surveyed five hospitals in the north-eastern

Table 17.1: Comprehensive approach to cardiac rehabilitation advocated by WHO
Secondary prevention
Relaxation
Education
Stress management
Psychosocial adjustment
Source: WHO, 1993

counties of England. They found that patient education post-MI is dependent largely on the provision of written information, and that nurses and other hospital staff do not routinely discuss topics such as exercise, diet, sexual activity, anxiety and stress with patients, either formally or opportunistically.

It is important not to rely too heavily on one means of communication. Fridlund (1994) and Salisbury (1996) suggest that rehabilitation post-MI should be carried out within a holistic nursing framework. However, as Lauri (1991) points out, a holistic nursing framework does not guarantee good nursing care, although it does help the nurse to keep sight of the person as a human being with body, mind and spiritual needs.

The cardiac rehabilitation programme can take many forms, including a home-based structure (Lewin *et al*, 1992). Thompson (1990) describes one example of this called *The Heart Manual*, which consists of six weekly sections that include education, a home-based exercise programme, and a tape-based relaxation and stress management programme. Patients who completed this programme had less contact with their GP during the following year, and significantly fewer readmissions to hospital in the first six months.

A similar type of programme is currently in use in more than 80 hospitals throughout the UK. The majority of units adopt a more hospital-based approach comprising the following risk factor modification strategies.

Exercise training

Since the 1950s it has been recognised that there is a positive correlation between increased physical activity and reduction in coronary artery disease (Wilson, 1988). Before 1950, bed rest for a minimum of three weeks following AMI was recommended (Certo, 1985), but such patients are now encouraged to mobilise within days of their infarct, in order to avert the harmful effects of prolonged bed rest (WHO, 1993; Jowett and Thompson, 1996).

The precise amount of activity advised   before discharge, following an uncomplicated MI, is described by Nutter *et al* (1972) as four metabolic equivalents (METS), which is equivalent to walking 50 yards or climbing an average flight of stairs. These researchers found that activity above this level during the first week of recovery can result in angina or malignant tachydysrhythmias.

In their overview of 22 randomised trials of exercise-based rehabilitation programmes, Horgan *et al* (1992) found that trials of exercise-based rehabilitation after MI in 4554 patients showed a 20% reduction in overall mortality. Exercise would therefore appear to be important in the reduction of mortality post-MI.

Table 17.2 shows the benefits of exercise training, as summarised by Pell (1977).

Groups of patients undergoing sustained training for longer than one year have shown increases in stroke volume, ejection fraction, myocardial contractility, left ventricular end-iastolic dimensions, posterior left ventricular wall thickness and left ventricular mass (Horgan *et al*, 1992). Hung *et al* (1994) argue that the increase in exercise capacity that occurs three to twenty six weeks after clinically uncomplicated MI results primarily from adaptations other than direct improvement in myocardial perfusion or left ventricular function.

Patients who participate in formal exercise programmes achieve their optimum functional state more rapidly than patients who do not (Hung *et al*, 1994), visit their doctor and the hospital less frequently (Ades *et al*, 1992) and are more likely to return to work (Bourdes *et al*, 1994). Exercise training can also be effective in long-term weight reduction and hypertension control (Laslett *et al*, 1987), both of which may provide additional benefits for cardiovascular morbidity and mortality.

Exercise may improve the symptoms of heart disease by promoting the development of a collateral circulation (arteries that grow up around a diseased vessel in order to bypass the problem area). Although there is conclusive evidence in animals that exercise stimulates collateralisation, there is no direct evidence yet that it has this effect in humans.

Flaws in experimental design include the use of small groups and low-intensity, short-term, exercise training programmes, and the inadequacy of coronary angiography for measuring collateral growth (Froozan and Forfar, 1996).

Table 17.2: Benefits of exercise training
A reduction in heart rate and blood pressure at rest and during exercise
Increased high-density lipoprotein cholesterol levels
Improved glucose tolerance in diabetic patients
Enhanced fibrinolysis in response to thrombotic stimuli
Improvements in electrocardiographic ST segment changes
Improvements in ejection fraction
A high ischaemic threshold
Increase in coronary collateral circulation
Source: Pell, 1997

Smoking cessation

Cigarette smoking is a widely recognised risk factor for the development of coronary artery disease (Saons, 1986) and continued smoking following MI doubles the risk of a recurrent cardiac event (Rosenberg *et al*, 1985). It is therefore important to incorporate smoking cessation techniques into all cardiac rehabilitation programmes.

Patients who attended classes in cardiac rehabilitation reported a 60% success rate in stopping smoking (Higgins and Schweiger, 1983); success rates in those who did not attend classes were lower (Siegel *et al*, 1988).

Management of hypertension

Patients who remain hypertensive post-MI have a greater risk of subsequent death than normotensive patients (Kannel *et al*, 1980). Treatment of hypertension following AMI has been demonstrated to reduce total mortality by 20% (Langford *et al*, 1986).

Management of hypercholesterolaemia

Treatment of hypercholesterolaemia significantly decreases the risk of MI and sudden cardiac death, as well as reducing mortality following MI (Canner *et al*, 1986). The 4S study (Scandinavian Simvastatin Survival Study Group, 1994) demonstrated that treatment of moderate hypercholesterolaemia with simvastatin in patients with angina or previous MI resulted in a 42% reduction in the risk of coronary death and a 30% reduction in total mortality. In addition, the need for myocardial revascularisation procedures was reduced by 37%.

Weight reduction

There have been no randomised controlled trials of weight reduction in MI survivors, but it has been recommended that patients who are more than 20% above the mid-range desirable weight would benefit from a weight-reduction programme (Siegel *et al*, 1988).

Psychological interventions

Thompson (1990) writes,

> *The experience of suffering a heart attack is virtually always frightening and painful, arousing intense distress in the patient and family, especially the spouse. Later, as the fear of death recedes, they are confronted with the consequences of physical impairment and the experience of surviving a sudden, life-threatening crisis. The patient and spouse, in particular, are likely to be faced with an uncertain future and worry about the patient's ability to resume work, the fulfilment of family obligations and the curtailment of activities that have been important sources of satisfaction and support.*

Research on the link between stress and coronary artery disease has focused mainly on the type A behaviour pattern, originally described by Friedman and Rosenman (1959) (*Table 17.3*). Besides being more prone to involvement in potentially stressful situations, people exhibiting type A behaviour are likely to have a greater catecholamine response to such

Table 17.3: Type A and type B behaviour patterns	
Type A behaviour	Being irritable, quick to anger, competitive and full of aggression
Type B behaviour	Being none of the above, but relaxed and unhurried

Table 17.4: Factors associated with a poor outcome of rehabilitation
A history of anxiety or depression
Lower educational level
Socioeconomic deprivation
Perceived health status
Perceived stress
Social isolation
Personality variables (eg. hypochondria)

situations. Brackett and Powell (1988) found that type A behaviour was an independent predictor of sudden cardiac death. Another study found that patients suffering social isolation and high levels of stress have four times the risk of death during the three years following MI (Ruberman *et al*, 1984).

Ruberman *et al* (1984) found that a poor outcome of rehabilitation was associated with the type A characteristics shown in *Table 17.4*. Research by Frasure-Smith (1991) indicates that patients who exhibit many of these characteristics are the very people who would benefit most from cardiac rehabilitation. Frasure-Smith (1991) pointed out that patients who reported high levels of stress symptoms in the hospital were at substantially increased long-term risk of both cardiac mortality and reinfarction. Programme participation decreased the long-term risk of cardiac mortality and AMI recurrence.

Evaluation of cardiac rehabilitation

The provision of cardiac rehabilitation programmes to cardiac patients seems justified in terms of cost-benefit (Levin *et al*, 1991; Oldridge *et al*, 1991). In the UK in the mid-1980s, coronary artery disease was estimated to cost £500 million and £1800 million in lost productivity. It also accounted for 11.6% of sick leave (Tunstall-Pedoe, 1991). As the cost of running a cardiac rehabilitation session is only £4–£15 per patient (Horgan *et al*, 1992), the financial benefits to be gained in terms of productivity and maintaining an occupational income by returning to work are clear.

In a Swedish study, 51.8% of patients who had undergone cardiac rehabilitation remained in active employment five years after AMI, compared with 27.4% of a control group (Levin *et al*, 1991). This was attributed to a reduction in factors such as anxiety, depression and recurrent cardiac events. The rate of readmission with cardiac disease, and hence the cost, was also lower in the patients who had been rehabilitated.

Other studies have confirmed a reduction in readmissions, shorter lengths of stay in hospital during readmission, fewer cardiac events and marginally lower costs following rehabilitation (Picard *et al*, 1989; Ades *et al*, 1992). However, neither of these was a randomised trial. Oldridge *et al* (1993) carried out an economic evaluation of cardiac rehabilitation using a randomised study design, and concluded that,

Brief cardiac rehabilitation initiated soon after AMI for patients with mild

to moderate anxiety or depression, or both, is an efficient use of healthcare resources and may be economically justified.

Lipkin (1991) found that 8–38% of patients do not return to work after MI although many of them seem physically capable of resuming employment. He suggests that the major beneficial effect of rehabilitation programmes may be the reassurance that patients get from close contact with paramedical staff.

Oldridge *et al* (1991) point out that the clinical effectiveness of rehabilitation in chronic diseases needs to be judged not only in terms of mortality and morbidity but also in terms of health-related quality of life, where it has also been shown to be worthwhile. Davies (1993) considers return to work to be a significant indicator of success following completion of cardiac rehabilitation and suggests that programmes should focus more on this goal.

The benefits of cardiac rehabilitation post-CABG are listed in *Table 17.5* (Skelton *et al*, 1994).

Table 17.5: Benefits of cardiac rehabilitation following coronary artery bypass grafting
Improves physical conditioning
Decreases musculoskeletal discomfort associated with surgery
Improves quality of life
Increases work capacity
Decreases the number of readmissions to hospital
Improves the mean scores for psychological distress

The role of the nurse in cardiac rehabilitation

Cardiac rehabilitation programmes use a multidisciplinary approach, relying on the skilled professional input from a dietician, physiotherapist, GP, cardiologist, pharmacist, social worker, occupational therapist, psychiatrist, health visitor and nurse. The nurse often acts as the coordinator of the service and will usually have the most frequent contact with the patient and his/her significant others. The post of specialist nurse in cardiac rehabilitation varies widely, ranging from the part-time unfunded enthusiast to the full-time G grade sister (Newens *et al*, 1995).

Nurses are important providers of information to patients in hospital. However, much of it takes the form of written information rather than one-to-one discussion, the exception being hospitals that have a dedicated rehabilitation nurse in post and a structured teaching programme for patients (eg. *The Heart Manual*).

Salisbury (1996) considers that effective rehabilitation programmes need to be holistic and address the physical, psychological and social needs of the patients, with the aim of empowering them to take control of the rehabilitative process by using their lay knowledge and social networks. She believes that working in partnership and empowering people are central to the practice of community nursing. The health visitor is ideally placed to make early contact once the patient has been discharged from hospital and to assess and construct individualised rehabilitation programmes with clients and their families, thus ensuring continuity of care.

Whatever the structure of cardiac rehabilitation programmes, it is clear that nurses play an important part. The new Green Paper *Our Healthier Nation*, published by the Government (Department of Health, 1998), describes two key aims for improving the health of the population:

- to improve the health of the population as a whole by increasing the length of people's lives and the numbers of years that people spend free from illness
- to improve the health of the worst off in society and to narrow the health gap.

The Green paper proposes targets on heart disease and stroke, accidents, cancer and mental health. The target for heart disease and stroke is,

> *To reduce the death rate from heart disease and stroke and related illnesses amongst people under 65 years by at least a further third.*

Since cardiac rehabilitation programmes have been proven to reduce mortality, they must be an important consideration when planning initiatives to help achieve this target. *Table 17.6* outlines the Government's proposed contract on heart disease and stroke. The wording in italics has specific relevance to cardiac rehabilitation and to the role of the nurse in such programmes.

Although the nurse's role is only a small part of a much larger picture, it is a crucial one and should be carried out by an experienced and well-trained professional (ie. a clinical nurse specialist).

Conclusion

Cardiac rehabilitation programmes may differ in content, but they share the same goal, ie. for the patients involved to feel some relief from symptoms and experience an enhanced quality of life. This is achieved through a combination of secondary prevention, relaxation, education, stress management and psychosocial adjustment.

The programme must incorporate an individualised approach so that it can be tailored to the specific needs of the patient. New advances in the treatment of cardiac conditions means that these needs are continually changing, eg. patients with heart failure are now included in such programmes.

Research has shown that cardiac rehabilitation has physical and psychosocial benefits for the patient, with additional cost benefits for the health service and economy through earlier return to work and decreased hospital admissions and GP visits.

Table 17.6: The Government's proposed contract on heart disease and stroke		
	Government and national players can:	**Local players and communities can:**	**People can:**
Social and economic	Continue to make smoking cost more through taxation Tackle joblessness, social exclusion, low educational standards and other factors that make it harder to live a healthier life	Tackle social exclusion in the community, which makes it harder to have a healthy lifestyle Provide incentives to employees to cycle or walk to work, or leave their cars at home	Take opportunities to better their lives and their families' lives, through education, training and employment
Enviro-mental	Encourage employers and others to provide a smoke-free environment for non-smokers	Through local employers and others, provide a smoke-free environment for non-smokers Through employers and staff, work in partnership to reduce stress at work Provide safe cycling and walking routes	Protect others from second-hand smoke
Lifestyle	End advertising promotion of cigarettes Enforce prohibition of sale of cigarettes to youngsters Develop healthy living centres Ensure access to, and availability of, a wide range of foods for a healthy diet Provide sound information on the health risks of smoking, poor diet and lack of exercise	Encourage the development of healthy schools and healthy workplaces Implement an integrated transport policy, including a national cycling strategy and measures to make walking more of an option *Target information about a healthy lifestyle on groups where people are at most risk*	Stop smoking or cut down, watch what they eat and take regular exercise
Services	*Encourage doctors and nurses and other health professionals to give advice on healthier living* Ensure catering and leisure professionals are retrained in healthy eating and physical activity	Provide help to people who want to stop smoking Improve access to a variety of affordable food in deprived areas *Provide facilities for physical activity and relaxation* and decent transport to help people get to them *Identify those at high risk of heart disease and stroke and provide high quality services*	Learn how to recognise a heart attack and what to do, including resuscitation skills Have their blood pressure checked regularly Take medicine as it is prescribed

* Italics indicate sections with specific reference to cardiac rehabilitation and the role of the nurse in such programmes

The Government's proposed contract on heart disease and stroke incorporates a clear incentive for hospitals to develop cardiac rehabilitation services. It is anticipated that such programmes will be available in all major district hospitals in the near future.

Key points

* Cardiac rehabilitation is the process by which patients with coronary heart disease are enabled to achieve their optimal physical, emotional, social, vocational and economic status.
* Cardiac rehabilitation should be carried out using a holistic framework, ensuring individualised care.
* Cardiac rehabilitation has been advocated for patients who have suffered a myocardial infarction, those who have undergone cardiac surgery and those suffering from heart failure and angina.
* Programmes should incorporate exercise training, smoking cessation, management of hypertension and hypercholesterolaemia as well as psychological interventions.

References

Ades PA, Huang D, Weaver MS (1992) Cardiac rehabilitation participation predicts lower rehospitalisation costs. *Am Heart J* **123**: 916–21

Bourdes H, De Backer G, Comchaire B (1994) Return to work after myocardial infarction: results of a longitudinal population based study. *Eur Heart J* **15**: 32–6

Brackett CD, Powell LH (1988) Psychological and physiological predictors of sudden cardiac death after healing of acute myocardial infarction. *Am J Cardiol* **61**: 979–83

Canner Pl, Berge KG, Wenger NK *et al* (1986) Fifteen-year mortality in coronary drug project patients: long-term benefit with niacin. *J Am Coll Cardiol* **8**: 1245–55

Certo CM (1985) History of cardiac rehabilitation. *Phys Ther* **65**(12): 1793–5

Chua T, Lipkin DP (1993) Cardiac rehabilitation should be available to all who would benefit. *Br Med J* **306**: 731–2

Coats JS, Adamopoulos S, Meyer TE (1990) Effects of physical training in chronic heart failure. *Lancet* **335**: 63–6

Davidson C, Reval K, Chamberlain DA (1995) A report of a working group of the British Cardiac Society: Cardiac rehabilitation services in the United Kingdom 1992. *Br Heart J* **73**: 201–2

Davies B (1993) Restoration of occupational capacity in post-cardiac patients. *Occup Health* **45**(10): 330–4

Department of Health (1998) *Our Healthier Nation: A Contract for Health. A consultation paper*. The Stationery Office, London

Fawcett J (1993) Heartfelt advice. *Nurs Times* **89**(27): 36–8

Frasure-Smith N (1991) In-hospital symptoms of psychological stress as predictors of long-term outcome after acute myocardial infarction in men. *Am J Cardiol* **67**: 121–7

Fridlund B (1994) A holistic framework for nursing care: rehabilitation of the MI patient. *J Holist Nurs* **12**(2): 204–17

Friedman M, Rosenman RH (1959) Association of a specific overt behaviour pattern with blood and cardiovascular findings. *JAMA* **169**: 1286–95

Froozan S, Forfar JC (1996) Exercise training and the collateral circulation: is its value underestimated in man? *Eur Heart J* **17**(12): 1791–5

Higgins C, Schweiger MJ (1983) Smoking termination patterns in a cardiac rehabilitation population. *J Cardiac Rehabil* **3**: 55–9

Horgan J, Bethell H, Carson P (1992) Working party report on cardiac rehabilitation. *Br Heart J* **67**: 412–8

Hung J, Gordon EP, Houston N *et al* (1994) Changes in rest and exercise myocardial perfusion and left ventricular function 3 to 26 weeks after clinically uncomplicated myocardial infarction: effects of exercise training. *Am J Cardiol* **54**: 943–50

Jones D, West R (1995) *Cardiac Rehabilitation*. BMJ Publishing Group, London

Jowett N, Thompson D (1996) *Comprehensive Coronary Care*. 2nd edn. Baillière Tindall, London

Kannel WB, Sorlie P, Castelli WP *et al* (1980) Blood pressure and survival after myocardial infarction: the Framingham study. *Am J Cardiol* **45**: 326–30

Langford HG, Stamler J, Wassertheil-Smoller S *et al* (1986) All cause mortality in the hypertension detection and follow-up program: findings for the whole cohort and for persons with less severe hypertension, with and without other traits related to the risk of mortality. *Prog Cardiovasc Dis* **29**(suppl 1): 29–54

Laslett L, Paumer L, Amsterdam EA (1987) Exercise training in coronary artery disease. *Cardiol Clin* **5**: 211–25

Lauri S (1991) Good nursing care. *Hoitotiede (J Nurs Sci)* **3**: 185–222

Levin LA, Perk J, Hedbeck B (1991) Cardiac rehabilitation — cost analysis. *J Intern Med* **230**: 427–34

Lewin B, Robertson IH, Cay EL *et al* (1992) Effects of self-help post myocardial infarction rehabilitation on psychological adjustment and use of health services. *Lancet* **329**: 1036–40

Lipkin DP (1991) Is cardiac rehabilitation necessary? *Br Heart J* **65**: 237–8

McGee HM, Horgan JH (1992) Cardiac rehabilitation programmes: are women less likely to attend? *Br Med J* **305**: 283–4

Newens A, Bond S, Priest J (1995) Nurse involvement in cardiac rehabilitation prior to hospital discharge. *J Clin Nurs* **4**: 390–6

Nutter DO, Schant RS, Hurst JW (1972) Isometric exercises and the cardiovascular system. *Mod Concepts Cardiovasc Dis* **41**: 11–5

Oberman A (1989) Does cardiac rehabilitation increase long-term survival after myocardial infarction? *Circulation* **80**: 416–18

Oldridge N, Gyatt G, Jones N (1991) Effects on quality of life with comprehensive rehabilitation after acute myocardial infarction. *Am J Cardiol* **67**: 1084–9

Oldridge N, Furlong W, Feeny D (1993) Economic evaluation of cardiac rehabilitation soon after myocardial infarction. *Am J Cardiol* **72**: 154–61

Pell J (1997) Cardiac rehabilitation: a review of its effectiveness. *Coronary Health Care* **1**: 8–17

Picard MH, Dennis C, Schwartz RG (1989) Cost benefit analysis of early return to work after uncomplicated myocardial infarction. *Am J Cardiol* **63**: 1308–14

Ruberman W, Weinblatt E, Goldberg JD *et al* (1984) Psychosocial influences on mortality after myocardial infarction. *N Engl J Med* **311**: 552–9

Rosenberg L, Kaufman DW, Helmrich SP *et al* (1985) The risk of myocardial infarction after quitting smoking in men under 55 years of age. *N Engl J Med* **313**: 1511–17

Salisbury C (1996) The role of health psychology post-MI. *Nurs Standard* **10**(39): 43–6

Saons DPL (1986) Cigarette smoking: health effects and cessation strategies. *Clin Geriatr Med* **2**: 337–45

Scandinavian Simvastatin Survival Study Group: The 4S Study (1994) Randomised trial of cholesterol lowering in 4444 patients with coronary heart disease. *Lancet* **344**: 1383–9

Siddiqui MA (1992) Cardiac rehabilitation and elderly patients. *Age Ageing* **21**: 157–9

Siegel D, Grady D, Browner WS *et al* (1988) Risk factor modification after myocardial infarction. *Ann Intern Med* **109**: 213–8

Skelton CE, McLweir A, Caye L *et al* (1994) Workload of an inpatient cardiac rehabilitation service in Edinburgh: a five year survey. *Clin Rehabil* **8**: 41–7

Thompson DR (1990) *Counselling the Coronary Patient and Partner*. RCN Research Series. Scutari Press, Harrow

Tunstall-Pedoe H (1991) The health of the nation: responses. Coronary heart disease. *Br Med J* **303**: 701–4

WHO (1993) Needs and action priorities in cardiac rehabilitation and secondary prevention in patients with coronary heart disease. In: Jowett N, Thompson D (1996) *Comprehensive Coronary Care*. 2nd edn. Baillière Tindall, London

Williams G (1993) A one-to-one relationship with lasting benefits: implementing primary nursing in a CCU. *Prof Nurse* September: 770–4

Wilson P (1988) Cardiac rehabilitation: then and now. *The Physician and Sports Medicine* **16**(9): 75–84

18

Cardiac rehabilitation following myocardial infarction

Mike Nolan and Janet Nolan

Coronary heart disease is the major cause of death in the UK, but cardiac rehabilitation programmes have tended to develop in an ad hoc and unsystematic way. This chapter considers some of the deficits in current practice and suggests ways in which nurses can contribute more fully to care in this area. The need for better training and the necessity to develop skills in psychological care are highlighted. The authors also emphasise the importance of giving greater attention to a number of areas such as family involvement, sexuality and gender issues, and community follow-up.

Coronary heart disease is the major cause of death in the UK and, although mortality has been declining in recent years, Britain still has one of the highest rates in the world (Thompson and Bowman, 1995). Cardiac rehabilitation, which emerged during the 1950s, initially focused primarily on early mobilisation. However, it has since evolved into a more comprehensive programme aimed at improving cardiovascular fitness and initiating and sustaining a range of lifestyle changes (Thompson and Bowman, 1995). While conclusive evidence on the benefits of cardiac rehabilitation is lacking (Amsterdam *et al*, 1994; Thompson and Bowman, 1995), studies suggest that major reductions in mortality and morbidity and improved quality of life can be achieved.

However, following an audit of services in England and Wales, Thompson and Bowman (1995) concluded that the present provision of cardiac rehabilitation was patchy and ad hoc, with programmes varying considerably. Most interventions relied on the personal motivation of individual staff members and focused largely on exercise and education. Individualised rehabilitation programmes were the exception, with most units utilising published information leaflets. Many programmes did not view psychological problems as part of their remit. Of the 199 centres claiming to offer cardiac rehabilitation, the majority were coordinated by a nurse (140 of 176 coordinators were nurses). It would therefore appear that there is considerable potential for nurses to have a significant impact in cardiac rehabilitation, at least in a hospital setting.

As an individualised rehabilitation programme has long been acknowledged as being the most successful approach to cardiac rehabilitation (Ashworth, 1984; Hentinen, 1986; Miller *et al*, 1989; Murray, 1989; Fridlund *et al*, 1991; Davidson, 1995; Lewin, 1995; Thompson, 1995) and as attention to psychological adjustment is vital (Lewin, 1995), it would appear that there is further scope for improvement in current practice.

Thompson (1995) suggested that attention to four areas is required if the present cardiac rehabilitation services are to be improved and meet the needs of patients and their families: closer coordination and liaison between rehabilitation services and aftercare arrangements; maximum use of self-help materials; better use of primary care; and greater emphasis on the impact of coronary disease on the family.

Table 18.1: Phases of cardiac rehabilitation
In hospital
Early post-discharge
Late post-discharge
Long-term follow-up
Source: Thompson and Bowman, 1995

It is recognised that cardiac rehabilitation comprises a number of phases (*Table 18.1*; Thompson and Bowman, 1995) and that there are gaps in provision both within and between phases. The initial post-discharge period between leaving hospital and the start of a rehabilitation programme, usually four to eight weeks, is known to be both stressful and poorly addressed (Thompson and Cordle, 1988; Webster and Christman, 1988; Thompson, 1995; Thompson *et al*, 1995; Waters, 1995), as is longer term follow-up (Bethell, 1995; Linden, 1995; Horgan and McGee, 1995; Thompson, 1995).

In addition to coordinating cardiac rehabilitation programmes, nurses are considered to have an important role (actual or potential) during the acute hospital period (Ashworth, 1984; Caunt, 1992; Hendrick, 1994; Mayor, 1994; Webb and Riggin, 1994) and subsequently in the community (Keckeisen and Nyamathi, 1990; Mayor, 1994; Jones and West, 1995; Keeling and Dennison, 1995; Thompson *et al*, 1995). It is important that nurses are aware of the gaps in existing services and have the knowledge and skills to address current deficits in order to make an optimal contribution to this client group.

An individual perspective

An individual approach to rehabilitation is seen to be essential yet there is a dearth of qualitative research in cardiac rehabilitation. This may help to explain why, despite extensive research, the adjustment process following myocardial infarction (MI) is poorly understood (Johnson, 1991; Thompson *et al*, 1995). There is general consensus in the literature that the aims of cardiac rehabilitation should extend beyond a simple reduction in mortality and morbidity and incorporate a 'plurality' of outcomes (West, 1995). These include not only clinical and economic outcomes (Horgan and McGee, 1995), a reduction in symptamology and improved function (Thompson and Bowman, 1995), but also an enhanced quality of life (Horgan and McGee, 1995; Kinney, 1995; Lewin, 1995; West, 1995). The inclusion of family carers, particularly spouses, in the rehabilitation process is also advocated (Hentinen, 1983; Derenowski, 1988; Miller *et al*, 1988; Ford, 1989; Roberts, 1989; Ben-Sira and Eliezer, 1990; Thompson *et al*, 1990).

The potential differences between professional perspectives and those of patients/carers is less well described in the literature on MI, possibly reflecting the dearth of qualitative research. Nevertheless, the limited literature available recognises that such perspectives may differ (Johnson and Morse, 1990) and that the goals of rehabilitation should be meaningful to individual patients (Malan, 1992).

The few studies that have adopted a qualitative and temporal approach reach conclusions remarkably similar to those in other chronic illnesses such as multiple sclerosis (MS), arthritis and spinal cord injury. Hawthorne (1991) stressed the importance of adopting a longitudinal dimension and advocated the use of the trajectory model (Corbin and Strauss, 1988, 1991). A temporal perspective was also highlighted by Ford (1989) who suggested that two years after MI men had relearned to 'listen to their bodies'. Ford suggested that this might explain non-compliance with treatment.

The most detailed qualitative study describing adjustment to MI is that of Johnson (Johnson and Morse, 1990; Johnson, 1991). It presents a model of the adjustment process comprising four phases, with the main aim being to regain control. These stages are seen as following a cyclical rather than a linear pattern. The four stages, each with a number of sub-processes, are: defending the self; coming to terms; learning to live; and living again.

Defending the self involves attempts to normalise or trivialise the initial symptoms of MI in order to deny the potential seriousness of events. However, once help is sought patients attempt to distance themselves from their circumstances and enter a period of unreality. *Coming to terms* involves facing one's own mortality and making sense of the infarction. In order for progress to be made, it is important to recognise limitations and look to the future. *Learning to live* is a process of preserving self, minimising uncertainty, and developing new guidelines for living. It is important that individuals have a sense of progress. According to Johnson (1991), they often look to professionals for reassurance that they are 'doing well'. In order to *live again* individuals have to accept their limitations, focus on the positive aspects of their situation, and attain a sense of mastery. Those who fail to achieve this balance 'abandon the struggle', seeing their situation as hopeless and insurmountable. Johnson acknowledges the need to develop and further refine this model, but it is consistent with much of the psychological literature on adjustment to MI which stresses the importance of correcting erroneous misconceptions and facilitating a sense of hope and control.

Taking a different focus and time scale, Thompson *et al* (1995) studied the first month post-infarction, for both the sufferer and the partner. They high-lighted the lack of information and advice received, particularly by the partner, and described how emotional reactions such as fear of another attack could lead to over protection of the sufferer. These authors considered that insufficient attention is given to the needs of both parties during the month following discharge. They advocate the development of 'novel' services, ie. systems of monitoring and support by community nurses, coronary care teams or drop-in centres. Thompson *et al* (1995) also argue for more qualitative in-depth studies on the effects of MI.

Ask the family

Developing an individual programme of rehabilitation involves not only the person affected but also the wider family. However, it is apparent that partners/ families are often not sufficiently involved in cardiac rehabilitation programmes (Thompson and Cordle, 1988; Thompson, 1989, 1991; Marsden and Dracup, 1991; Jones, 1995; Thompson *et al*, 1995). In addition to providing social support, spouses and family members, including children (Hilgenberg *et al*, 1992), have their own emotional and support needs (Hilgenberg and Crowley, 1987; Verderber *et al*, 1990; Wastlick *et al*, 1991; Malan, 1992). Families require an outlet for their own fears and concerns (Marsden and Dracup, 1991; Hilgenberg *et al*, 1992) and benefit from good, honest advice (Lewin, 1995).

In the immediate post-infarction period, family members need to be prepared for seeing their relatives for the first time in the coronary care unit (CCU) (Hentinen, 1983; Jones, 1995), and will require reassurance and empathy to cope with this distressing experience (Marsden and Dracup, 1991). This early support should continue and result in systematic input throughout the rehabilitation period (Thompson and Cordle, 1988). As the sufferer recovers, attention should be focused on family dynamics (Wastlick *et al*, 1991), ways of coping (Verderber *et al*, 1990) and levels of distress, eg. by using the family APGAR scale (Hilbert, 1994). Dynamics such as over-protectiveness (Wastlick *et al*, 1991; Lewin, 1995) need further exploration, for although it is often suggested that families can 'wrap patients in cotton wool' (Rolland, 1988; Lewin, 1995), there have been few empirical studies investigating this phenomenon (Hilgenberg *et al*, 1992).

In terms of family caregiving generally, there is a need for more sophisticated models which better capture the dynamic nature of family interactions (Kahana and Young, 1990; Nolan *et al*, 1996). This need has been identified in relation to MI with Young and Kahana (1994) highlighting the current, rather impoverished models of caregiving which pay insufficient attention to the dyadic interactions that occur. While a number of authors suggest that nurses are in a unique (Marsden and Dracup, 1991) or key (Schigoda and Hook, 1991) position to assist family carers, little evidence in support of this role has emerged to date.

Schigoda and Hook (1991) described a 'Take Heart Programme', based on small group work which was intended to clarify perceptions of the MI, explore alternative coping strategies, and facilitate social support. In the UK, Thompson and colleagues have demonstrated the effectiveness of a simple nurse-led intervention aimed at sufferers and partners which resulted in improvements in a number of areas (Thompson, 1989; Thompson and Webster, 1989; Lewin, 1995), such as reduced anxiety and depression that were apparent for up to six months (Thompson *et al*, 1990; Thompson, 1991). The programme started early, within 24 hours of admission, included both partners and focused on specific sources of anxiety; it also incorporated a structured plan for the early resumption of activity (Lewin, 1995). Studies such as these, however, appear to be the exception and it is clear from most of the literature that family members are rarely involved as active participants in rehabilitation following MI.

Other areas in need of attention

Aspects of rehabilitation, such as sexuality, are also relatively neglected. This is an area in which there are a number of misconceptions (Lewin, 1995) and in which patients and their partners have many anxieties. However, they often do not raise their concerns with professionals (Amsterdam *et al*, 1994). Lewin (1995) suggested that doctors often avoid such issues and that junior doctors are likely to give misleading advice. Others argue that nurses are in an 'ideal' position to address worries concerning sexuality (Boykoff, 1989). Sexuality is rarely addressed adequately in basic training (Briggs, 1994) and consequently, although nurses may provide written information about sexuality (Newens *et al*, 1995; Thompson and Bowman, 1995), this is often generic rather than specific (Thompson and Bowman, 1995). Newens *et al* (1995) suggest that only one in 10 patients has a discussion relating to his/her sexual concerns. Thompson and Bowman (1995) discovered that of the 25 units they audited, none had procedures for formally assessing the sexual needs of the patient or his/her partner.

Gender is also an area in which disparities exist. Most of the studies on recovery from MI relate to men (Jones, 1995), with interventions being based primarily on such evidence (Cochrane, 1992). Little is known about the needs of women post-infarction (Conn *et al*, 1991; Cochrane, 1992; Amsterdam *et al*, 1994; Thompson, 1995) and they receive less support than men (Hamilton, 1991; Folta and Potempa, 1992) despite experiencing higher levels of morbidity and mortality (Amsterdam *et al*, 1994). Women have differing physiological reactions to MI (Conn *et al*, 1991; Hawthorne, 1991; Folta and Potempa, 1992), are often older, widowed, or single and may have greater co-morbidity than men (Hamilton,1991; Rankin, 1995). Furthermore, women may be under greater pressure than men to recommence their domestic responsibilities (Webb and Riggin, 1994). Certain groups of women, eg. young post-partum females, pose rare though considerable challenges for rehabilitation (McHugh and Taubman, 1990).

Older men are another potentially disadvantaged group and there is evidence of ageist practice in cardiac rehabilitation (Newens *et al*, 1995; Thompson and Bowman, 1995). The literature also suggests that the rehabilitation needs of those from ethnic minorities have not been given serious consideration (Thompson, 1995).

Clearly there are a number of potential areas within cardiac rehabilitation services across the spectrum of care that could be improved. These range from hospital services through to long-term follow-up and include specific areas such as supporting families and sexuality, and certain groups of people such as women, older men and ethnic minorities. The literature indicates where improvements can be made and how nurses can contribute.

Current knowledge of the nurse's role

Although unequivocal evidence in favour of cardiac rehabilitation is lacking, there is, nevertheless, as noted earlier, relatively strong support in terms of the benefits provided. While early rehabilitative efforts focused largely on ambulation, and exercise still figures prominently (Thompson and Bowman, 1995), far greater attention is now given to a range of psychological and behavioural components aimed at improving quality of life and reducing risk factors. While multidisciplinary teamwork is important (Horgan and McGee, 1995), the nurse's role in coordinating rehabilitation is well established, and there are also emerging roles which relate to different components of rehabilitation at all stages of the process, eg. education and information giving, counselling and psychological support, and behavioural change. These generic aspects will be considered before the more specific nursing roles, in particular, phases of rehabilitation.

Lewin (1995) considers that psychological interventions post-infarction should begin as soon as possible and be guided by a number of principles:

- the reduction of misconceptions in a believable and sympathetic manner
- interventions should be based on a lay understanding of illness
- patients and families should be given honest and realistic advice
- particular attention should be given to the benefits of cognitive behavioural therapy.

Lewin advocated that, ideally, specialist help from a psychologist should be provided, but recognised that in its absence medical and nursing staff are best placed to deal with a number of issues, particularly misconceptions and false beliefs. This, Lewin argued, should become a routine part of care. However, he also considered that more intensive cognitive behavioural approaches are needed if life-style and behavioural changes (eg. giving up smoking or maintaining a diet) are to be achieved. Lewin, while acknowledging the expertise of psychologists in this latter area, nevertheless concluded by stating:

> ... research suggests that a good deal of psychological distress could be mitigated without the need for specialist psychologists' input *if* the routine management of MI was designed in such a way as to optimize psychological as well as physical recovery.

Psychological care is an area in which nurses, having the most prolonged and consistent contact with patients could, as Thompson (1989) has described, have a significant input. However, to achieve this requires not only that nurses recognise this as being an important area of care, but also that they have the necessary knowledge and skills to address psychological needs.

The notion of reducing uncertainty, fear and negative emotional responses by reversing misconceptions and creating a realistic set of perceptions is an important part of psychosocial care. Many authors therefore advocate a major role in the provision of education and information. Amsterdam *et al* (1994) contend that patients' fear of death is higher than the actual risk of death, and that this can lead to a negative perception of future prospects. As others point out, this can result in patients 'abandoning the struggle' (Johnson and Morse,1990; Johnson, 1991). Indeed, nurses may have a more negative perception of patients' potential recovery and relay such a perception to them (McCauley *et al*, 1992).

Unfortunately, however, the information and education given to patients is often vague and imprecise (Farrell *et al*, 1985; Murray, 1989) and can be given in an inappropriate way or at an inappropriate time (Farrell *et al*, 1985). Rather than the individualised approach to information giving advocated, the quality and quantity of information provided is often limited, relying primarily on written sources (Newens *et al*, 1995).

Similarly, although nurses are considered to have a major role in the psychological support of patients and carers post-infarction (Hentinen, 1986; Packa, 1989; Conn *et al*, 1992), empirical evidence suggests that this is rarely realised. Newens *et al* (1995) question whether nurses are adequately trained to adopt such roles, highlighting a lack of knowledge and training in risk factors and likely symptoms post-infarction (Newens *et al*, 1996). Ashworth (1984) stressed the importance of nurses being skilled in communication and problem-solving, and Webber (1994) advocates that a thorough appreciation of group dynamics is required. Others argue for a detailed understanding of the psychophysiological triggers to behaviour (Medich *et al*, 1991), or note the lack of attention given to self-help skills and social support in nurse training (Hildingh *et al*, 1995). It is apparent that there are several areas in which the education and training of nurses fails to prepare them adequately to adopt a proactive role in the psychological aspects of rehabilitation post MI. This may help to explain why most nurse-centred programmes do not see psychological care as part of their remit.

Passage through the acute healthcare system often involves a series of transfers between different care environments, and it is argued that nurses have a key role to play in easing such transitions so that stress is reduced (Glick, 1986; Jenkins and Rogers, 1995). Glick (1986) advocates the use of therapeutic touch, whereas Jenkins and Rogers (1995) provide a detailed protocol directed specifically at transfers between CCU and other wards. This is consistent with the coordinating aspect of the nursing role, which is recognised by many nurses as being one of their key contributions (Murray, 1989; Davidson, 1995; Thompson and Bowman, 1995). Other more specific aspects include exercise therapy, which requires a detailed knowledge of physiology (Folta and Potempa, 1992; Davidson, 1995) and relaxation therapy (Hase and Douglas, 1987).

Cardiac rehabilitation is not confined to acute care settings and, as stated earlier, is generally considered to comprise the four stages highlighted in *Table 18. 1*. Jones (1995) suggests that nurses have a role to play in easing the transition from the in-hospital phase to the early post-discharge phase. However, Thompson and Bowman (1995) found that seventeen of the twenty five units they audited had no routine contact with district nurses and health visitors. Moreover, the early convalescence period between hospital discharge and rehabilitation is a stressful period in which there is little support (Thompson and

Cordle, 1988; Webster and Christman, 1988; Thompson *et al*, 1995; Waters, 1995), leading some to call for the development of innovative and 'novel' services (Thompson *et al*, 1995).

One such initiative is the use of telephone follow-up (Keckeisen and Nyamathi, 1990; Amsterdam *et al*, 1994) with Keeling and Dennison (1995) describing a pilot study in which cardiac specialist nurses, who had previously been involved with the patient in hospital, maintained telephone contact post-discharge. Evaluation suggested that the service had great potential, with patients and carers valuing the opportunity to discuss their worries, concerns and queries with an acknowledged expert. The authors consider that more work is needed to develop and fully evaluate such a service.

One initiative of proven benefit is the *Heart Manual*, a self-instructional package developed by Lewin and colleagues (Lewin *et al*, 1992). It comprises six weekly sessions focusing on education, home-based exercise, relaxation and self-help treatments for psychologically distressing events such as anxiety or panic attacks. Patients using this package were found to have significantly better psychological adjustment, less contact with their GPs, and fewer hospital readmissions than the control group. The intervention was found to be particularly successful with individuals who were anxious or depressed at the time of discharge. Average costs were estimated at between £30 and £50 per patient. Another trial with the same package reached similar conclusions regarding the efficacy and cost-effectiveness of the intervention (Linden, 1995).

Poor long-term follow-up of individuals and families post-infarction is common (Bethell, 1995; Horgan and McGee, 1995; Thompson, 1995) and it is suggested that health visitors may have a crucial role to play in this area of rehabilitation (Salisbury, 1994, 1995; Jones and West, 1995). Such a role could include providing detailed knowledge of community resources, education, counselling, and the development of coping skills (Salisbury, 1994, 1995) and information, relaxation, stress management and behavioural modification (Jones and West, 1995). Apart from the study of Jones and West (1995), which found no significant difference between subjects and controls, descriptions of such initiatives are rare.

Conclusions

It is clear that despite considerable potential for nurses gaps and tensions are apparent in current rehabilitation practice in MI. Authors suggest that nurses are in an 'ideal' position to develop a more comprehensive role, but few specific interventions are described and these are rarely systematically introduced and/or evaluated. Moreover, the authors acknowledge that developing an expanded role requires detailed knowledge in a number of areas, together with the development of high levels of skill. Yet current education and training, especially for non-specialist roles, is often described as inadequate.

This is an area that merits attention as recent work has reaffirmed the potential roles that nurses might fulfil in a variety of contexts. Zeechan *et al* (1999) for example demonstrate that with sufficient training nurses are well able to undertake a number of diagnostic related procedures such as exercise stress testing. From a more overtly therapeutic perspective Lisspers *et al* (1999) describe an innovative rehabilitation programme comprising a four-week residential component followed by regular follow-ups from a specialist nurse. This initiative demonstrated significantly improved outcomes in terms of both physiological (blood lipiots, exercise and Body Mass Index) and psychological (Type A behaviour) parameters. Similarly, Johnston *et al* (1999) tested the efficiency of an inpatient nurse counsellor who offered a rehabilitation programme for both MI sufferers and their partners. Participants, compared to a control group, showed better knowledge of MI, reduced anxiety and depression and higher levels of satisfaction. Shifting the focus to the community the role of the practice nurse was highlighted by Jolly *et al* (1998) who suggested that the challenge for the future is for practice nurses to pay more attention to assisting people post MI to sustain lifestyle changes.

All of the above demonstrate the significant potential for greater nursing involvement and as the nurse consultant role develops cardiac rehabilitation is an area in which there is scope for innovative and flexible nurse-led programmes, which needs to be systematically evaluated.

Key points

* Cardiac rehabilitation has been established for nearly fifty years, but evidence for its effectiveness is equivocal.
* Most of the coordinators of cardiac rehabilitation programmes are nurses but such programmes are often not individualised and tend to focus primarily on exercise and education, with less attention being paid to psychological concerns.
* The needs of family carers and early rehabilitation in the community are neglected areas of practice.
* Despite some qualitative studies of the experience of myocardial infarction, knowledge in this area is lacking and adjustment poorly understood.
* Nurses have a potentially significant, but relatively under-developed role in addressing many current deficits.

References

Amsterdam EA, Cadieux RJ, Debusk RF *et al* (1994) Cardiac rehab: still a good idea? *Patient Care* **28**: 24–9, 33–4, 37–40

Ashworth PM (1984) Staff-patient communication in coronary care units. *J Adv Nurs* **9**: 35–42

Ben-Sira Z, Eliezer R (1990) The structure of readjustment after heart attack. *Soc Sci Med* **30**: 523–36

Bethell HJN (1995) Community-based cardiac rehabilitation. In: Jones D, West R eds. *Cardiac Rehabilitation*. BMJ Publishing Group, London: 167–83

Boykoff SL (1989) Strategies for sexual counselling of patients following a myocardial infarction. *Dimens Crit Care Nurs* **8**: 368–73

Briggs LM (1994) Sexual healing: caring for patients recovering from myocardial infarction. *Br J Nurs* **3**(16): 837–42

Caunt JE (1992) The changing role of coronary care nurses. *Intensive Crit Care Nurs* **8**: 82–93

Cochrane BL (1992) Acute myocardial infarction in women. *Crit Care Nurs Clin North Am* **4**: 279–89

Conn VS, Taylor SG, Abele PB (1991) Myocardial infarction survivors: age and gender differences in physical health, psychosocial state and regimen adherence. *J Adv Nurs* **16**: 1026–34

Conn VS, Taylor SG, Casey B (1992) Cardiac rehabilitation program participation and outcomes after myocardial infarction. *Rehabil Nurs* **17**: 58–63

Corbin JM, Strauss A (1988) *Unending Work and Care Managing Chronic Illness at Home*. Jossey-Bass, San Francisco

Corbin JM, Strauss A (1991) A nursing model for chronic illness management based upon the trajectory framework. *Sch Inq Nurs Pract* **5**(3): 155–74

Davidson C (1995) Cardiac rehabilitation in the district hospital. In: Jones D, West R, eds. *Cardiac Rehabilitation*. BMJ Publishing, London:144–66

Derenowski JM (1988) The relationship of social support systems, health locus of control, health value orientation, and wellness motivation in the postmyocardial infarction patient during three phases of rehabilitation. *Progress in Cardiovasc Nurs* **3**: 143–52

Farrell J, Booth E, Hayburne T (1985) Telling it straight. *Nurs Mirror* **160**(18): 51–2

Folta A, Potempa KM (1992) Reduced cardiac output and exercise capacity in patients after myocardial infarction. *J Cardiovasc Nurs* **6**: 71–7

Ford JS (1989) Living with a history of a heart attack: a human science investigation. *J Adv Nurs* **14**: 173–9

Fridlund B, Hogstedt B, Lidell E *et al* (1991) Recovery after myocardial infarction. Effects of a caring rehabilitation programme. *Scand J Caring Sci* **5**: 23–32

Glick MS (1986) Caring touch and anxiety in myocardial infarction patients in the intermedicate cardiac care unit. *Intensive Care Nurs* **2**: 61–6

Hase S, Douglas A (1987) Effects of relaxation training on recovery from myocardial infarction. *Aust J Adv Nurs* **5**: 18–27

Hamilton GA (1991) The importance of systematic inquiry in nursing research: an example; women and recovery from acute myocardial infarction. *Vard I Norden Nursing Science and Research in the Nordic Countries* **11**: 5–7

Hawthorne MH (1991) Using the trajectory framework: reconceptualizing cardiac illness. *Sch Inq Nurs Pract* **5**: 185–95

Hendrick JA (1994) The challenge of myocardial infarction in accident and emergency nursing. *Accid Emerg Nurs* **2**: 160-6

Hentinen M (1983) Need for instruction and support of the wives of patients with myocardial infarction. J Adv Nurs 8: 519–24

Hentinen M (1986) Teaching and adaptation of patients with myocardial infarction. *Int J Nurs Studies* **23**: 125–38

Hilbert GA (1994) Cardiac patients and spouses: family functioning and emotions. *Clin Nurs Res* **3**: 243–52

Hildingh C, Fridlund B, Segesten K (1995) Cardiac nurses preparedness to use self-help groups as a support strategy. *J Adv Nurs* **22**(5): 921–8

Hilgenberg C, Crowley C (1987) Changes in family patterns after a myocardial infarction. *Home Healthcare Nurse* **5**: 26–7, 30–2, 34–5

Hilgenberg C, Liddy KG, Standerfer J *et al* (1992) Changes in family patterns six months after a MI. *J Cardiovasc Nurs* **6**: 46–56

Horgan J, McGee HM (1995) Cardiac rehabilitation: future directions. In: Jones D, West R, eds. *Cardiac Rehabilitation.* BMJ Publishing, London: 244–57

Jenkins DA, Rogers H (1995) Transfer anxiety in patients with MI. *Br J Nur* **4**(21): 1248–52

Johnson JL (1991) Learning to live again: the process of adjustment following a heart attack. In: Morse JM, Johnson LJ, eds. *The Illness Experience Dimensions of Suffering.* Sage, Newbury Park, California

Johnson JL, Morse JM (1990) Regaining control: the process of adjustment after myocardial infarction. *Heart Lung* **19**: 126–35

Johnston M, Foulkes J, Johnston DW *et al* (1999) Impact on patients and partners of inpatient and extended cardiac counselling and rehabilitation: A controlled trial. *Psycosom Med* **61**(2): 225–233

Jolly K, Bradley F, Sharp S *et al* (1998) Follow up course in general practice of patients with myocardial infarction or angina pectoris: initial results of the SHIP trial. *Fam Pract* **15**(6): 548–555

Jones D (1995) Influences on spouses and influences in spouses. In: Jones D, West R, eds. *Cardiac Rehabilitation.* BMJ Publishing Group, London: 227–43

Jones D, West R (1995) A multi-centre randominzed controlled trial of psychological rehabilitation. In: Jones D, West R, eds. *Cardiac Rehabilitation.* BMJ Publishing Group, London: 207–26

Kahana E, Young R (1990) Clarifying the caregiving paradigm: challenges for the future. In: Biegel DE, Blum A, eds. *Ageing and Caregiving: Theory, Research and Policy.* Sage, Newbury Park, California: 76–97

Keckeisen ME, Nyamathi AM (1990) Coping and adjustment to illness in the acute postmyocardial infarction patient. *J Cardiovasc Nurs* **5**: 25–33

Keeling AW, Dennison PD (1995) Nurse-initiated telephone follow-up after acute myocardial infarction: a pilot study. *Heart Lung* **24**(1): 45–9

Kinney MR (1995) Assessment of quality of life in recovery settings. *J Cardiovasc Nurs* **10**: 88–96

Lewin B, Robertson IH, Cay EL *et al* (1992) Effects of self-help post-myocardial infarction rehabilitation on psychological adjustment and use of health services. *Lancet* **339**: 1036–40

Lewin B (1995) Psychological factors in cardiac rehabilitation. In: Jones D, West R, eds. *Cardiac Rehabilitation.* BMJ Publishing Group, London: 83–108

Linden B (1995) Evaluation of a home-based rehabilitation programme for patients recovering from acute myocardial infarction. *Intensive Crit Care Nurs* **11**: 10–9

Lisspers J, Hofmanbang C, Nordlander R *et al* (1999) Multifactorial evaluation of a program for lifestyle behavior change in rehabilitation and secondary prevention of coronary artery disease. *Scand Cardiovasc J* **33** (1): 9–16

Malan SS (1992) Psychosocial adjustment following myocardial infarction: current views and nursing implications. *J Cardiovasc Nurs* **6**: 57–70

Marsden C, Dracup K (1991) Different perspectives: the effect of heart disease on patients and spouses. *AACN Clin Issues Crit Care Nurs* **2**: 285–92

Mayor S (1994) Heartbeat. *Nurs Times* **90**(40): 18

McCauley KM, Lowery BJ, Jacobsen BS (1992) A comparison of patient/nurse perceptions about current and future recovery status. *Clin Nurse Spec* **6**: 148–52

McHugh MJ, Taubman MR (1990) Postpartum myocardial infarction: a rehabilitation challenge. *J Cardiovasc Nurs* **4**(4): 57–63

Medich C, Stuart EM, Deckro JP *et al* (1991) Psychophysiologic control mechanisms in ischemic heart disease: the mind-heart connection. *J Cardiovasc Nurs* **5**: 10–26

Miller P, Wikoff R, McMahon M *et al* (1988) Influence of a nursing intervention on regimen adherence and societal adjustments postmyocardial infarction. *Nurs Res* **37**: 297–302

Miller P, McMahon M, Garrett MJ *et al* (1989) A content analysis of life adjustments post infarction. *West J Nurs Res* **11**: 559–67

Murray PJ (1989) Rehabilitation information and health beliefs in the post-coronary patient: do we meet their information needs? *J Adv Nurs* **14**: 686–93

Newens AJ, Bond S, Priest J (1995) Nurse involvement in cardiac rehabilitation prior to hospital discharge. *J Clin Nurs* **4**: 390–6

Newens AJ, McColl E, Bond S *et al* (1996) Patients' and nurses' knowledge of cardio-related symptoms and cardiac misconceptions. *Heart Lung* **25**(3): 190–9

Nolan MR, Grant G, Keady J (1996) *Understanding Family Care: A Multidimensional Model of Caring and Coping.* Open University Press, Buckingham

Packa DR (1989) Quality of life of cardiac patients: a review. *J Cardiovasc Nurs* **3**: 1–11

Rankin SH (1995) Going it alone — women managing recovery from acute myocardial infarction. *Fam Community Health* **17**: 50–62

Roberts SL (1989) Cognitive model of depression and the myocardial infarction patient. *Progress in Cardiovasc Nurs* **4**: 61–70

Rolland JS (1988) A conceptual model of chronic and life threatening illness and its impact on families. In: Chilman CS, Nunnally EW, Cox FM, eds *Chronic Illness and Disabilities.* Sage, Beverley Hills, California: 17–68

Salisbury H (1994) Health visitor's role in cardiac rehabilitation. *Health Visit* **67**(8): 262–4

Salisbury H (1995) Maintaining lifestyles change after myocardial infarction. *Health Visit* **68**(11): 460–3

Schigoda MG, Hook ML (1991) 'Take heart...' — developing support sessions for families of acutely ill cardiac patients. *AACN Clin Issues Crit Care Nurs* **2**: 299–306

Thompson DR (1989) A randomized controlled trial of in-hospital nursing support for first time myocardial infarction patients and their partners: effects on anxiety and depression. *J Adv Nurs* **14**: 291–7

Thompson DR (1991) Effect of in-hospital counselling on knowledge in myocardial infarction patients and spouses. *Patient Educ Counselling* **18**: 171–7

Thompson DR (1995) Cardiac rehabilitation: how can it be improved? (editorial). *J Psychosom Res* **39**: 519–23

Thompson DR, Cordle CJ (1988) Support of wives of myocardial infarction patients. *J Adv Nurs* **13**: 223–8

Thompson DR, Bowman GS (1995) *An audit of Cardiac Rehabilitation Services in England and Wales.* NHS Executive, Leeds

Thompson DR, Webster RA (1989) Effect of counselling on anxiety and depression in coronary patients. *Intensive Care Nurs* **5**: 52–4

Thompson DR, Webster RA, Meddis R (1990) In-hospital counselling for first-time myocardial infarction patients and spouses: effects on satisfaction. *J Adv Nurs* **15**: 1064–9

Thompson DR, Ersser SJ, Webster RA (1995) The experiences of patients and their partners 1 month after a heart attack. *J Adv Nurs* **22**: 707–14

Verderber A, Shively M, Fitzsimmons L (1990) Coping and heart disease. *J Cardiovasc Nurs* **5**: 74–8

Wastlick LA, Anderson KH, Claire E (1991) Family protective thinking about cardiac events: nursing interventions to promote maintenance of family health behaviours. *Wisconsin Med J* **90**: 438–40

Waters J (1995) The end result... ensuring that heart patients get vital long-term health monitoring. *Nurs Times* **91**: 14–5

Webb MS, Riggin OZ (1994) A comparison of anxiety levels of female and male patients with myocardial infarction. *Crit Care Nurse* **14**: 118–24

Webber KS (1994) The role of a health care professional in the evaluation of a self-help group. *Can J Cardiovasc Nurs* **5**(2): 30–3

Webster KK, Christman NJ (1988) Perceived uncertainty and coping: post myocardial infarction. *West J Nurs Res* **10**: 398–9

West R (1995) Evaluation of rehabilitation programmes. In: Jones D, West R, eds *Cardiac Rehabilitation*. BMJ Publishing Group, London: 184–206

Young RF, Kahana E (1994) Caregiving issues after a heart attack: perspectives of elderly patients and their families. In: Kahana E, Biegel DE, Wykle ML eds *Family Caregiving Across the Lifespan*. Sage, Thousand Oaks, California: 262–84

Zecchin RP, Chai YY, Roach KA *et al* (1999) Is nurse-supervised exercise stress testing safe practice? *Heart Lung* **28**(3): 175–185

Section 4: Developing nursing skills and effective practice in cardiovascular nursing

19

Central venous cannulation

Dorothy A Gourlay

This chapter addresses a learning experience involving the insertion of central venous cannulae, for both the assessment of a patient's internal environment in relation to the need for medical intervention and the administration of medical treatment. The issues explored highlight the important uses of such cannulae and stress the potential problems which may be encountered during insertion of the cannulae or when they are used for the administration of drug therapy.

Daily experience, whether gained through formal teaching sessions or prompted by clinical incidents, allows the nurse to increase his/her personal level of knowledge and understanding of practical aspects of patient care.

One such clinical incident concerned a patient undergoing elective surgery for bilateral renal revascularisation. This required the insertion of a central venous cannula for intraoperative monitoring of central venous pressure (CVP) and the administration of dopamine in order to maximise renal perfusion for the duration of the procedure. Unfortunately, anaesthetic staff were unable to insert a multi-lumen cannula into either internal jugular vein, and so two separate single-lumen central venous cannulae were inserted into the right and left distal basilic veins.

This chapter will discuss the three main issues highlighted by the above incident:

1. Central venous pressure: the term CVP will be defined and the various mechanisms that control it and the value of CVP measurement will be outlined.
2. Administration of drugs through a central venous catheter: the reasons why some drugs are given through a central venous catheter as the route of choice, and not through the same catheter as that used for CVP measurement will be explained.
3. Routes of entry available for the insertion of central venous catheters: the advantages and disadvantages associated with each route will be discussed, together with recent research advocating specific choices.

Central venous pressure

CVP is most often measured from a catheter inserted into the surperior vena cava. This measurement not only reflects pressures from the right side of the heart, but also monitors the venous return to the heart, thus providing an overview of the cardiac efficiency and circulatory status of the patient (Rainbow, 1993).

Of prime importance is the right ventricular end-diastolic pressure reading, the normal range of which is 3–11 cmH$_2$O (0–8 mmHg) (Aitkenhead and Smith, 1990). This pressure is regulated by a number of factors: venous return, the compliance and competence of the heart, circulating volume and venous tone.

Venous return

Although essentially similar to arteries, veins lack the same elasticity and contractility, and rely heavily on the presence of valves to prevent gravitational backflow of blood. The action of these valves, assisted by skeletal muscle contraction, ensures the return, or milking, of venous blood to the heart.

The negative pressure created within the chest cavity during inspiration is another important aid to venous return. The corresponding increase in pressure within the abdomen causes the squeezing of venous blood from the abdominal veins into the thoracic veins (Anagnostakos and Tortora, 1984). During intermittent positive-pressure ventilation, however, there is no negative inspiratory pressure within the thoracic cavity, and therefore no corresponding assistance to venous return is given. Such sustained positive pressure can be expected to raise the CVP by 5cmH$_2$O (2 mmHg) (Rainbow, 1993).

Similarly, intrathoracic pressure can be increased by the presence of:

- a pneumothorax
- a mediastinal tumour
- cardiac tamponade
- a change in the position of the patient (Lett, 1983).

All of these will reduce venous return to the heart to a certain degree, and thus lead to an increase in CVP.

Compliance and competence of the heart

If the venous return to the heart is slow, as in an immobile patient in whom venous return is not being aided by skeletal muscle contraction in the lower limbs, the heart responds by pumping harder to compensate for this. If venous return was then to increase, eg. during initial rehabilitation exercises and then later during more strenuous exercise, a larger volume of blood than normal would enter the right atrium, causing a subsequent increase in pressure.

The resultant distension of the atrium causes an increase in heart rate. This is known as the Bainbridge reflex. If, however, the heart muscle has been damaged in any way, such as following an infarction, the expected and required competency of ventricular contraction is compromised, and stroke volume decreases. Compensatory mechanisms will then attempt to increase the strength and rate of contraction and salvage the situation (Anagnostakos and Tortora, 1984).

This compensatory action is regulated by autonomic control (*Figure 19.1*), particularly the right atrial reflex. The initiating baroreceptors are located in the superior vena cava and within the right atrium. An increase in venous pressure results in the stimulation of the cardio-acceleratory centre, causing an increase in heart rate (the Bainbridge reflex).

Any cardiac impairment will disturb the balance within these chains of control. For example, in heart block, when electrical impulses passing between the atria and ventricles are blocked, causing arrhythmias, the potential for missed ventricular beats is high. In such cases, cardiac output decreases, and any compensatory mechanism fails to achieve its desired result. In myocardial infarction, the physical ability of the heart to increase the strength of contractions in order to cope with increased blood volume is reduced. In such cases, CVP measurements alone may not be sufficient to provide an accurate assessment of cardiac function. In normal cardiac function, left ventricular function is often comparable to right ventricular function as reflected by the CVP. However, in heart failure, a more accurate picture of the disparity between the two ventricles can be obtained from a catheter inserted in the pulmonary artery, and this clearer view of left ventricular filling pressures is sometimes required to enable assessment of the patient's condition, and to plan interventional care (Adams and Cashman, 1991).

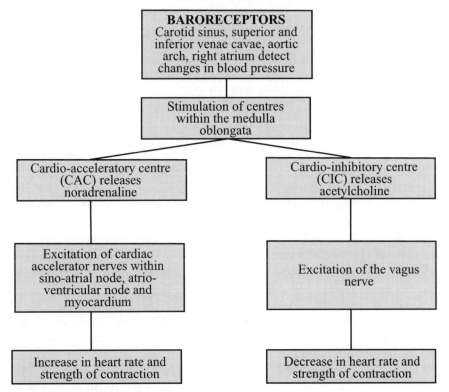

Figure 19.1: Autonomic control: regulation of heart rate and strength of contractions (adapted from Anagnostakos and Tortora, 1984)

Circulating volume

Circulatory shock may occur as a result of cardiac failure, haemorrhage or histamine release, all of which lead to a reduction in both circulating blood volume and tissue perfusion. A drop in CVP will be observed before the compensatory mechanisms of vasoconstriction and water retention take place (Anagnostakos and Tortora, 1984).

Venous tone

Venous tone is controlled by the vasomotor centre within the medulla oblongata. The vasomotor centre continually stimulates the smooth muscle of blood vessel walls, causing a certain degree of vasoconstriction. This vasomotor tone ensures the maintenance of peripheral resistance and thereby maintains blood pressure at a near-constant level (Anagnostakos and Tortora, 1984).

Peripheral resistance is controlled by the increase or decrease in sympathetic impulses from the vasomotor centre in response to the triggering of baro-receptors in the carotid sinus and aortic arch.

Atkinson *et al* (1987) explain the significance of venous tone to the overall circulating blood volume. They claim that half the total blood volume is accommodated within the venous system, whereas only 15% is contained within the arterial system. Thus, vasodilation resulting from a decrease in sympathetic activity from the vasomotor centre will increase the circulatory capacity. Even with a normal circulating volume, such an effect (often resulting from the excessive use of vasodilating drugs, or from septicaemia) will cause a fall in CVP, indicating a decrease in blood flow and in tissue oxygenation (Manley, 1991).

The measurement of right-sided heart pressures was not used clinically until 1910 (Atkinson *et al*, 1987). In 1931, the insertion of a central venous catheter for the more accurate measurement of right ventricular end-diastolic pressure was pioneered, and the first polythene catheters were used in 1945 (Atkinson *et al*, 1987).

Central venous catheterisation is thus a relatively long-standing technique, but there is still a need for this invasive technique if, as Aitkenhead and Smith (1990) claim,

The best clinical indication of cardiac function is the state of the peripheral circulation.

In circulatory shock, easily observed signs are paleness, clammy skin, cyanosis of the extremities, and a rapid and feeble pulse. Another accurate clinical sign which may be overlooked is the engorgement of neck veins (Black, 1987). Palpation of the external jugular vein, together with measurement of the heart rate, blood pressure and urine output, can provide a great deal of information about the patient's condition.

In the specific incident described above, patient dehydration (most probably due to preoperative fasting) almost certainly contributed to the difficulties in attempting to insert an internal jugular cannula, as the vein was unusually threadlike and difficult to palpate. However, in this particular case, the knowledge that the patient was suffering from a low circulating volume as a result of fasting was not sufficient reason for not inserting a central venous cannula. Observable, physiological changes, together with the patient's prolonged fasting times prompted the infusion of a daily basal requirement of 30–40 ml/kg of water and 1 mmol/kg of sodium (Adams and Cashman, 1991) without the need to measure CVP.

As revascularisation of the kidneys involves clamping the abdominal aorta while the surgeon attempts grafting work on the renal and mesenteric arteries, the patient needs to be systemically heparinised to maintain adequate circulation and perfusion. Heparinisation together with the vascular hazards associated with this type of surgery increases the risk of surgical haemorrhage, as well as placing a strain on cardiac output. Accurate measurement of CVP is therefore of vital importance in assessing the adequacy of intravenous fluid replacement and any change in cardiac competency (Atkinson *et al*, 1987).

Similarly, if postoperative haemorrhaging should occur, CVP measurement will indicate a reduction in circulating volume before a fall in blood pressure, thereby enabling early intervention to take place (Rainbow, 1993).

If haemorrhaging were to occur, rapid intravenous fluid replacement would most probably be the initial treatment of choice, carrying with it the risk of acute circulatory overload, which can be easily detected by means of CVP measurement. A raised CVP, accompanied by engorgement of neck veins and a decrease in arterial pressure, indicates cardiac overloading. The potential risk of pulmonary oedema can be avoided by stopping the infusion and commencing appropriate intravenous drug treatment, eg. frusemide (Atkinson *et al*, 1987).

Lett (1983) stresses the importance of paying particular attention to pressure trends, rather than to absolute pressure measurements. This is reiterated by Aitkenhead and Smith (1990), who state that observations of the response of the CVP to small fluid challenges gives a much more valuable insight into the condition of the patient than a single reading.

Such a challenge is usually prescribed by medical staff but carried out by nursing staff. It usually comprises the rapid infusion of 100–200 ml of 0.9% sodium chloride over a period of 10–15 minutes, and can be used effectively as a diagnostic tool.

An elevated CVP may indicate either cardiac impairment or hypovolaemia due to decreased sympathetic activity. In the former case, a fluid challenge will sustain the elevated CVP, whereas in the hypovolaemic patient the extra fluid increases the heart rate, causes vasodilatation, and consequently decreases the CVP. The correct diagnosis can not be made and the correct intervention taken (Aitkenhead and Smith, 1990). It is therefore clear that,

The central vein serves as the route of information which is essential for the scientific management of many patients in anaesthesia.

(Rosen *et al*, 1992)

In such a capacity, CVP measurement is particularly useful in:

- massive blood or fluid replacement
- acute circulatory failure

- unstable cardiovascular dynamic states
- anuria and oliguria (Lett, 1983).

Administration of drugs through a central venous cannula

Some drugs such as cytotoxic and anti-cancer drugs, eg. dactinomycin and doxorubicin, can be very irritant and can cause local tissue damage when given through a peripheral venous cannula. Localised reactions include inflammation, pain, redness and swelling of the veins used for administration. If the drug infiltrates the surrounding tissues, necrosis and ulceration of these tissues will follow. If such drugs are to be used for long-term therapy, it is recommended that they are administered via a central venous catheter (Malpas and Wrigley, 1992).

Some drugs that are used only for short-term therapy may have a similar local effect, caused by stimulation of autonomic activity as well as their own irritant tendencies (Rainbow, 1993). One such example is the inotrope adrenaline, a cardiac stimulant which also assists in central perfusion and increases blood pressure by causing peripheral vasoconstriction. If given peripherally in large continuous doses, such drugs would be trapped within a collapsed vein, causing localised pain and tissue damage without delivering any desired systemic effect.

Similarly, in an emergency, the physiological response to acute haemorrhage causes peripheral veins to constrict in order to maintain central blood volume and blood pressure. Any intravenous agent administered on such an occasion would therefore be trapped peripherally, and must then be given centrally in order to have its effect. In both cases, the desired effects of the drugs can only be realised if the drugs are administered through a central venous catheter (Rosen *et al*, 1992).

In the prompting incident, the inotrope, dopamine was administered in order to maximise renal perfusion for the duration of surgery. For this purpose, a small dose (2 µg/kg/min) was administered by continuous infusion, in a controlled manner, using an automatic syringe pump. This method of administration was used to avoid the drug being given as a bolus injection, which would stimulate the beta receptors in the cardiac muscle to increase the contractility of the heart, causing excessive strain — especially in cardiac failure — and increasing vasoconstriction (*British National Formulary*, 1995). The use of a separately inserted central venous cannula allows for the continuous uninterrupted administration of dopamine, and does not affect the CVP trace measured from the left peripheral catheter.

During the initiating procedure the anaesthetist was concerned that the CVP tracing was 'damped' because of a partial blockage of the catheter (*Figure 19.2*: cf. *Figure 19.3* of normal tracing). He therefore flushed the catheter with 0.9% sodium chloride in order to clear the blockage. If the dopamine infusion had been administered through the same catheter, he would have inadvertently given the patient a bolus injection, hence negating the controlled continuous infusion.

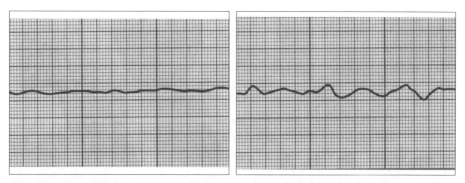

Figure 19.2: A 'damped' central venous pressure tracing (taken from a print-out)

Figure 19.3: A 'normal' central venous pressure tracing (taken from a print-out)

If the CVP is to be monitored in the ward postoperatively, it is likely that a fluid manometer will be the measuring device available. This in itself causes a multitude of problems for nursing staff if it has been decided to use one cannula for both the measurement of CVP and the administration of non-inotropic drugs. Manley (1991) suggests that such usage should be limited to the administration of only prescribed, safe, bolus injections or intermittent, rather than continuous infusions.

If the carer ensures that strict attention is paid to the fact that such a drug is delivered directly into the venous system, eg. into a port between the manometer and the patient, with no possibility of potential backflow of the drug into the manometer system, then bolus injection will be avoided when the manometer column drops later during the reading of the CVP. In such cases, it is also important to check carefully that each drug is compatible with the central line infusion fluid.

Routes of entry available for the insertion of central venous catheters

Rainbow (1993) is one of many authors to applaud recent advances in cannulae design. The fairly recent use of multilumen devices, particularly for neck and subclavian insertion, allows the concurrent and safe administration of drugs as well as simultaneous fluid replacement and CVP measurements. Such advances also avoid the multiple venepunctures that are necessary for the safe use of single lumen catheters (Rosen *et al*, 1992).

A major change in direction over the past twelve years is the increasingly favoured choice of the internal jugular vein for central catheterisation, primarily due to the development of new, safer cannulation techniques. However, Rosen *et al* (1992) and Abi-Nader (1993) both advocate the use of peripheral venous cannulae for short operative procedures.

Unfortunately, the venous system is extremely variable. There is considerable risk of injury to anatomical structures in a situation where catheterisation might normally be relatively easy given fairly constant anatomy. The doctor who wishes to combine minimum hazard with maximum certainty of success needs to be familiar with different routes of catheterisation: it is not sufficient to learn just one technique (Rosen *et al*, 1992).

Before choosing an entry point for central venous cannulation (*Table 19.1*) medical staff must assess the patient, taking into account a number of factors. These include:

- the length of time the cannula is expected to be in situ
- what it will be used for: drug administration, blood sampling, pressure measurement, intravenous infusion, total parenteral nutrition
- is the vein of choice in good condition.

These factors, combined with practical knowledge and expertise, will determine the choice of route and the catheter used (Rosen *et al*, 1992).

It is important for nurses to be aware of the advantages and disadvantages of central venous cannulation, so that they can exercise patient advocacy when alternative sites of entry are being considered.

Conclusion

This overview of the mechanisms that regulate CVP has outlined the causes of changes in CVP, as well as the use of CVP measurement to detect not only falling circulatory volume, but also circulatory overloading, which is always possible in a shocked patient who is being given a rapid infusion. Such improved knowledge increases not only professional confidence but also personal accountability at work.

The discussion of drug administration via a central venous catheter has highlighted the need for vigilance on the part of the nurse when administering any infusion via the catheter. In order to maintain personal accountability and ensure safe practice, any member of staff not practised in such procedures must acknowledge their limitations and observe such procedures before becoming involved themselves (UKCC, 1992). On the whole, especially where inotropic infusions are involved, medical staff are closely involved with their use.

In either situation, the experienced nurse must use his/her position as the patient's advocate to ensure that there is no possibility of the inadvertent administration of a bolus of a drug. This is especially important if pressures are being monitored by means of a fluid-filled manometer. If an infusion is given through the same lumen as that being used for CVP measurements, the three-way tap to facilitate this must be located between the patient and the manometer tubing (Rainbow, 1993).

Patient advocacy should also be implemented when:

- multiple stab wounds are being inflicted during attempts to cannulate a vein
- signs of cannula misplacement are present
- trauma has been caused during insertion, eg. pneumothorax or cardiac tamponade.

A great deal of literature has been published on central venous cannulation, opening up a whole host of areas for further research. Notably, a large number of the most recent publications and research articles cover venous thrombosis and infection rates related to central venous cannulation.

Both topics include research into the use of the most recently manufactured catheters, and further reading of the available literature is recommended, not only to increase the nurse's personal knowledge and capacity as an educator, as well as his/her competency as a nurse, but also as it will increase both the nurse's and the patient's confidence during the perioperative experience.

Key points

* The normal range for central venous pressure (CVP) is 3–11 cmH$_2$O (0–8 mmHg).
* CVP can be expected to rise by 5 cmH$_2$O (2 mmHg) when patients are intubated and artificially ventilated using intermittent positive-pressure ventilation.
* Accurate and repeated measurement of CVP is vital in assessing the adequacy of intravenous fluid replacement and any change in cardiac competency.
* Central venous drug administration allows the safe, long-term and short-term administration of cytotoxic drugs.
* The use of multilumen or separate single-lumen cannulae reduces the chances of recording an inaccurate CVP and of inadvertently administering a bolus of harmful substances.
* Risk assessment must be carried out, and patient advocacy should be evident when the routes of cannulae insertion are debated.

Table 19.1: Indications for the various routes of entry of central venous cannulae

Route of entry	Advantages	Disadvantages
Distal arm (basilic vein, cephalic vein)	Avoids many of the major complications associated with other routes (Rosen *et al*, 1992)	Misplacement of cannulae is reported to occur in 60% of cases (Aitkenhead and Smith, 1990)
		Phlebitis and sepsis occur if cannulae are left in situ for prolonged periods (Aitkenhead and Smith, 1990)
		Not well tolerated by patients (Woodrow, 1992
Proximal arm (axillary vein, basilic vein, cephalic vein)	Useful when peripheral areas have been subjected to venepuncture, burned or even covered with plaster of Paris (Rosen *et al*, 1992)	Veins are not always easy to locate. Cunitz *et al* (1994) suggest the use of Doppler ultrasound to facilitate location
		20% of patients experience transient paraesthesia following cannula insertion (Taylor and Yellowlees, 1990)
Chest (supraclavicular and infraclavicular subclavian veins)	Allows for secure fixation of the cannula to the chest wall: ideal for long-term enteral feeding (Rosen *et al*, 1992)	Risk of pneumothorax or haemothorax, perforation of the pericardium, haemorrhagic shock and air embolism (Rainbow, 1993)
	The only route of access available for cannulation in a patient suffering from circulatory collapse (Rosen *et al*, 1992)	
Neck (external and internal jugular veins)	Use of the internal jugular vein facilitates 90% correct catheter placement (Rosen *et al*, 1992)	'Through the needle' rather than a Seldinger technique of cannula insertion may facilitate immediate and massive bleeding into the pleural space (Bruckner *et al*, 1986)
		Repeated trauma may result in thrombosis, causing unsightly swelling and pain (Davis, 1991)
		Risks associated with chest entry apply
Leg (femoral vein)		Central venous pressure readings are less accurate (Woodrow, 1992)
		High risk of infection
		Extreme pain if the femoral nerve is damaged
		Restricts patient movement
		Risk of venous thrombosis and pulmonary embolism (Adams and Cashman, 1991)
Scalp	Avoids the use of surgical cut-down techniques in neonates (Rosen *et al*, 1992)	

References

Abi-Nader JA (1993) Peripherally inserted central venous catheters in critical care patients. *Heart Lung* **22**(5): 428–33

Adams AP, Cashman JN (1991) *Anaesthesia, Analgesia and Intensive Care.* St Edmunsbury Press, Suffolk

Aitkenhead AR, Smith G (1990) *Textbook of Anaesthesia.* 2nd edn. Churchill Livingstone, Edinburgh

Anagnostakos NP, Tortora GJ (1984) *Principles of Anatomy and Physiology.* 4th edn. Biological Sciences Textbooks, New York

Atkinson RS, Alfred Lee J, Rushman GB (1987) *A Synopsis of Anaesthesia.* 10th edn. John Wright and Sons, Bristol

Black A (1987) Monitoring in anaesthesia: standards. *Br J Hosp Med* **38**(1): 71–3

British National Formulary: No 30 (1995) British Medical Association and Royal Pharmacological Society of Great Britain

Bruckner JC, Forster A, Gamulin Z *et al* (1986) Multiple complications after internal jugular vein catheterization. *Anaesthesia* **41**(4): 408–12

Cunitz G, Hoer H, Schregel W *et al* (1994) Doppler-guided puncture of the axillary vein in ICU patients. *Br J Anaesth* **72** (suppl 1): 13

Davis CL (1991) Upper extremity venous thrombosis and central venous catheters. *Crit Care Nurse* **11**(8): 16–22

Lett Z (1983) *Anaesthesia.* Hong Kong University Press, Hong Kong

Malpas JS, Wrigley PFM (1992) Safe administration of anti-cancer drugs. *Hosp Update* **18**(7): 546–49

Manley K (1991) Central venous pressure: what, why, how? *Surg Nurse* **4**s(5): 10–13

Rainbow C (1993) *Monitoring of the Critically Ill Patient: Patient Problems and Nursing Care.* Butterworth-Heinemann, Oxford

Rosen M, Latto IP, Shang NGW (1992) *Handbook of Percutaneous Central Venous Catheterization.* 2nd edn. WB Saunders, London

Taylor B, Yellowlees I (1990) Central venous cannulation using the infraclavicular axillary vein. *Anesthesiology* **72**(1): 55–8

UKCC (1992) *Code of Professional Conduct for the Nurse, Midwife and Health Visitor.* 3rd edn. UKCC, London

Woodrow P (1992) Monitoring central venous pressure. *Nurs Stand* **6**(33): 25–9

Bibliography

Bakker NC, Corsten SA, de Lange JJ *et al* (1994) Central venous catheter placement using the cavafix-certodyn SD catheter. *Br J Anaesth* **72**(suppl 1): 14

Rosen M, Latto IP, Shang NGW (1981) *Handbook of Percutaneous Central Venous Catheterization.* WB Saunders, East Sussex

20

Blood and blood transfusion reactions: I

Martyn Bradbury and Jeremy Pope Cruickshank

Blood transfusion is a well-established mode of treatment for many disorders. This chapter examines the therapeutic indications for blood replacement and provides a framework for transfusion practice.

To the practising nurse, the use of blood and blood products is now commonplace. Indeed, their use has revolutionised the management of many conditions, while enabling other therapeutic techniques such as cardiac, liver and bone marrow transplantation to develop.

This does not, however, mean that blood transfusion is without risk, and as many as 5% of patients who receive a transfusion react in some form to the transfused components (Urbaniak, 1990).

Historical perspectives

The first faltering steps towards our present understanding of blood transfusion almost certainly predate William Harvey's description of the circulation in 1628. Indeed, it is possible that the first transfusion may have occurred in 1492 when Pope Innocent VIII received blood from three luckless young men — all four died following the procedure (Marshall and Bird, 1983).

These early experiments in blood transfusion frequently involved the transfer of blood from one animal to another. However, animal-to-human transfusions were also made and, in 1667, Richard Lower made the first recorded transfusion of blood to a human in England — the donor being a sheep (Lower and King, 1667).

Given our current understanding of blood cell antigens and blood incompatibility, it is unsurprising that patients frequently died following these early attempts at blood transfusion. Death following blood transfusion from either a human or animal donor became so prevalent that in 1670 all blood transfusions were outlawed both in Britain and France (Marshall and Bird, 1983).

As a result, the existence of blood incompatibilities between different species was not recognised until 150 years later. At this time, the physician and obstetrician James Blundell (1828) revived interest in the use of blood transfusion by successfully treating postpartum haemorrhage with blood taken from his assistants.

Apart from Joseph Lister's descriptions of sepsis in 1867, it was not until the turn of the century that the next major breakthrough occurred. In 1900, the Nobel prize winner, Karl Landsteiner, became the first to describe the ABO system of blood groups, and in 1914 the first transfusion of citrated blood was made by Luis Agote in Buenos Aires.

Ironically, though, the major impetus for the development of blood transfusion technology was the demand for blood made during the First and Second World Wars.

The chronology of events was as follows:

1917: American combatants received the first stored blood

1927: M, N and P blood groups were discovered

1940: The Rhesus system described by Landsteiner and Wiener

1945: Coombs *et al* described the antihuman globulin test to detect red-cell antigens (Coombs' test).

Additionally, the increasing demands for blood and blood products meant that there was a greater need for the coordination of transfusion activity. Thus, in 1946 the National Blood Transfusion Service was founded. This is currently responsible for the collection, screening and supply of over 2 000 000 units of donated blood each year (Garwood and Knowles, 1998).

Blood grouping

Many of the catastrophic outcomes associated with the early attempts at blood transfusion can now be attributed to incompatibility between the antigenic properties of the donor's blood and the antibody status of the recipient.

A major aspect of present-day transfusion is therefore ensuring that a good cross-match exists between the donor and recipient. Approximately 400 red blood cell group antigens have been identified (Hoffbrand and Pettit, 1993), although from a clinical perspective the most significant of these are the ABO and rhesus systems.

In addition to these two major systems, other less significant groups include Kell, Kidd, Duffy, Lewis, Li, Lutheran, M, N and P.

The ABO system

The ABO characteristics of the red blood cell are determined genetically by three genes: A, B and O. Approximately six months after birth, naturally occurring antibodies begin to appear in the blood; the antigenic challenge probably arises in response to antigens on the gut flora that resemble the naturally occurring AB blood group antigens (Linch, 1994).

Given this, and the fact that lymphocytes normally produce antibodies to non-self antigens, the antigen/antibody profile shown in *Table 20.1* is usually present for the ABO blood group.

Table 20.1: Blood groups			
Blood group	**Antigen present**	**Antibody present**	**% of people (Caucasian)**
AB	A + B	None	3
A	A	Anti-B	42
B	B	Anti-A	8
0	0	Anti-A and anti-B	47

Rhesus

This complex system is genetically determined and comprises five common antigens: C, D, E, c and e. Of these, the D antigen is the most significant, with approximately 85% of the Caucasian population and 95% of black individuals possessing the antigen. These individuals are therefore classed as being rhesus D positive.

Antibodies to the rhesus antigens rarely occur naturally and are therefore only found in individuals who have become sensitised following pregnancy or previous mismatched transfusion.

Finally, it must be remembered that while red cell antigen/antibody reactions are of the greatest clinical significance, other specific antigen/antibody reactions can also occur for leucocytes and platelets. When an antigen/antibody reaction occurs in response to blood transfusion, it is primarily mediated via the IgM and IgG immunoglobulins (antibodies). These antibodies are also responsible for activating the complement cascade and it is this which leads to many of the physiological responses associated with the more severe transfusion reactions.

Complement

This complex group of nine plasma proteins ordinarily functions by 'complementing' the body's normal immune response. When activated, a cascade of reactions is initiated that is analogous to the clotting cascade (*Figure 20.1*). The result of this chain reaction is the formation of biologically active substances such as C3b, C7, C8 and C9. These bring about cell death by:

- opsonization, ie. coating of the antigen so that it can be phagocytosed by macrophages and neutrophils
- cell lysis via enzymatic disruption of the cell membrane.

Additionally, active complement fragments are also formed, eg. C3a and C5a. These substances act as anaphylatoxins, causing smooth muscle contraction, platelet aggregation, histamine release and vasodilatation.

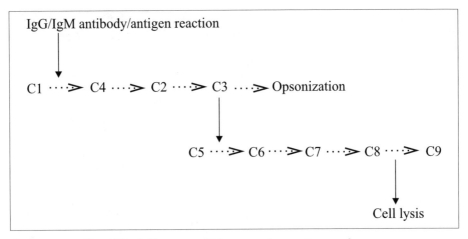

IgG/IgM antibody/antigen reaction

C1 ···▷ C4 ···▷ C2 ···▷ C3 ···▷ Opsonization

C5 ···▷ C6 ···▷ C7 ···▷ C8 ···▷ C9

Cell lysis

Figure 20.1: Simplified diagram of the complement cascade

Indications for blood transfusion

There are a variety of clinical situations in which the transfusion of blood or its constituent parts is desirable. These indications can be subdivided according to the following need:

- reduced circulatory volume, eg. hypovolaemia, haemorrhage, shock
- decreased oxygen carrying capacity, eg. anaemia
- deficiency of a specific blood constituent, eg. white blood cells, platelets, clotting factors, immunoglobulins.

When considering whether blood products should be used, it is vitally important to bear in mind the potentially harmful side-effects that may result. Additionally, blood is a scarce resource and, as such, only the portion of blood that is actually required should be transfused (*Table 20.2*). Finally, the circumspect use of blood is also advantageous for a variety of clinical and economic reasons, as it ensures that:

- maximum use can be made of each unit of donated blood
- greater concentrations of the desired blood component are given than would be the case with whole blood
- over-expansion of the recipient's circulation is reduced
- transfusion of potentially harmful materials is minimised.

The transfusion of whole blood should therefore be reserved for situations where both hypovolaemia and hypoxia are concurrent, ie. haemorrhage.

As it is the registered nurse who is primarily responsible for initiating the blood transfusion, it is essential that he/she adheres strictly to locally agreed policies and procedures when administering the prescribed blood component. It is with reference to these local policies that the following principles for safe transfusion practice and the PACK mnemonic (see overleaf) is offered.

Table 20.2: Blood and principal blood components available for transfusion		
Product	**Primary indication**	**Notes**
Whole blood	Substantial traumatic or surgical blood loss	Stored whole blood contains reduced platelet and clotting factor concentrations
Packed red cells		Diuretic frequently given to prevent circulatory overload in the elderly
Frozen red cells	Decreased oxygen carrying capacity due to reduced haemoglobin or red cell count	Increased shelf-life, therefore useful for rarer blood groups
Washed red cells		Surface antigen removed to reduce the risk of anaphylaxis
Pooled platelets	Thrombocytopenia	As platelets are derived from multiple blood units there is an increased risk of reaction. Prophylactic steroids and antihistamines may be used
White-cell concentrates	Acute leukaemia Aplastic anaemia Neutropenia <0.5 x 10º/litre in patients who are not responding to antibiotics (Hoffbrand and Pettit, 1993)	Rarely used. Tissue typing is necessary to prevent incompatibilities Prophylactic steroids and antihistamines may be used
Fresh frozen plasma	Hypocoagulability	Needs to be used within half an hour of thawing in order to preserve clotting factors
Cryoprecipitate	Hypocoagulability	Should be thawed at 37ºC

PACK: the crucial steps in safe transfusion practice

(P): Patient and pre-transfusion checks

The 1997–1998 SHOT report identifies eight cases where blood samples, for cross match, were taken from the wrong patient or were mislabelled (Williamson *et al*, 1999). This led to the transfusion of incompatible blood products and major morbidity in at least one patient. Therefore, in guarding against the risk of such a potentially catastrophic outcome it is essential that patient and pre-transfusion checks begin at the point of blood sample collection. As such, blood samples should only be collected from the patient once their identity has been verified both verbally (whenever possible) and against the patient's record/identity bracelet. Blood bottles must be labelled in full at the patient's bedside after the sample has been collected and include the patient's surname, first name, date of birth, gender, patient identification number and signature of the staff member taking the sample (BCSH, 1999). The practice of prior labelling of sample bottles and/or labelling of bottles remote from the patient should be avoided. Whenever possible, it is important that a full medical and nursing assessment is made prior to transfusion in order to identify factors which may increase the likelihood of transfusion-related complications. This will necessarily include questioning regarding any current medication that the patient is taking and any history of pregnancy, transfusion or transplantation (Contreras and Mollison, 1998). Routine blood transfusion should, ideally, be performed during daylight hours when the patient will normally be awake and therefore able to report any abnormal symptoms. In addition, the increased numbers of specialist staff and services available will ensure that any complications can be dealt with promptly and efficaciously.

Blood for transfusion should not be removed from temperature controlled storage until a maximum of 30 minutes before the commencement of transfusion. In those instances where the transfusion is not commenced within this time window the blood must be discarded because of the risk of bacterial proliferation (McClelland, 1996). With this in mind, it is sensible to ensure that a full explanation of the transfusion procedure is given prior to the removal of the blood product from storage. An opportunity should also be given for the patient to raise any questions or concerns he/she might have. Patient consent, verbal rather than written, can then be obtained.

Errors in the collection of blood from the blood bank/storage were identified by the SHOT report as the most common site of first error and led to one patient fatality (Williamson *et al*, 1999). It is therefore important that those members of staff, whether qualified or unqualified, who collect blood from storage are aware of their responsibilities and receive training in respect of local policies. Checking should, as a minimum, include checking of the blood product details against the blood request form, patient notes, patient identification label or prescription chart. In cases where a telephone request for blood collection is made, details of the patient's surname, first name, date of birth and patient identification number must be given so they can be recorded on a blood collection slip (BCSH, 1999). Last, the blood register should be completed in full, as per local policy, once the blood has been removed from storage.

(A): Asepsis and apparatus

In order to negate the risk of bacterial contamination it is vital that strict aseptic technique is observed throughout the setting up procedure. Attention should be paid to the cannula site; a clear dressing should be used to ensure early detection of extravasation and inflammation (Clarke, 1997). Blood should be administrated through an appropriately designed intravenous giving set which incorporates a 170 micron filter to remove micro aggregates formed during storage (Davies and Williamson, 1998). Additional in line blood filters are also available and these may be indicated in accordance with local policy, or where multiple units of blood are to be given. Due to the potential risk of haemolysis, glucose solutions must never be administered immediately before or after a unit of blood. No other infusion solutions or drugs should be added to any blood component. The blood administration set should be primed with physiological saline (0.9% sodium chloride) and venous patency verified before the commencement of transfusion. McClelland (1996) maintains that there is no evidence that the warming of blood is beneficial to the patient if the infusion is given slowly. However, the rapid transfusion of large volumes of cold blood increases the chances of ventricular fibrillation (Ravel, 1995) and may cause cardiac arrest (McClelland, 1996). For this reason a proprietary blood warmer may be indicated where the rate of transfusion is greater than 50ml/kg/hour or when blood is administered via a central line. As direct heat can cause the blood to haemolyse it is important to note that blood and blood components must not be warmed artificially by improvisations, such as placing the blood unit into hot water, on a radiator or in a microwave (Davies and Williamson, 1998). Administration sets should be routinely replaced on the completion of blood transfusion and after a maximum of twelve hours in patient's who receive multiple blood transfusions (BCSH, 1999).

(C): Checking and clerical procedures

The failure to adequately verify the identity of the patient before transfusion is cited as the 'single most important cause contributing to incorrect transfusions' (Williamson *et al*, 1999). Ironically, this is also the final opportunity to prevent the administration of an incorrect blood product and as such it is imperative that the checking procedure is both robust, accurate and does not compound errors that have been made in earlier parts of the blood transfusion process. In the clinical situation it is generally recommended, and accepted best practice, for the registered nurse and one other to check the blood product immediately prior to transfusion (Bradbury and Cruickshank, 1995a; McClelland, 1996; Contreras and Mollison, 1998). However, this practice has recently been questioned in so far that it may lead to a diffusion of responsibility, where each checker relies on the other to spot errors. Given this, a recommendation has been made that it may be more appropriate for one registered general nurse to carry out the checking procedure (BCSH, 1999). This recommendation is also in line with professional guidelines pertaining to the administration of medicines (UKCC, 1992). In either case, it is vital that all checking procedures are carried out at the patients' bedside (see *Table 20.3*)

A visual check of the blood should be made at this point and the haematologist alerted if there is any loss of blood container integrity, if there are any air bubbles present or if there is any abnormal discoloration or clotting of the blood. The blood unit details must then be checked against the prescription, cross match/blood compatibility form, patient notes and patient identity (Jamieson *et al*, 1997). Again, this checking should include verbal and documentary verification of the patient's identity whenever possible. A set of baseline observations — temperature, pulse, respiration (TPR), and blood pressure (BP) should then be taken before the commencement of the transfusion.

Table 20.3: An overview of the checking procedure

All checking procedures must be perfomed at the patient's bedside.
Confirm patient consent for transfusion.

Verify patient's identity against the:
- transfusion compatibility report form
- compatibility label on the blood unit
- prescription chart
- patient notes.

Ensure blood group and blood unit numbers on unit for transfusion unit are identical to those on the blood transfusion compatibility report form.

Check expiry date and perform visual check on blood unit.

Record patient baseline observations.

Complete documentation.

Withhold blood if any discrepancies or abnormality found.

(K): Keeping vigilant and keeping accurate records

It is important that the nurse remains vigilant and observes for the development of any adverse reactions both during and after the completion of blood transfusion. Huntly and Rawlinson (1999) report that as little as 5–10 mls of incompatible blood can initiate an immediate haemolytic reaction. These potentially life threatening reactions account for over 50% of deaths from blood transfusion (Murphy, 1998) and most commonly occur within 10–15 minutes of commencing transfusion (Davies and Williamson, 1998). In order to minimise this risk it is important that the patient is closely observed during this period. This will, ideally, necessitate the nurse remaining with the patient and titrating the transfusion to run at a slower rate during this time. An additional set of observations, TPR and B/P, should also be recorded at this time. Local policy and procedure will largely determine the timing of further observations. Suffice to say there is little research evidence regarding the optimum frequency for any subsequent observations. However, given that the pulse is easily accessible and rapidly reflects changes in the patient's condition, it would seem circumspect to record the pulse every 15 minutes for the first hour of each transfusion. Additional observations, TPR and BP should be taken when there is a significant alteration in pulse rate, or when other signs and symptoms become manifest (*Table 20.4*).

A full set of observations should also be routinely recorded following the completion of each

Table 20.4: Potentially adverse signs and symptoms include:

Headache	Nausea and vomiting
Palpitations	Pain
Shortness of breath/ dyspnoea	Pyrexia
Dizziness	Tachycardia
Rash	Hypotension
Pruritus	Oliguria
Haemoglobinuria	Spontaneous bleeding

transfused unit of blood. In addition to these observations it is important that the nurse remains alert to the early signs of renal impairment and disseminated intravascular coagulation (DIC) as evidenced by haemoglobinuria, oliguria, anuria and spontaneous bruising/bleeding. In those instances where a serious adverse reaction is suspected, the transfusion should be stopped and 0.9% physiological saline infused to maintain venous patency (McClelland, 1996; BCSH, 1999). A further set of observations must be recorded and the medical staff informed immediately so that resuscitative measures can be initiated as required. The haematologist should also be informed and the unit of blood retained for investigation. Comprehensive and accurate records relating to the blood being transfused and any adverse reactions should be detailed in the nursing notes in a manner which complies with both local and national guidelines (UKCC, 1998). Details of the transfusion should also be entered in the patient's medical records and the transfusion slip retained for future reference. Finally, while some doubts have been expressed about the validity of retaining blood containers post transfusion (BCSH, 1999), it would still seem prudent to retain these for a period of 48 hours in case any delayed transfusion reaction should develop (Glover and Powell, 1996). Again, local policies will dictate the exact procedure to be followed.

Conclusion

The beginning of the twentieth century heralded an era from which much has been learnt about the physiology of blood, its transfusion and the reduction of risks associated with its administration. However, it is important to remember that blood transfusion involves the transfer of living tissue from one individual to another. It therefore follows that the procedure is not without inherent risk of complication. Unfortunately, this risk is often compounded by human error, which can result in the transfusion of incorrect and incompatible blood products. In safeguarding patients against such risks it is essential that rigorous pre-transfusion and patient identification checks are instituted before the transfusion of blood and that nurses are aware of the complications associated with blood transfusion and their management.

Key points

* Blood should only be given when the therapeutic benefits outweigh the associated risks.
* Failure to verify the identity of the patient is the single most important cause of incorrect blood transfusion.
* Particular attention must be given to the procedure and methods for collecting blood from storage.
* It is essential that rigorous checking procedures are followed in all cases.

References

Bradbury M, Cruickshank JP (1995) Blood & Blood Transfusion 1. *Br J Nurs* **4**(14): 814–817

British Committee for Standards in Haematology (1999). The Administration of Blood & Blood Components and the Management of Transfusion Patients. *Transfus Med* **9**(3): 227–238

Clarke A (1997). The Nursing Management of Intravenous Drug Therapy. *Br J Nurs* **6**(4): 200–206

Contreras M, Mollison PL (1998) Testing before transfusion and blood ordering policies. In: Contreras M (ed) *ABC of Transfusion.* 3rd edn. BMJ Books, London

Davies SC, Williamson LM (1998) Transfusion of red cells. In: Contreras M (ed) *ABC of Transfusion.* 3rd edn. BMJ Books, London

Garwood PA, Knowles SE (1998). Supply and demand of blood and blood components. In: Contreras M (ed) *ABC of Transfusion.* 3rd edn. BMJ Books, London

Glover G, Powell F (1996) Blood Transfusion. *Nurs Standard* **10**(21): 49–54

Hoffbrand AV, Pettit JE (1993) *Essential haematology.* 3rd edn. Blackwell Scientific Publications, Oxford

Huntly BJP, Rawlison S (1999) Blood Transfusion. *Surgery* **17**(2): 45–47

Jamieson EM, McCall JM, Blythe R *et al* (1997) *Clinical Nursing Practices.* Churchill Livingstone, Edinburgh

Linch DC (1994) Haematological Disorders. In: Souhami RL, Moxham J (ed) *Textbook of Medicine.* 2nd edn. Churchill Livingstone, Edinburgh

Lower R, King E (1667) An account of the experiment of transfusion, practised upon a man in London. *Phil Trans* **2**: 557–64

Marshall M , Bird T (1983) *Blood Loss & Replacement.* Edward Arnold Publications, London

McClelland DBL (ed) (1996) *Handbook of Transfusion Medicine.* HMSO, London

Murphy MF (1998) Haematological disease. In: Parveen K, Clark M (ed), *Clinical Medicine.* 4th edn. WB Saunders, Edinburgh

Ravel R (1995) *Clinical Laboratory Medicine: Clinical application of laboratory data.* 6th edn. Mosby, St Louis

Williamson LM, Lowe S, Love E *et al* (1999) *Serious Hazards of Transfusion* (SHOT) *Annual Report 1997–1998.* The Serious Hazards of Transfusion Steering Group, Manchester

United Kingdom Central Council for Nursing, Midwifery, & Health Visiting (1992) *Standards for the Administration of Medicines.* UKCC, London

United Kingdom Central Council for Nursing, Midwifery, & Health Visiting (1998) *Guidelines for Records & Record Keeping.* UKCC, London

Urbaniak SJ (1990) Adverse Effects of Transfusion. In: Ludlam C (ed) *Clinical Haematology.* Churchill Livingstone, Edinburgh

21

Blood and blood transfusion reactions: 2

Martyn Bradbury and Jeremy Pope Cruickshank

This chapter describes the immediate complications of blood transfusion and offers guidelines for their nursing management.

When considering the complications of blood transfusion it is convenient to divide them into those that occur immediately, and those in which the onset of symptoms is delayed for days, weeks, months or even years. In addition to this chronological classification, it is useful to further subdivide complications into those that have an immune aetiology and those with a non-immune origin (*Table 21.1*).

This chapter will consider these complications and, more specifically, the immediate complications of blood transfusion. *Table 21.2* lists the complications that may appear later or in association with multiple transfusion.

Table 21.1: Onset and aetiology of complications associated with blood transfusions		
	Immune	**Non-immune**
Immediate	Acute haemolytic reaction	Bacteraemia/septic reaction
	Febrile reactions	Circulatory overload
	Allergic reactions	
	Transfusion-related acute lung injury	
Delayed	Delayed haemolytic reaction	Transmission of infection
	Post-transfusion purpura	Haemosiderosis

Management of immediate transfusion reactions

Acute haemolytic reaction (AHR)

This is a potentially fatal reaction that usually results from the transfusion of incompatible ABO or rhesus blood groups. It is characterised by the destruction of donor red blood cells (RBCs) (haemolysis) within the circulation (intravascular haemolysis) or by macrophages within the reticulo-endothelial system (extravascular haemolysis).

When haemolysis occurs it is primarily mediated by surface antigens on the donor RBCs which bind with the recipient's IgM and IgG antibodies. The resultant antigen/antibody complex then activates complement causing:

- haemolysis of donor RBCs (*Figure 21.1*)

- smooth muscle contraction
- degranulation of mast cells and the release of vasoactive substances, eg. histamine, bradykinin and serotonin
- the release of anaphylatoxins, eg. C3a, C5a.

The clinical picture that results varies greatly from patient to patient, but is largely governed by:

- the strength of the recipient's antibody titre
- the nature of the antigenic challenge
- the volume of blood transfused
- the clinical condition of the patient before transfusion
- whether haemolysis occurs within the intra- or extravascular compartment.

Table 21.2: Complications associated with transfusions or multiple transfusions
Air embolus
Hypothermia
Citrate toxicity
Haemosiderosis
Hypocoagulation
Thrombophlebitis
Graft *vs* host disease
Infection transmission
Delayed haemolytic reaction
Pulmonary micro-embolisation
Metabolic changes, eg. hypo/ hyperkalaemia

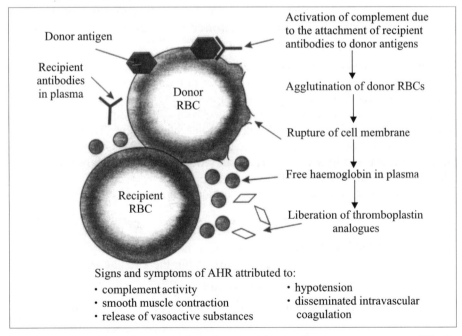

Figure 21.1: Events associated with acute haemolytic reaction (simplified). RBC=red blood cell; AHR=acute haemolytic reaction

Intravascular haemolysis: This is the most catastrophic form of haemolytic reaction and carries a mortality rate of up to 10%. It is nearly always due to ABO incompatibility and is associated with the full activation of complement. As such, the onset of symptoms is usually rapid and classically develops within the first thirty minutes of transfusion when the patient complains of pain over the infusion site, increasing restlessness and anxiety, headache, flushing of the face, urticaria and nausea/vomiting.

In addition, the release of vasoactive substances leads to vasodilation, with a subsequent drop in blood pressure and tachycardia. In severe cases, this progresses to profound hypotension and circulatory collapse. Pyrexia and rigor are also common and the patient may complain of dyspnoea and chest/lumbar pain.

This elaborate scenario is further complicated by the concurrent lysis of RBCs which liberates thromboplastin-like substances into the plasma. These thromboplastin analogues activate the clotting cascade and initiate the subsequent development of disseminated intravascular coagulation (DIC). This serious complication presents as bruising and persistent bleeding from wounds and injection/venepuncture sites.

In addition, the presence of haemoglobin within the plasma leads to haemoglobinaemia and the development of jaundice. Ultimately, this 'free' haemoglobin appears in the urine causing the passage of port wine-coloured urine (haemoglobinuria).

The precipitation of haemoglobin within the renal tubule has also been widely implicated in the development of acute tubular necrosis and renal failure. However, this is now considered to be an unlikely cause (Schroeder, 1999) as renal function is more likely to be jeopardised by ischaemia and hypotension, vasoconstriction and DIC (Contreras and Hewitt, 1999).

Extravascular haemolysis: This tends to be associated with rhesus antibodies that do not activate complement fully. The symptoms therefore tend to be mild and are frequently delayed until several days after the completion of transfusion. When extravascular haemolysis occurs immediately, the symptoms are also mild and less dramatic than those of intravascular haemolysis. These symptoms develop at least one hour after the transfusion has commenced and tend to be limited to fever and hyperbilirubinaemia, with an absence of any transfusion-related haemoglobin rise.

It should be noted that other non-immune causes of red cell lysis exist, including:

- mixing blood with an incompatible solution,eg. 5% dextrose (McClelland, 1996)
- incorrect freezing or warming of blood
- the prolonged or improper storage of blood.

Table 21.3 gives a review of the rationale and principles of management of AHR.

Table 21.3: Management of acute haemolytic reaction

Principles of management	Rationale
Obtain detailed history before transfusion. Report previous transfusions or pregnancies	Sensitisation to red blood cell antigens increases in patients who have had previous exposure to blood products or who have been pregnant
Ensure that local policies are adhered to regarding the verification and administration of blood for transfusion	The most common cause of a transfusion reaction is human error in handling the blood sample or in initiating the transfusion (Williamson *et al*, 1999)
Ask the patient to report any unusual feelings that evolve during or following the transfusion	These initial tacit feelings may indicate an impending acute reaction
Remain with the patient for the first 15 minutes following the commencement of transfusion, which should initially be run at a slow rate. If the patient is left alone at any time ensure that the call bell is within easy reach	Severe reaction is more likely to arise during this period. Just 5–10mls of incompatible blood can cause an acute haemolytic reaction (Huntly and Rawlinson, 1999).
Prompt assessment: record vital signs — blood pressure, pulse, temperature, respiratory rate, depth and rhythm. Stop transfusion if acute haemolytic reaction is suspected and obtain medical assistance	Early detection of acute haemolytic reaction. Detection of shock Limits opportunity for further incompatibility
Change intravenous infusion administration set. Assess cannula site, exchange blood unit for physiological saline (0.9% sodium chloride). Give slowly	To maintain patency of intravenous infusion. Observe for signs of thrombophlebitis
Initiate prescribed resuscitative measures (*Table 21.6*)	Maintenance of blood pressure, treatment of shock
Keep blood unit, notify laboratory and return unit	Required by the laboratory for reanalysis and rematching
Review/recheck transfusion documentation	To establish any clerical errors. Remember that another patient may be involved in the mismatch
Strict fluid balance. Use of prescribed diuretics. Monitor effectiveness	Early detection of renal failure. There is around 10% chance of developing oliguria or anuria (Hughes-Jones and Wickramasinghe, 1996)
Assist in obtaining further blood sample from patient	Reanalysis of blood to detect the extent of haemolysis. Results of these analyses should help to confirm the appearance of haemolysis and to identify whether this was due to an initial 'missed' incompatibility test or a clerical error (Contreras and Hewitt, 1999)
Obtain urine specimen and perform urinalysis. Send the initial specimen of urine to the laboratory for analysis	Urinalysis is performed to detect haemoglobinuria and for microscopy. As haemoglobinuria is often transient, it is vital to collect the first urine voided by the patient
The patient may require cardiac monitoring. Continue to monitor vital signs	Prompt detection of life-threatening cardiac arrhythmias
Observe for signs of bleeding, especially from wounds or venepunctures	May indicate the development of disseminated intravascular coagulation (Firkin *et al*, 1989)

Febrile reactions

Febrile reactions are the most common form of transfusion reaction. They are usually mild and present some 30–90 minutes after transfusion has commenced. The cause is an immune response to surface antigens on the donor white blood cells (human leucocyte antigen) or, more rarely, platelets.

Subsequent release of endogenous pyrogens effects the central control of temperature and leads to pyrexia. Frequently, this may be the only presenting symptom, but the patient may also complain of chills, rigor, headache and flushing of the face. However, it is important to note that there is no concomitant fall in blood pressure or lumbar pain.

Table 21.4 gives a review of the rationale and principles of management of febrile reaction.

Table 21.4: Management of febrile reactions	
Principles of management	**Rationale**
Ascertain history from patient regarding previous transfusions/pregnancy	Reactions are more likely to occur in multiparous or previously transfused patients (Contreras and Hewitt, 1999)
Prompt assessment. Stop infusion if in any doubt. Keep vein open. Report to medical staff	The possibility of a haemolytic reaction should always be considered when fever occurs (Schroeder, 1999)
If there is only a mild rise in temperature, the infusion will usually be recommenced at a slower rate	Allows for the cautious continuation of transfusion and prevents wastage of blood caused by the premature termination of the transfusion. The immune response is proportionate to the number of incompatible cells and the rate at which they are transfused (Hoffbrand and Pettit, 1993)
Monitor vital signs — record temperature, pulse and blood pressure at least hourly	Continuing vigilance is vital as it is difficult to distinguish between simple febrile reactions and the pyrexial responses that may have been initiated by infections or an acute haemolytic reaction
Administration of prescribed anti-pyretics (aspirin may be the chosen drug unless contraindicated). Note: administration of these medications prophylactically may potentially mask the febrile effects caused by an acute haemolytic reaction	Antipyretic agent used to reduce temperature
Report any severe febrile reaction to the laboratory. Return unit to the laboratory	Those patients who require a transfusion but have a sensitivity to white cells or platelets may receive future transfusions which are depleted of white cells, eg. filtered and washed red cells (McClelland, 1996)

Allergic reactions

Allergic reactions occur in about 1% of all transfusions and range from milder urticarial reactions to potentially life-threatening anaphylaxis.

Urticaria: This reaction is most commonly seen in patients who have become sensitised by previous transfusions or pregnancy. Several mechanisms may account for this allergic response, but it is usually initiated by anti-IgA antibodies within the recipient's plasma that react with some, but not all, IgA subtypes within the transfused plasma/blood.

This, plus a normally low antibody titre, means that the allergic response is mild and characterised by mast cell degranulation and the release of histamine. Vasodilation and increased capillary permeability therefore ensue, leading to the characteristic swelling known as hives or weals. There may also be generalised itching, rash, fever, nausea and vomiting. *Table 21.5* gives a review of the rationale and principles of the management of urticarial reaction.

Table 21.5: Management of urticarial reactions	
Principles of management	**Rationale**
Check with the patient whether he/she has previous allergic reactions during or following a blood transfusion	Urticarial reactions are more common in patients who have been sensitised by previous transfusion or pregnancy
If no accompanying fever, slow the rate of the transfusion	Assists in alleviating the symptoms while allowing the patient to continue with the transfusion. Patients may require prophylactic administration of antihistamines and/or steroids
If fever appears, stop transfusion	Prevents any futher risk of incompatibility
Seek medical support. Keep vein open	To maintain venous access
Monitor vital signs	Detection of any abnormalities
Administration of antihistamines, eg. chlorpheniramine. Monitor for side-effects which include drowsiness, dizziness and hypotension	Urticaria responds effectively to antihistamines as a result of their blocking action on the H_1 receptor sites. By blocking the access of released histamine to H_1 receptor sites, the allergic response is inhibited (Hopkins, 1999)
Observe intravenous site for signs of irritation, redness and/or swelling	Chlorpheniramine can induce phlebitis if given intravenously

Anaphylaxis: Unlike urticaria, this potentially fatal complication usually presents in patients who have had no previous exposure to a blood transfusion. The patient is classically IgA-deficient, but in this case the antibody (anti-IgA) titre is high and reaction occurs against all IgA subtypes.

Transfusion of donor blood that is rich in IgA initiates a systemic hypersensitivity response, with the activation of complement and the release of anaphylatoxins. These act on mast cells, polymorphonuclearcytes and smooth muscle in order to promote the inflammatory response (Playfair, 1996). In addition to the symptoms already outlined for urticaria, the patient can progress rapidly towards full circulatory collapse, with marked hypotension, tachycardia, chest pain and cardiac failure.

Additionally, the release of vasoactive substances, eg. histamine, leads to an increase in vascular permeability within the lungs, gastrointestinal (GI) tract and circulation (Urbaniak, 1990).

As a consequence, vomiting and other GI disturbances can occur. More importantly, angio-oedema and bronchospasm can lead to acute respiratory embarrassment with dyspnoea, wheezing and cyanosis. At its most severe, the above scenario will be terminated by cardiopulmonary arrest. *Table 21.6* gives a review of the rationale and principles of management of anaphylaxis.

Table 21.6: Management of anaphylactic reactions		
Principles of management	**Rationale**	
Obtain full transfusion history from patient	As anaphylaxis is generated by a reaction involving recipient antibody to donor IgA and not red blood cell incompatibility, it is difficult to predict precisely the likelihood of an anaphylactic reaction. Nevertheless, a thorough transfusion assessment is essential	
Stop infusion and seek assistance	To prevent further reactions which can be escalated by the rate of transfusion and strength of antibody titre	
Keep vein open — use of intravenous fluids. Monitor vital signs	To maintain patency of the intravenous infusion, the circulatory volume and to treat hypotension. Detection of abnormalities	
Reassure patient	To provide psychological support	
Administer prescribed oxygen therapy; nurse upright	To maintain airway and allow for maximal chest expansion	
Drug regime prescribed	Epinephrine (Adrenaline)	Promotes bronchodilatation and opposes hypotension through its vasoconstrictive properties (Trounce, 1997)
	Salbutamol	Nebulised bronchodilator
	Hydrocortisone Antihistamines	Steroids are powerful anti-inflammatory drugs. Hydrocortisone induces vasoconstriction and decreases capillary permeability by suppressing the activity of kinins and the release of histamine (Goldfien, 1998)
	Aminophylline	Smooth muscle relaxant properties have a bronchodilating effect that assists in the alleviation of bronchospasm
Assist in the obtaining of blood samples from the patient. Keep all used blood units	Blood samples analysed for IgA deficiency and anti-IgA (McClelland, 1996). Patients who require subsequent IgA-free blood components may benefit from transfusion of washed red cells or frozen red cells (Hoffbrand and Pettit, 1993)	

Cardiac pulmonary oedema (circulatory overload)

This most frequently occurs in association with multiple or rapid transfusion of whole blood. Patients who are at particular risk include the elderly, the very young or those with chronic anaemia or pre-existing cardiac/pulmonary disease.

The increased volume (hypervolaemia) leads to hypertension and a bounding pulse. Cardiac failure may ensue, causing elevation of the jugular venous pressure, congestion within the pulmonary vasculature and the development of pulmonary oedema. The patient will develop a dry cough, increasing dyspnoea and cyanosis, with the resultant hypoxia leading to increasing confusion and restlessness.

Table 21.7 gives a review of the rationale and principles of the management of cardiac pulmonary oedema.

Table 21.7: Management of cardiac pulmonary oedema (circulatory overload)	
Principles of management	**Rationale**
Assess patient for risk factors	To detect any potential risk groups
Transfusion may need to be given over a longer period (4–6 hours). Packed cells will usually be prescribed	To reduce the likelihood of cardiac pulmonary oedema
Monitor vital signs	To enable the early detection of abnormalities
If signs/symptoms appear, stop infusion. Seek medical support. Keep vein open	To reduce any further risk of overload
Use of oxygen as prescribed. Nurse in an upright position	To reduce hypoxia and alleviate dyspnoea
Aminophylline may be prescribed	Effective in stimulating respiration by reducing smooth muscle spasm, especially in the bronchioles
Opiates may be prescribed. Monitor for any associated respiratory depression	To reduce anxiety (anxiolytic effect) and decrease peripheral resistance, thereby diverting blood flow from the pulmonary circulation to the peripheral circulation
Intravenous diuretics may be administered, eg. frusemide (may also be given prophylactically)	To promote renal diuresis and prevent hypervolaemia
Monitor urine output, maintain accurate fluid balance	To monitor effectiveness of diuretics. Assessment of positive or negative fluid status
Spend time with the patient, reassure and give careful explanations	Good interpersonal skills integral to this situation to alleviate undue anxiety
Transfusions should ideally be given during daytime hours	Patient will tend to be awake and this will facilitate monitoring

Non-cardiac pulmonary oedema: transfusion-related acute lung injury

This rare but serious complication is characterised by lung damage, pulmonary oedema and hypoxia. It tends to be seen in multiparous women and is usually precipitated by antibodies within the transfused blood that react with the recipient's granulocytes. The exact mechanism by which the resultant antibody/antigen complex initiates pulmonary oedema is uncertain, but the agglutination of granulocytes and activation of complement within the pulmonary vaculature has been suggested as a likely cause (Schroeder, 1999).

From a clinical perspective, the patient will develop chills, fever, hypotension and chest pain. The most serious manifestations, however, are those associated with the development of pulmonary oedema, including dyspnoea, cyanosis and cough.

Table 21.8 gives a review of the rationale and the principles of management of non-cardiac pulmonary oedema.

Table 21.8: Management of non-cardiac pulmonary oedema (transfusion-related acute lung injury)	
Principles of management	**Rationale**
Stop transfusion, keep vein open. Use of intravenous fluids	Prevents further opportunity for incompatibility. To maintain cardiac output and blood pressure
Use of prescribed oxygen therapy. Pulse oximetry/measurement of blood gases. Nurse in an upright position	To detect for and monitor the degree of hypoxia
May require assisted ventilation	To maintain oxygen saturation
Monitor vital signs — pulse, blood pressure, temperature and respiratory rate, depth and rhythm	Prompt detection where pulmonary oedema is provoked by volume overload
Diuretics only effective if fluid overload is detected	Diuretics increase diuresis and are effective in fluid overload. Should be avoided in cases of non-cardiac pulmonary oedema (Urbaniak, 1990)
Administration of high doses of steroids	Steroids potentially block aggregation of granulocytes in the pulmonary capillaries, thus reducing the opportunity for vascular injury (Schroeder, 1999)

Septic reaction

With modern infection control techniques this complication is now extremely rare. However, the potential for bacterial contamination still exists during the donation, processing, storage and administration of blood and blood products. Fortunately, many of the microorganisms that may infect blood, eg. *staphylococcus epidermidis*, are destroyed by a combination of the citrate that is added to prevent clotting and the subsequent storage of blood at 4–8°C. In contrast, however, some faecal contaminants such as the pseudomonads and Gram-negative coliforms are readily able to multiply at low temperatures by utilising citrate as an energy source.

If transfused into a patient, these microorganisms can produce septicaemia and symptoms associated with the release of bacterial endotoxins. The onset of symptoms is therefore rapid, with endotoxic/bacteraemic shock and a clinical picture similar to that associated with acute haemolysis.

Table 21.9 gives a review of the rationale and principles of the management of septic reaction.

Table 21.9: Management of septic reaction	
Principles of management	**Rationale**
Preventive measures should embrace stringent aseptic technique during the donation and administration of the blood	Prevention of contamination and hence the transfer of microorganisms
Blood must always be stored in a temperature-controlled environment. It must not be removed from storage until thirty minutes before use (McClelland, 1996)	An increase in blood temperature can promote bacterial growth
Inspect the unit before commencement of the transfusion. Observe for gas bubbles, clots or a change in colour (beware of purplish colour) (Brunner and Suddarth, 1992)	May strongly indicate that blood contamination or haemolysis has taken place. Gram-negative bacteria can multiply at 4–8°C or at room temperature using the citrate that has been added to the blood for its source of energy. This can lead to clot formation within the stored blood (Contreras, 1998)
Notify laboratory. Provide necessary details and return unit	For reanalyses of the unit and the batch
If reaction does occur seek medical support, stop transfusion. Change giving set, keep vein open with physiological saline (0.9% sodium chloride)	To prevent further risk of contamination and maintain venous access
Monitor signs, measure fluid balance	To monitor urinary output and to detect abnormalities
Assist the doctor in obtaining blood cultures	Detection of the causal organism in the septicaemic reaction
Administration of large doses of broad-spectrum antibiotics (beware allergies to antibiotics in the patient)	Effective against Gram-positive and Gram-negative organisms
Use of steroids (hydrocortisone)	Inhibits the inflammatory process
Use of sympathomimetic drugs (vasopressors), eg. dobutamine hydrochloride	Drugs act on the autonomic nervous system, increasing cardiac contractility and renal perfusion. Used to correct haemodynamic imbalance

Conclusion

The transfusion of blood and blood products has enabled therapeutic medicine to progress rapidly and now offers patients a relatively safe and effective treatment option. It must be remembered, however, that blood transfusion involves the transfer of living tissue from one individual to another. As such, the nurse must be aware that there are small but significant and potentially catastrophic risks associated with the transfusion of blood and blood products. These risks, however, can be minimised through comprehensive nursing assessment and vigilant monitoring of patients who are receiving a blood transfusion.

Key points

* Transfusion reactions vary, ranging from acute to delayed and immune or non-immune.
* Blood transfusion involves the donation of living tissue from one person to another.
* As little as 5–10 mls of incompatible blood can precipitate an acute haemolytic reaction.
* The risks associated with transfusion can be minimised through adequate nursing assessment and close observation.

References

Brunner LS, Suddarth DS (1992) *The Textbook of Adult Nursing*. Chapman & Hall, London

Contreras M (ed) (1998) *ABC of Transfusion*. 3rd edn. BMJ Publishing, London

Contreras M, Hewitt PE (1999) *Clinical Blood Transfusion, in Postgraduate Haematology*. 4th edn. (eds Hoffbrand AV, Lewis MS, Tuddenham EGD). Butterworth Heinmann, Oxford

Goldfien JA (1998) Adrenocorticoidsteroids and adrenocortical antagonists. In: Katzung BG (ed) *Basic and Clinical Pharmacology*. 7th edn. Appleton & Lange, Stamford

Firkin F, Chesterman C, Penington D *et al* (eds) (1989) *De Gruchy's Clinical Haematology in Medical Practice*. 5th edn. Blackwell Science, Oxford

Hoffbrand AV, Pettit JE (1993) *Essential Haematology*. 3rd edn. Blackwell Science, Oxford

Hopkins SJ (1999) *Drugs and Pharmacology for Nurses*. 13th edn. Churchill Livingstone, London

Hughes-Jones NC, Wickramasinghe SN (1996) *Lecture Notes on Haematology*. 6th edn. Blackwell Science, Oxford

Huntly BJP, Rawlinson S (1999) Blood Transfusion. *Surgery* **17**(2): 45–47

McClelland B (ed) (1996) *Handbook of Transfusion Medicine*. 2nd edn. HMSO, London

Playfair JHL (1996) *Immunology at a glance*. 6th edn. Blackwell Science, Oxford

Urbaniak SJ (1990) Adverse effects of transfusion. In: Ludlam C (ed) *Clinical Haematology*. Churchill Livingstone, Edinburgh: 449–59

Schroeder ML (1999) Principles and Practice of Transfusion Medicine. In: Lee GR, Foerster J, Lukens J *et al* (eds) *Wintrobe's Clinical Hematology*. 10th edn. Williams & Wilkins Publishing, Baltimore

Trounce J (1997) *Clinical Pharmacology for Nurses*. Churchill Livingstone, London

Williamson LM, Lowe S, Love E *et al* (1999) Serious Hazards of Transfusion (SHOT) *Annual Report 1997–1998*. The Serious Hazards of Transfusion Steering Group, Manchester

22

Use of pulmonary artery flotation catheters in the coronary care unit

Charles G Bloe

As critical care nurses strive towards holistic patient care they must now interpret parameters previously regarded as the domain of the physician. The interpretation and understanding of results derived from pulmonary artery flotation catheters are important skills that are outlined in this chapter.

In the critically ill patient, clinical observations and routinely measured cardiovascular parameters such as pulse, blood pressure and central venous pressure (*Table 22.1*) are of limited value as they may not accurately reflect left ventricular function (Forrester *et al*, 1971; Eisenberg *et al*, 1984). However, in the coronary care unit this knowledge is often essential for optimal treatment.

Insertion of a pulmonary artery flotation catheter (PAFC or Swan-Ganz catheter) allows the measurement of cardiac output and other important indices of cardiovascular function, which makes possible the assessment of left ventricular performance (Swan *et al*, 1970). The balloon-tipped, and consequently flow-directable, catheter (*Figure 22.1*) is inserted into the right (venous) side of the circulation.

This chapter describes clinical situations in the coronary care unit in which the use of a PAFC may be considered and outlines the nursing responsibilities.

Haemodynamic basics

Cardiac output (CO) is the volume of blood pumped by the heart each minute. A more meaningful expression of CO is the cardiac index (CI), which relates CO to body size. Cardiac index is calculated as CO divided by body surface area. The two main determinants of CO are heart rate (HR) and stroke volume (SV).

$$CO = HR \times SV$$

Heart rate

Arrhythmias and extremes in HR can reduce CO. As HR increases under normal circumstances, eg. exercise, CO rises to meet the increased oxygen demands of the body. Excessive tachycardia reduces ventricular filling time and CO may fall, eg. as in ventricular tachycardias. Generally, as HR decreases, SV increases to maintain CO. However, the diseased myocardium may be unable to increase SV and CO may fall, eg. as in myocardial infarction with heart block.

Table 22.1: Normal values of cardiovascular parameters	
Heart rate	60–100 beats/min
Stroke volume	60–130 ml
Cardiac output	5–8 litres/min
Cardiac index	>2.7 litres/min/m^2
Pulmonary vascular resistance	100–200 dyn.s/cm^{-5}
Systemic vascular resistance	1800–2500 dyn.s/cm^{-5}
Right atrial pressure (mean)	0–7 mmHg
Right ventricular pressure	15–25 mmHg (systolic) 1–7 mmHg (diastolic)
Pulmonary arterial pressure	15–25 mmHg (systolic) 6–12 mmHg (diastolic)
Pulmonary capillary wedge pressure (mean)	6–12 mmHg

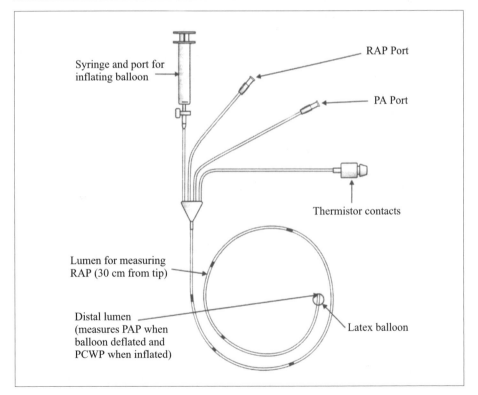

Figure 22.1: Diagram of thermodilution pulmonary artery flotation catheter. RAP=right atrial pressure; PA=pulmonary artery; PAP=pulmonary artery pressure; PCWP=pulmonary capillary wedge pressure

Stroke volume

SV is the volume of blood ejected by the heart at each beat. It is determined by preload, afterload and myocardial contractility.

Preload: Preload is the volume of blood in the ventricles at the end of diastole just before the onset of ventricular contraction, ie. the ventricular end-diastolic or filling pressure. Starling's law states that heart muscle responds to increased stretch by exerting an increased force of contraction such that the more the heart is filled in diastole the greater is the force of contraction in systole, resulting in increased CO (*Figure 22.2*). This is rather like a fully inflated balloon recoiling more vigorously than a partially inflated one. However, overstretching will lead to a reduced CO and the development of pulmonary congestion and oedema, just as an overinflated balloon will burst. The optimal left ventricular filling pressure in acute myocardial infarction is 14–18 mmHg (Crexells *et al*, 1973).

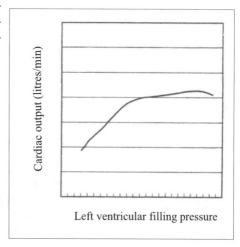

Figure 22.2: Starling's or ventricular performance curve. The optimal filling pressure is that which results in maximal cardiac output, which is most efficient in the range near the peak of the curve

Afterload: Afterload is the resistance against which the ventricles are pumping. It depends on three factors:

1. Systemic vascular resistance. This reflects left ventricular afterload, ie. the resistance the left ventricle must overcome in order to open the aortic valve and eject blood into the systemic circulation.

2. Pulmonary vascular resistance. This reflects right ventricular afterload, ie. the resistance the right ventricle must overcome in order to eject blood into the pulmonary circulation

3. Blood viscosity. An increase in blood viscosity will increase afterload.

In general, increasing afterload will reduce CO.

Myocardial contractility: Myocardial contractility refers to the pumping power of the ventricles.

Haemodynamic parameters recorded by a PAFC

Figure 22.3 demonstrates those haemodynamic parameters that may be recorded by a PAFC.

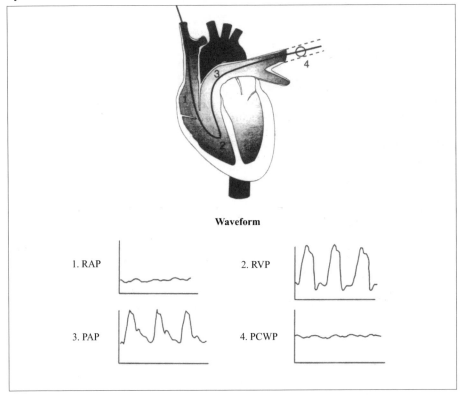

Figure 22.3: Passage of a pulmonary artery flotation catheter (PAFC) through the right heart into the wedge position and the associated haemodynamic waveform changes. RAP=right atrial pressure; RVP=right ventricular pressure; PAP=pulmonary artery pressure; PCWP=pulmonary capillary wedge pressure

Right atrial pressure

Right atrial pressure is often referred to as central venous pressure, but is more accurately defined as right ventricular end-diastolic pressure or right ventricular preload, and is an indication of right ventricular function. Accurate prediction of left ventricular pressure from right atrial pressure is difficult as there is not always a consistent relationship between the two (Forrester *et al*, 1971). For example, in the case of left ventricular infarction the left ventricular filling pressure may be elevated secondary to impaired function but the right atrial pressure may remain normal, at least initially. Conversely, in right ventricular infarction the right atrial pressure may be elevated and this may not necessarily reflect the presence of impaired left ventricular function.

Right ventricular pressure

The pressures within the right ventricle are only recorded during catheter insertion.

Pulmonary artery pressure

Pulmonary artery pressure is essentially the same as pulmonary venous pressure, ie. the pressure within the pulmonary vasculature.

Pulmonary capillary wedge pressure

The determination of pulmonary capillary wedge pressure (PCWP) remains a principal use of a PAFC. PCWP is measured when the balloon is inflated and floats into the pulmonary circulation, impacting in a small branch of the pulmonary artery and occluding the blood flow. As there are no valves between the pulmonary artery and the left heart, the pressure transmitted retrogradely from the left side is recorded from a lumen distal to the balloon. In the absence of mitral valvular or pulmonary vascular disease, PCWP closely approximates left atrial and ventricular filling pressures and therefore provides an indirect means of determining how well the left ventricle is functioning (Forrester *et al*, 1971).

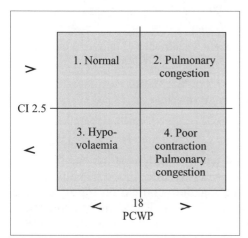

Figure 22.4: Classification of patients with acute myocardial infarction clinically and by pulmonary artery flotation catheterisation. Source: Forrester et al (1976). CI=cardiac index; PCWP= pulmonary capillary wedge pressure

Clinical conditions resulting in a rise or fall in recorded pressures

The main clinical conditions that bring about a rise or fall in the recorded pressures are outlined in *Table 22.2*.

Forrester *et al* (1976) categorised patients with acute myocardial infarction into four haemodynamic subsets (*Figure 22.4*) which, on the basis of clinical assessment alone, may be difficult to differentiate. As each requires a quite different treatment regimen, pulmonary artery flotation catheterisation can provide invaluable diagnostic information.

Reduced cardiac output

A reduced cardiac output can be due to either left ventricular dysfunction (subset 4) or hypovolaemia (subset 3).

Table 22.2: Clinical conditions resulting in a rise or fall in recorded pressures	
Raised right atrial or right ventricular pressure	Right ventricular dysfunction, eg. right ventricular infarction
	Volume overload
	Tricuspid or pulmonary valvular stenosis or regurgitation
	Pulmonary hypertension
	Congestive cardiac failure
	Vasoconstriction
Decreased right atrial or ventricular pressure	Hypovolaemia, eg. dehydration, haemorrhage
	Vasodilatation
Raised pulmonary artery pressure	Left ventricular failure
	Pulmonary hypertension
	Mitral stenosis
	Left-to-right shunts, eg. atrioventricular septal defects
Decreased pulmonary artery pressure	Hypovolaemia
	Vasodilatation
Raised pulmonary capillary wedge pressure	Left ventricular failure, eg. left ventricular infarction
	Mitral stenosis
Decreased pulmonary capillary wedge pressure	Hypovolaemia

Left ventricular dysfunction: Myocardial contractility and cardiac output may be reduced as a consequence of left ventricular muscle destruction. Typically such patients are in cardiogenic shock. After systole, blood remains in the ventricle. During diastole the blood entering the ventricle on top of what is already there leads to increased filling pressures and pulmonary congestion, which are reflected by a raised PCWP. Treatment is aimed at reducing PCWP and improving cardiac output by the use of vasodilators, diuretics and inotropes.

Hypovolaemia: In hypovolaemia, reduced circulatory volume and filling pressures are reflected in reduced PCWP and cardiac output. Treatment is aimed at increasing PCWP and improving cardiac output by the use of volume expansion.

Pulmonary congestion and oedema

Pulmonary congestion and oedema can be due to either left ventricular failure (subset 2) or increased capillary permeability.

Left ventricular failure: In the coronary care unit pulmonary oedema is most commonly due to acute myocardial infarction or ischaemia. Increased left ventricular filling pressure in the failing heart increases pressure within the pulmonary capillary system. When PCWP increases to a critical degree (usually 18–20 mmHg) fluid is forced out into the alveolar spaces, resulting in pulmonary congestion and oedema. Treatment is aimed at reducing PCWP and improving cardiac output using vasodilators and diuretics.

Increased capillary permeability: In this situation, pulmonary oedema results from leakage of fluid through the capillary membranes into the alveolar spaces, ie. adult respiratory distress syndrome. PCWP can be normal or even low. Such cases are rare in the coronary care unit.

Potential complications and nursing care

Patients with a PAFC in situ will, by their very nature, require intensive nursing care. The main requirements of care are to recognise, interpret and act upon significant changes in the waveforms and parameters outlined previously and also to be vigilant regarding early identification of potential complications. Evidence suggests that serious complications are in fact quite rare (Shah *et al*, 1984). However, they can arise and the more important ones are outlined in *Table 22.3* together with the main nursing considerations.

Contraindications

There are few absolute contraindications to the use of a PAFC. While the following are considered to be relative contraindications, a PAFC should only be used when the benefit clearly outweighs the potential risks:

1. The presence of a prosthetic tricuspid or pulmonary valve.
2. Coagulopathy
3. Left bundle-branch block.
4. An endocardial pacemaker in situ.

Conclusion

The use of a PAFC in the context of acute myocardial infarction remains controversial. An analysis of such usage by Gore *et al* (1987) failed to demonstrate any overall benefit. Perhaps not surprisingly, the frequency of use of PAFCs in British coronary care units remains low, with more than half of all units not using them at all (Singer and Bennett, 1989). However, as a diagnostic aid employed in conjunction with other clinical information it is generally accepted that the PAFC may lead to more appropriate treatment regimens.

Table 22.3: Serious complications and nursing considerations

Problem	Possible causes	Nursing considerations
Anxiety	Usually seriously ill; fear of unknown	Help allay fears by explaining procedure and rationale to patient and relatives
Haemorrhage	Arterial puncture	Observe insertion site Observe for signs of haemorrhage Caution post-thrombolysis
Cardiac arrhythmias	Ventricular ectopy common during insertion due to valvular or endocardial irritation	Continuous ECG monitoring during and post insertion. Defibrillator or resuscitation equipment at hand during insertion
	New right bundle-branch block may develop in up to 5% of cases	Consider using PAFC with temporary pacing lumen in patients with left bundle-branch block
	Catheter knotting	Consider use of X-ray imaging during insertion Advance catheter slowly
	Arrhythmias more common if using ice-cold injectate	Room temperature injectate safer (slightly less accurate)
Air embolism	Balloon rupture (usually no adverse effect unless right-to-left shunt)	Stop balloon inflation if no resistance met Aspiration of blood from inflation port will confirm Observe for dyspnoea, chest pain, cyanosis
Pneumothorax or haemothorax	More common with subclavian insertion	Consider internal jugular insertion Encourage patient to remain still during insertion Observe for dyspnoea, chest pain, cyanosis Chest X-ray after insertion
Infection	Mainly localised at insertion site	Strict asepsis during insertion and at bag and line changes

Infection contin.	Rarely septicaemia or endocarditis	Observe for and report signs of local or systemic infection Minimise catheter manipulation and line disconnections Use closed injectate set for cardiac output measurement Ensure catheter never remains in situ > 72 hours Prompt removal of catheter if sepsis apparent Send catheter tip for culture
Pulmonary embolism	Clot formation in terminal lumen	Maintain pressure of 300 mmHg through transducer Never flush blocked line; always attempt to aspirate
Pulmonary artery infarction	Balloon inflation within smaller vessel	Routinely display pulmonary artery pressure on monitor to identify catheter migration
	Spontaneous wedging (migration of catheter into smaller vessel)	Never inflate balloon in presence of PCWP waveform
	Prolonged balloon inflation	Deflate balloon once confirmed PCWP is obtained Never leave balloon inflated more than 15 seconds Use minimum amount of air to obtain PCWP Be able to identify overwedging (spuriously high values with loss of trace above scale) Partial withdrawal of catheter if spontaneously wedging or overwedging
Inaccurate recordings	Fluctuations in waveform with respirations	Avoid monitors that calculate averages Monitors with graph and cursor to identify end respiratory point are better If latter unavailable, pulmonary artery diastolic pressure at end respiratory point may be used
	Effect of back rest position on recorded values	Recordings of PCWP and cardiac index should be made with patient in same position; evidence suggests that back rest positions up to 30° yield more accurate measurements* Keep transducers at mid-axilla, fourth intercostal level

PAFC = pulmonary artery flotation catheter; PCWP = pulmonary capillary wedge pressure; *data from Cline and Gurka (1991)

Key points

* Cannulation of the left ventricle for pressure monitoring purposes is both difficult and dangerous.

* Pulmonary arterial flotation catheters (PAFCs) allows indirect determination of left ventricular function by cannulation of the venous circulation.

* Cardiac output is determined by heart rate, preload, afterload and myocardial contractility.

* PAFCs are principally used for determination of pulmonary capillary wedge pressure and cardiac output.

* In the coronary care unit, pulmonary arterial flotation catheters are predominantly used to determine the aetiology of reduced cardiac output and pulmonary oedema.

References

Cline JK, Gurka AM (1991) Effect of backrest position on pulmonary artery pressure and cardiac output measurements in critically ill patients. *Crit Care Nurs* **18**(5): 383–9

Crexells C, Chatterjee K, Forrester JS *et al* (1973) Optimal level of filling pressure in the left side of the heart in acute myocardial infarction. *N Engl J Med* **289**(24): 1263–6

Eisenberg PR, Jaffe As, Schuster DP (1984) Clinical evaluation compared to pulmonary artery catheterisation in the haemodynamic assessment of critically ill patients. *Crit Care Med* **12**: 549–53

Forrester JS, Diamond G, McHugh TJ *et al* (1971) Filling pressures in the right and left sides of the heart in acute myocardial infarction: a reappraisal of central venous pressure monitoring. *N Engl J Med* **285**: 190–3

Forrester JS, Diamond G, Chatterjee K *et al* (1976) Medical therapy of acute myocardial infarction by application of haemodynamic subsets. *N Engl J Med* **295**: 1404

Gore JM, Goldberg RJ, Spodick DH *et al* (1987) A community wide assessment of the use of pulmonary artery catheters in patients with acute myocardial infarction. *Chest* **92**: 721–7

Shah KB, Rao TLK, Laughlin S *et al* (1984) A review of pulmonary artery catheterisation in 6245 patients. *Anesthesiology* **61**: 271–5

Singer M, Bennett ED (1989) Invasive haemodynamic monitoring in the United Kingdom. *Chest* **95**: 623–6

Swan HJC, Ganz W, Forrester J *et al* (1970) Catheterization of the heart in man with the use of a flow directed balloon tipped catheter. *N Engl J Med* **283**: 447–51

23

An introduction to the reading of electrocardiograms

Philip Woodrow

This chapter introduces the basic principles of reading electrocardiograms (ECGs) for nurses who are unfamiliar with reading them. The ECG records cardiac electrical activity as a graph; interpretation is illustrated here by sinus rhythm. A single ECG lead (lead II) is used throughout this chapter. Atrial fibrillation is described to show a contrasting dysrhythmia. Specific nursing care is suggested for patients being monitored or having ECGs taken.

As ECG monitoring in hospital is most often used when patients are suffering from heart disease, the ECGs seen in practice are likely to include abnormalities. However, these can be identified once the principles of the normal ECG are understood. This chapter is only an introduction to the subject. Like most aspects of care, understanding ECGs improves with practice. Readers should therefore use this chapter to obtain an understanding of the initial principles of interpretation, and then practise interpretation by relating these principles to the ECGs of patients in their care.

Interpretation is an advanced skill; practitioners who are unfamiliar with ECGs should not try to memorise everything they see and read about ECGs, but should focus on recognising the normal ECG, so that they can confidently recognise when an ECG is abnormal and seek assistance, even if they are unable to identify what the abnormality means.

An ECG is a graph of the electrical activity of the heart. It is therefore a two-dimensional picture of something that occurs in three dimensions. This means that the nurse needs to translate what is seen on paper to what is happening in the patient's heart. Thus, before translating, the nurse needs to become familiar with the language of ECGs.

Unlike standard mathematical graph paper, the large squares on ECG graph paper are divided only a further five times on each axis (making a total of 25 small squares in each large square). Each of the small squares measures 1mm x 1mm (Schamroth, 1990). As the ECG records at a constant speed (normally 25mm/s; Schamroth, 1990) the timing of the various stages of electrical activity can be read relatively easily. At 25mm/s, 25 small squares, or 5 large squares, are covered every second. So one large square represents 0.2 seconds, and one small square 0.04 seconds (Armstrong, 1985), as illustrated below.

Normally, electrical activity in the heart initiates muscle contraction. In this chapter, and for reading most ECGs, this will be assumed, although electrical and muscular activity can be uncoordinated (electro-mechanical dissociation is a dangerous, but relatively rare condition). Provided that there is no dissociation between electrical and muscular activity, muscle activity (contraction) will follow electrical stimulus. Muscle contraction causes the chambers of the heart to contract. Atrial contraction completes ventricular filling, while ventricular contraction results in the systolic phase of the cardiac cycle. Once active muscle contraction is complete, passive muscular relaxation initiates the diastolic phase of the cardiac cycle, which lasts until the next muscular contraction.

Diastole is the gap between systoles, so that tachycardias reduce the amount of diastolic time in the cycle. The subendocardial left ventricular muscle is perfused only during diastole (Ganong, 1997). Consequently, tachycardias inevitably reduce left ventricle muscle perfusion, at the same time as oxygen consumption by the left ventricular muscle is increased. If demand continues to exceed supply, the muscle will become ischaemic; if ischaemia persists, muscle will infarct.

Baseline of the ECG

When there is no electrical activity to record, the ECG will show a straight line, termed the isoelectric line (*Figure 23.1*). If this persists, the patient, having no electrical activity in his/her heart, has no cardiac muscle contraction. Since systole is absent, the patient is therefore in **asystole**. This is a cardiac arrest situation, so the resuscitation policy should be followed: the arrest (crash) call should be made and basic life support commenced.

Machines displaying ECGs, ie. monitors, will not record electrical activity if, for any reason, there is a break in the connection to the monitor (commonly a lead becoming disconnected from the patient, or drying of conduction gel). For example, the monitor of a patient carrying out normal activities of living (such as drinking a cup of tea) may appear to show asystole, so the nurse should always look at the patient as well as the monitor. ECGs are an adjunct to patient care, not a substitute for it.

The height of the isoelectric line on the graph is not significant, but can be adjusted to enable the complete ECG trace to be viewed.

The heart is three-dimensional, but the ECG has only two dimensions. So, in order to show a clearer picture of electrical activity, views are taken from a variety of places (or **leads**, see below). The same activity will therefore give a different picture from different leads. Some of these leads are **unipolar** (from one point only), and some are **bipolar** (travelling between two points).

Electrical activity of the heart will be recorded on the graph as movement away from the baseline. A rise from the baseline is called a **positive deflection**, and a fall a **negative deflection**. A positive deflection (*Figure 23.2*) means that electrical activity is following the same direction of flow as a bipolar lead, or travelling towards a unipolar lead. A negative deflection (*Figure 23.3*) is shown when the current goes in the opposite direction to a bipolar lead or away from a unipolar lead.

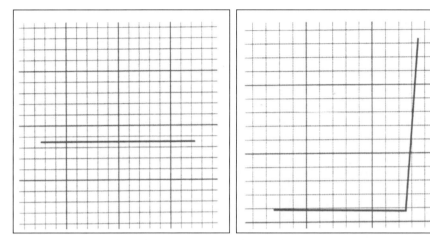

Figure 23.1: An isoelectric line   **Figure 23.2: A positive deflection**

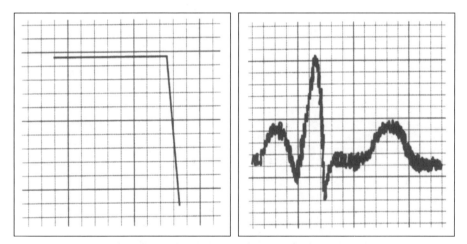

Figure 23.3: A negative deflection   **Figure 23.4: Artefact**

As the ECG is attached to the body by electrodes, it will record any electrical activity inside (or sometimes outside) the body. All body muscles move by electrical impulses. So, if a patient is shivering, there is much (non-cardiac) rapid muscle movement. This will be recorded on the ECG as a jagged line, or **artefact** (*Figure 23.4*). Artefact is anything appearing on the ECG trace that is not of cardiac origin. Artefact can usually be easily identified by its incongruity with other information shown on the trace. For example, *Figure 23.4* appears to show normal sinus rhythm, with the whole trace blurred by a jagged line. A jagged isoelectric line is often seen with atrial fibrillation (AF) (discussed later), but with AF the QRS complex would appear normal. The jaggedness here is therefore not a result of cardiac electrical activity; it is artefact.

Action potential

Some 1% of cardiac cells, unlike any other muscle cells, can initiate electrical impulses (Marieb, 1995). This ability to initiate impulses is called **automaticity**, and is a useful homeostatic safeguard against failure of the normal conduction mechanism. Normally, impulses originate from the sino-atrial (SA) node, controlled by the sympathetic and parasympathetic nervous systems. Electrical impulses spread through muscle cells owing to changes of ions between the intracellular and extracelluar fluid. The overall movement of these ions is referred to as an **action potential** (*Figure 23.5*), as ions move in or out of the cell at different electrical voltages. The voltages, although significant physiologically, are so small that they are measured in millivolts (thousandths of a volt).

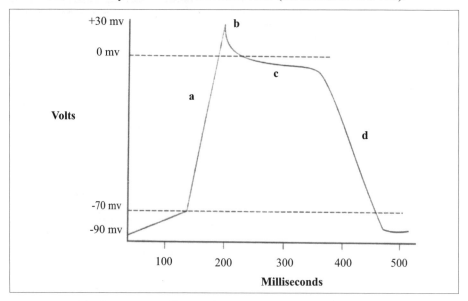

Figure 23.5: Action potential of a single cardiac muscle fibre.
a) rapid depolarisation — influx via fast sodium channel
b) fast calcium channel open
c) plateau — slow calcium channel open
d) rapid depolarisation — potassium channnel open

The action potential is the potential for action created by the balance between electrical charges of different ions on either side of the cell membrane. When there is no electrical activity present, the resting action potential of the heart is about -90mv (Ganong, 1997; Marieb, 1995). The three main ions involved with action potential are sodium, potassium and calcium. Intravascular levels of about 140mmol/litre of sodium and 4.0mmol/litre of potassium are reversed in the intracellular fluid. The high concentration of intracellular potassium makes the membrane of the resting cell more permeable to potassium than to other ions (Withington, 1997), so that potassium leaks slowly (and passively) from the intracellular fluid into the extracelluar space.

The first channel to open is the sodium channel, which enables ions from the sodium-rich extracelluar fluid to enter the sodium-poor intracellular fluid. Calcium then enters the cell via two channels: the fast or transient calcium (-40mv) and slow or long-lasting calcium (-30mv) channels (Ganong, 1997; Marieb, 1995). As the names suggest, the fast or transient calcium channel is open for a very brief time, giving the action potential graph its characteristic peak, but the slow calcium channel remains open for about 300–400 milliseconds (Withington, 1997), creating the subsequent plateau (*Figure 23.5*). The plateau phase (or absolute refractory period) prevents cardiac muscle from responding to further stimulus, thus ensuring coordinated contraction (Withington, 1997). The force of contraction is determined largely by the amount of intracellular calcium, so that the length of the plateau also influences contractile strength of the muscle fibre (Withington, 1997) which in turn determines stroke volume, and thus blood pressure.

The last channel to open is the potassium channel; at +8mv, ions from the potassium-rich intracellular fluid move across to the potassium-poor extracellular fluid. Voltage continues to rise until +30mv is reached. The transient change away from the resting negative charge is called **depolarisation** (Marieb, 1995). This whole process lasts only milliseconds (Marieb, 1995); the return to the resting charge of -90mv is called **repolarisation**.

ECG leads

An ECG lead refers to the view from which a graph is recorded. The word 'lead' should not be confused with the number of electrodes (and wires) used to make a recording (only 10 electrodes are used to record a 12-lead ECG).

Leads are divided into two main groups: limb leads and chest leads. To record a full 12-lead ECG, 10 electrodes are placed on the body. While each of the six chest electrodes records one lead each, the four limb electrodes record six different views of cardiac electrical activity. There are a number of ECG leads (12 are standardly used in the UK). The six limb leads show a vertical picture of electrical activity; the six chest leads surround the heart from the right atrium (chest lead 1) to the left atrium (chest lead 6), indicating horizontal perspectives. Confusingly, some texts refer to the chest leads by the prefix 'C', whereas others use 'V'; the prefixes are, however, interchangeable.

Understanding all 12 leads is an advanced skill; nurses who are unfamiliar with taking or reading ECGs are advised to focus on one commonly used lead. Once one lead is understood, the principles can then be applied to the other leads. Understanding all 12 leads enables the three-dimensional electrical activity of the heart to be deduced from the two-dimensional graph.

Monitors that do not offer a choice of lead, or texts that do not identify which lead is shown, normally use lead II. Lead II is the limb lead read from the right arm (red electrode) to the left foot (black or green electrode). This assumes that the electrodes have been placed correctly; machines will not correct human error. Nurses taking and reading ECGS should check electrode placement, as misplaced leads are fairly common. When most monitors were only capable of reading lead II, electrodes were often deliberately misplaced to gain readings of other leads; now that most monitors offer a choice of leads displayed, deliberate misplacement is unnecessary and potentially confusing, but unfortunately is still often practised. To aid correct placement, electrodes are colour coded. The sequence can be memorised as similar to a traffic light (right arm=red, left arm=yellow, left leg=green or black). When recording 12-lead ECGs, a fourth limb electrode (black) is placed on the right leg (the green electrode being placed on the left leg).

The picture of electrical activity in the heart remains constant at any point on the limb. An electrode placed on the right wrist will show the same waveform as one placed on the right elbow or right shoulder. So the electrical picture taken by lead II is effectively right shoulder to left neck of femur. This follows the main direction of flow (**vector**) of electrical activity in the heart: SA node, to atrio-ventricular (AV) node, and down the bundle of His (also called the atrioventricular bundle). As lead II is closest to the normal heart's own vector (*Figure 23.6*), it is the most appropriate lead for standard monitoring, the usual default lead of most monitors, and the lead used throughout this chapter.

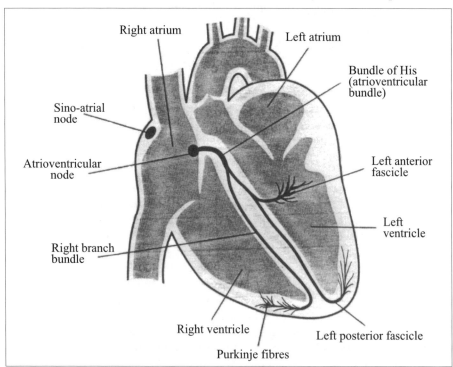

Figure 23.6: Diagrammatic representation of the normal electrical conduction pathways in the heart

The normal heart

In health, conduction of electrical impulses in the heart (*Figure 23.6*) starts at the SA node (Boltz, 1994) and spreads through the muscles of the atria (there are also some specialised atrial bundles of conduction fibres). As the SA node is near the top right-hand corner of the heart, the direction of the impulses is from the right shoulder towards the left leg. This is the same direction that lead II follows, so a positive deflection occurs. This first positive deflection, representing atrial depolarisation, is labelled the P wave (*Figure 23.7*). Because impulses spread from muscle fibre to muscle fibre, rather than through specialised conduction

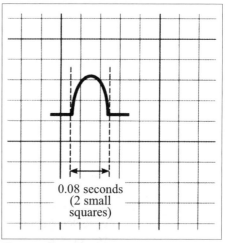

Figure 23.7: P wave

tissue, conduction is relatively slow in relation to the small muscle mass of the atria. This makes a normal P wave appear broad in relation to its height: a normal P wave lasts 0.08 seconds (Marieb, 1995) (2 small squares wide).

The ECG graph returns to the isoelectric baseline as electrical conduction is briefly delayed at the **AV node**. This slowing is measured on the ECG by the distance from the start of the P wave to the start of the R wave, called the **PR interval** (*Figure 23.8*). The PR interval will normally last between 0.12 and 0.2 seconds (3–5 small squares) (Hampton, 1997a). The Q wave, a negative deflection, is not always seen on ECGs. Its absence does not usually indicate a problem. A normal Q wave (less than 1 small square wide; Wark, 1997) is caused by electrical activity moving across the muscle fibres of the septum (depolarisation). An enlarged Q wave suggests an infarction (Hampton, 1997b).

The **atrioventricular bundle** or **bundle of His** is a specialised collection of conduction fibres, through which the electrical impulse is conducted more quickly than it was conducted across the atria. The direction of the impulse is similar to that in lead II, so the deflection is strongly positive (*Figure 23.8*). From the AV node onwards, all electrical activity seen takes place in the ventricles. The bundle of His divides into two branches: **a right bundle branch** and **a left bundle branch**. As the left ventricular muscle mass is larger than the right, the left branch further divides into the anterior (front) and posterior (rear) **fascicles** (fascicle = branch) (*Figure 23.6*) (Wilson, 1983).

The main direction of flow of current remains towards the left leg for most of the time; however, towards the end of the impulse, distal fibres of the branches, called **Purkinje fibres**, allow conduction to spread rapidly throughout the ventricular muscle mass, causing a final negative deflection of the RS line below the isoelectric line.

The S wave completes electrical impulses through the muscle. Despite the size of muscle mass covered, the specialised conduction pathway has allowed the impulse to pass quickly through the ventricular muscle mass. A normal QRS width lasts 0.12 seconds (within 3 small squares) (Hampton, 1997a) (*Figure 23.8*). Comparing this with the P wave or PR interval illustrates the speed of ventricular impulses. This speed enables co-ordinated contraction of the large ventricular muscle mass, ensuring an effective output (stroke volume, felt by the pulse). After the S wave the ECG should return to the isoelectric line.

A final impulse recorded by the ECG is the repolarisation of the ventricular muscle, representing the return of a -90mv charge as the muscle relaxes before the next electrical impulse. On the ECG, repolarisation is represented by the T wave (*Figure 23.9*). A normal T wave should be positive, and is separated from the S wave by a brief return to the isoelectric line. The T wave is shaped much like a P wave, only slightly larger; a normal T wave lasts 0.16 seconds (Marieb, 1995) (4 small squares). The length of

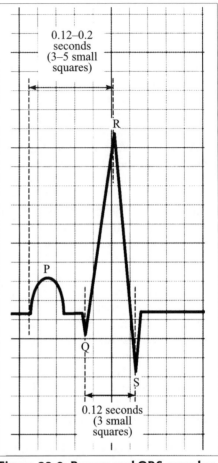

Figure 23.8: P wave and QRS complex, showing the PR interval

time between the S and T waves (ST segment) is unimportant, but if the isoelectric line does not look normal between the S and the T wave (it can appear raised or depressed; *Figure 23.10*), there is a problem with depolarisation, commonly due to infarction, ischaemia or abnormal potassium (or other electrolyte) levels.

Sinus rhythm

The description above has followed a single complex of the ECG. A pattern of complexes is called a rhythm. A pattern repeating the complexes is referred to as **sinus rhythm**, the normal rhythm originating from the SA node. For nursing staff who are unfamiliar with reading ECGs an important first step is to be able to recognise this rhythm, so that anything different can be identified as abnormal.

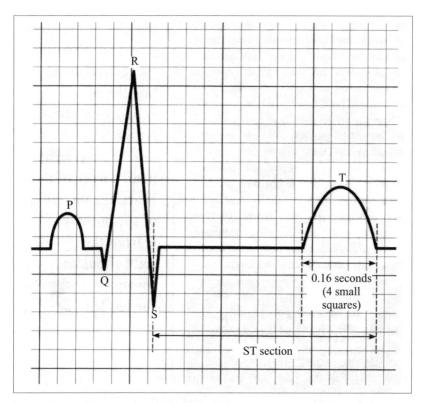

Figure 23.9: Normal sinus rhythm complex: P wave, QRS and T wave

The ECG provides much information in a relatively small space. To help interpret this information a logical system is recommended. The simplest systems start at the beginning of the complex (the P wave), and work through each stage in turn, just as the description above has worked step by step through the complex. At each stage, nurses should ask whether the complex looks normal or not (*Table 23.1*).

For a rhythm to be regular, the complex will appear at regular intervals on the ECG trace, with a regular distance betwccn any two identical parts of different complexes. Regularity is best measured by taking a prominent place (the R wave is usually easiest) on two complexes, and seeing whether this distance is repeated between all complexes. This can be done by tracing the RR interval on scrap paper, then moving the marked paper one or more complexes along the trace.

With practice, many abnormalities can be differentiated. For staff who have not yet developed these more advanced skills, the ability to recognise that some abnormality is present, and so alert more experienced staff, is a valuable and appropriate contribution to care.

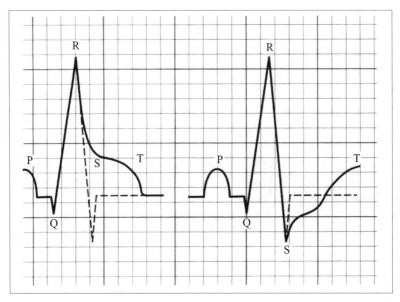

Figure 23.10: Depressed and elevated ST segments (normal ST segment shown by dotted line)

Abnormal rhythms may be normal for individual patients, or represent a pathological change in rhythm. As ECGs will usually be recorded to confirm or rule out cardiac disease, in practice a disproportionate number of ECGs taken show some abnormality. Any rhythm that deviates from sinus rhythm may be described as an abnormality. However, not all 'abnormal rhythms' are pathological, so they will usually only be treated if symptoms cause problems. To illustrate variance from normal sinus rhythm, AF is now described.

Atrial fibrillation

AF is the most common dysrhythmia requiring medical treatment (Donovan and Hockings, 1997). Fibrillation is uncoordinated contraction of muscles, so AF is caused by uncoordinated contraction of atrial muscle. As the SA node fails to coordinate atrial muscle contraction, impulses are initiated at other foci in the atria (owing to the automaticity of cardiac muscle). With some dysrhythmias, this may cause another specific focus to coordinate contraction; with AF, firing of various atrial foci causes a number of different impulses of various strengths. The atrial rate will often be very rapid — Ganong (1997) cites rates of 300–500 causing the atrial muscle to 'quiver'. The 'quivering' causes the ECG baseline to appear as either a fine wave or a straight line (increasing the size, sometimes called the 'gain', of the ECG may reveal the uneven baseline).

Relatively few of these rapid impulses will reach and fire the AV node; Ganong (1997) cites ventricular rates of 80–160 as common). Those that do pass the AV node will be irregularly spaced. Provided that there is no other cardiac pathology, conduction from the AV node will be normal, causing each QRS complex to appear normal. However, there will not usually be any pattern to the frequency of QRS complexes (and hence ventricular contractions) on the ECG.

Following the guide for reading ECGs (*Table 23.1*), the ECG will appear as irregular, and irregularly irregular (*Figure 23.11*). The overall rate may be fast, normal or slow, but will usually be irregular and may be volatile. Monitors displaying pulse rates will show constantly changing figures, and the pulse will feel irregular. P waves will be absent, but QRS complexes and T waves will be normal.

AF affects many people and is often caused by cardiac disease. It becomes increasingly common with advancing age (Donovan and Hockings, 1997), but may also be induced by other conditions, such as hypothermia below 34°C (Aun, 1997). Provided that the ventricular rate is near normal and the person remains asymptomatic ('controlled AF'), medical intervention is unlikely. AF may be controlled well with drugs; digoxin is the drug of choice for chronic AF (Donovan and Hockings, 1997). Recent onset, but persistent, AF (lasting more than 36 hours) may be treated by cardioversion (Donovan and Hockings, 1997).

The abbreviation 'AF' should not be confused with **atrial flutter**, which is a different, and usually more sinister, dysrhythmia.

Table 23.1: Reading the electro-cardiogram (ECG)
Are the electrodes correctly placed (red = right arm, yellow = left arm, green/black = left leg)?
Is there a clear baseline (isoelectric line)?
Can P waves be seen?
Are the P waves within two small squares?
Are the P waves positive?
Is there one P wave before every QRS?
Is the PR interval 3–5 small squares?
Is the QRS positive?
Is the QRS within 3 small squares?
Does the isoelectric line return between the S and the T?
Is the T wave positive?
Is the T wave contained within 4 small squares?
Is the RR interval regular?

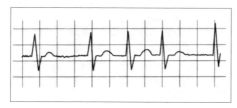

Figure 23.11: Atrial fibrillation

Caring for the patient

As with any procedure, the ECG should be explained to the patient before it is recorded. It is worth stressing to patients that the machine records electrical activity already in the heart; it does not put electricity into their body. Most patients are likely to be satisfied with this explanation, and some may be familiar with having their ECG recorded; however, if the patient still appears anxious, he/she may be reassured by seeing the nurse place the electrodes on herself to show that it is harmless.

Adhesive electrodes are designed to stay in place despite movement by patients. While this reduces the likelihood of displacement, it also makes them potentially uncomfortable to remove, particularly if stuck to body hair. It may therefore be necessary to remove body hair in areas where electrodes are to be placed. Continuous monitoring limits the patient's mobility. It may be safe to disconnect the patient from the monitor for short periods (such as to go to the bathroom), but if unsure seek advice. Medical treatment may rely on maximising rest for the patient. A clear plan of nursing care should be made and used so that all members of the nursing team (including the patient) understand what should and should not be done; the patient should, whenever possible, be involved in drawing up this plan of care. Anyone who is unsure of the patient's needs and limitations should seek advice.

In the past, ECG monitoring was initiated by doctors. But expansion of nursing roles empowers many nurses to decide whether or not to record ECGs. Like any observation, recording a single ECG or initiating continuous monitoring is only justified if the information will benefit diagnosis, treatment or care of the patient; no observation should be 'routine'. With continuous monitoring the benefits of potential medical information from the ECG should be weighed against anxiety caused to the patient by being monitored, and the restrictions placed on the patient's mobility by being attached to a machine. A single ECG recording does not cause serious problems with immobility, although it may still create anxiety.

A 12-lead ECG can provide much information about cardiac electrical activity, and is valuable if the nurse suspects there may have been a significant change in cardiac conduction or if the effects of drugs and other medical interventions need to be monitored. A 12-lead ECG gives more information than most continuous bedside monitors, and can therefore usefully clarify significant changes seen in monitored waveforms.

Continuous monitoring is useful where concern over cardiac instability (or potential cardiac instability) outweighs problems of anxiety and immobility caused by the monitor to the patient. The appropriateness of monitoring each patient should thus be individually assessed by the nurse planning each patient's care. Patients with acute or unstable cardiac conditions are likely to benefit from close monitoring. As with any other nursing or medical observations, the usefulness of information is limited by how effectively it is used.

The monitor itself is a potential source of danger to the patient and others. Because it uses electricity (even though it does not put electricity into the patient), it should be kept away from water, and inspected for safety (such as damaged wires from the mains). Many monitors are also relatively heavy, and should not be placed where they could fall on a patient or anyone else; the top of a bedside locker or table may not be a suitable place for a monitor. Particular caution should be used with patients suffering from confusional states, where pulling of wires may cause the monitor to follow. Even the lightest ECG monitor can cause considerable harm.

Conclusion

The attraction of mastering the reading of ECGs may obscure a holistic patient focus. For nursing, the technical skill is only an adjunct to care. Therefore, nurses should consider the impact that recording an ECG will have on their patients. Like any other aspect of care, recording an ECG is only justified if the benefits to the patient outweigh the burdens.

Nurses who are unfamiliar with reading ECGs should initially gain confidence by understanding and recognising normal sinus rhythm. They should develop their knowledge so that they may recognise the common arrest rhythms, followed by the rhythms that commonly lead to these arrest situations. However, such advanced skills are beyond the scope of this chapter. Nurses who are unfamiliar with reading ECGs should consult their colleagues if they have concerns about the trace, or do not understand what to look for with a particular patient.

Recognising abnormal ECGs is largely a skill of understanding and applying knowledge of abnormal physiology. There are a number of reliable texts that will help nurses to further their knowledge, and study days and courses are frequently advertised. There are many ways to continue to extend understanding of ECGs. A clear understanding of the basic principles, and taking every opportunity to apply existing knowledge to practice, should give the nurse a reliable foundation for future development.

Key points

* The electrocardiogram (ECG) is a two-dimensional diagram representing three-dimensional electrical activity in the heart.
* Lead II is the standard lead for understanding the principles of ECGs.
* A logical framework assists interpretation of the information.
* Applying the principles to other leads and rhythms is an advanced skill.
* The ECG is a useful adjunct to care, but it should be remembered that the patient is always more important than the monitor.

References

Armstrong M (1985) *Electrocardiograms: A Systematic Method of Reading Them.* Wright and Sons, Bristol

Aun C (1997) Thermal disorders. In: Oh T (ed) *Intensive Care Manual.* 4th edn. Butterworth-Heinemann, Oxford: 630–40

Boltz M (1994) Nurse's guide to identifying cardiac rhythms. *Nursing* **94** 24(4):54–8

Donovan K, Hockings B (1997) Cardiac arrhythmias. In: Oh T (ed) *Intensive Care Manual.* 4th edn. Butterworth-Heinemann, Oxford: 67–93

Ganong W (1997) *Review of Medical Physiology.* 18th edn. Appleton and Lange, Connecticut

Hampton J (1997a) *The ECG Made Easy.* 5th edn. Churchill Livingstone, Edinburgh

Hampton J (1997b) *The ECG in Practice.* 3rd edn. Churchill Livingstone, Edinburgh

Marieb E (1995) *Human Anatomy and Physiology.* 3rd edn. The Benjamin/Cummings Publishing Company, Redwood City, California

Schamroth L (1990) *An Introduction to Electrocardiography.* 7th edn. Blackwell Scientific, Oxford

Wark K (1997) Electrocardiography, defibrillation, pacing and pacemakers. In: Goldhill D, Withington S (eds) *Textbook of Intensive Care.* Chapman and Hall Medical, London: 313–24

Wilson V (1983) *Cardiac Nursing.* Blackwell Scientific, Oxford

Withington P (1997) Cardiovascular physiology. In: Goldhill D, Withington S (eds) *Textbook of Intensive Care.* Chapman and Hall, London: 237–43

24

Blood pressure measurement: rational and ritual actions in clinical nursing and midwifery

David O'Brien and Maria Barrell

There is a prevailing wisdom that the taking and recording of arterial blood pressure is a non-problematic nursing activity. Closer scrutiny reveals that the practices surrounding the taking and recording of blood pressure are subject to rational and ritual actions that have considerable significance for nursing practice.

Observation of nurses and midwives taking and recording blood pressure reveals a strange mixture of rational scientific actions laced with rituals that seem divorced from clinical decision making.

Blood pressure may be defined as the force exerted by blood against the walls of the vessels in which it is contained (Pritchard and David, 1988). It is determined by a number of factors, most significantly cardiac output, peripheral resistance, elasticity of vessels and hormonal and chemical control mechanisms.

Variation in blood pressure occurs as a result of age, exercise, emotional state, weight, gender and race. It is also influenced by the health status of the individual and as such is recognised as a major assessment observation in nursing. Consequently, the appropriate and accurate measurement and recording of blood pressure is a core nursing and midwifery skill.

There is a common assumption that nurses and midwives can easily master the taking and measuring of blood pressure in the early weeks of their professional education and that it is a procedure that does not need to be readdressed. Contemporary research suggests that, far from being unproblematic, the taking and recording of blood pressure is a complex nursing activity that draws upon knowledge of physiological, psychological and social sciences.

The practitioner is required to perform the skills involved competently in a variety of clinical settings, while initial teaching is usually classroom based (or completely absent). An added complexity are the rituals, custom and practice that have traditionally determined who has their blood pressure taken, when and how frequently.

Measuring and recording blood pressure

Most major introductory nursing texts offer at least an introduction to the importance of blood pressure measurement in the nursing assessment (Hinchliff *et al*, 1993; Brunner and Suddarth, 1992), while others have more substantial discussion (Sorensen and Luckmann, 1986; Boore *et al*, 1987; Royle and Walsh, 1992).

Similarly, articles in a number of journals are primarily concerned with ensuring accurate measurement and recording of blood pressure (Petrie *et al*, 1986; Draper, 1987; Jewell, 1987; Hill and Grim, 1991; Jolly, 1991; Cook, 1996). There is a range of factors that enhance the accuracy of blood pressure measurement and recording (*Table 24.1*).

Table 24.1: Factors that enhance the accuracy of arterial blood pressure measurement and recording	
Patient	Sitting or lying for at least three minutes
	No clothing on arm
	Arm supported level with heart
	Psychologically calm
	No recent smoking or alcohol consumption
Equipment	Bladder cuff: Croft and Cruikshank (1990) recommend that the cuff should cover at least 80% of the arm circumference. Drawing upon the recommendations of the American Heart Association, Brunner and Suddarth (1990) and Andersen and Bergsten (1982) stress the importance of matching cuff dimensions to the patient's arm circumference
	Sphygmomanometer calibrated 6-monthly
	Sphygmomanometer and stethoscope regularly maintained
	Stand-mounted sphygmomanometer preferred (mobile with a vertical mercury column)
Observer	No hearing deficit (if present a special stethoscope may be used)
	Understanding of what constitutes a consistent, accurate technique
	Good initial education
	Opportunities for updating and practice
Technique	Patient's arm must be adequately supported
	Detect point of maximum pressure over brachial artery (may be marked lightly with a felt pen)
	Cuff should be fitted firmly and comfortably and be well secured
	Centre of cuff bladder should be placed over brachial artery
	Lower edge of cuff bladder should be 2–3 cm above marked site

Auscultatory measurement technique

Based on the principles established in *Table 24.1*, the following method of auscultatory measurement is recommended:

1. Inflate the cuff for 3–5 seconds until brachial pulsation ceases (this is the estimated systolic pressure — do not use a stethoscope

2. Deflate the cuff and place the stethoscope over the marked site. The stethoscope must not be pressed firmly or come in contact with the cuff, otherwise diastolic pressure can be greatly underestimated

3. Inflate the cuff rapidly to 30mmHg above the estimated systolic blood pressure

4. Deflate the cuff 2–3mmHg every second, noting the point at which clear repetitive tapping sounds first appear for two consecutive beats — this is the systolic pressure

5. The point at which these sounds finally disappear is the diastolic pressure. If these sounds do not disappear, the point of muffling (Korotkoff phase 4) should be used to estimate diastolic pressure. This method is used routinely in pregnancy (De Swiet and Shennan, 1996)

6. The blood pressure should be recorded to the nearest 2mmHg.

(NB. Korotkoff sounds are audible, using a stethoscope, following the release of pressure on the compressed brachial artery. These were first described by Korotkoff in 1905.)

Potential sources of variation and error

Variation and error can occur because of characteristics in four major areas: the observer, the patient, the technique and the equipment (Boore *et al*, 1987; Jewell, 1987).

Observer

The observer may have either hearing or cognitive deficits that influence blood pressure measurement. Cognitive deficits are a result of poor initial education. Feher *et al* (1992) found that in a sample of qualified doctors, 43% did not know the extent to which the arm should be covered with the cuff bladder, 61% did not know the occasions for using Korotkoff 4 sounds for measuring diastolic blood pressure, and 59% were prepared to round the reading to the nearest 5–10mmHg.

Similar problems were noted by Kemp *et al* (1993) in their study of 100 nurses. They found that 40% claimed to have had no formal training in the technique, 75% had had no further update in the technique since qualification, only 4% had received updates within the past year, and 50% admitted to occasional estimation of systolic, diastolic or both. The authors concluded that knowledge of blood pressure measurement and technique is poor and is probably related to inadequate training.

Patient

Certain patient characteristics are positively correlated with potential errors in blood pressure measurement. Physical and physiological variables include excessive heat, cold, constrictive clothing and a full bladder. Behaviours associated with alterations in blood pressure include smoking, alcohol consumption and brisk physical activity. Psychosocial variables include anxiety, excitement and stressful lifestyle (Jewell, 1987).

Technique

Poor technique is another potential source of measurement error and this includes excessive stethoscope pressure (giving an artificially low diastolic pressure), excessively fast or slow deflation of the cuff, non-support of the patient's arm (giving false high systolic pressure), repeating blood pressure measurement before one minute has elapsed, and not applying the cuff firmly and evenly in the correct position. Incorrect cuff width is also associated with errors in measurement (Maxwell, 1982; Anderson and Bergsten, 1982; Brunner and Suddarth, 1990; Croft and Cruickshank, 1990).

Errors arising from faulty equipment are common. Conceicao *et al* (1976) found that almost half the sphygmomanometers in a teaching hospital group had defects and that maintenance was poor. The correct calibration of sphygmomanometers is clearly essential for accurate recording and, in this respect, it is suggested that aneroid sphygmomanometers are less robust than mercury ones. Cuffs that are too short are associated with an over estimation of blood pressure in tall and obese patients.

Blood pressure measurement as ritual behaviour

Ritualistic and non-rational actions by clinical nursing staff have been observed by several authors (Menzies, 1960; Chapman, 1983; Kilgour and Speedie, 1985; Walsh and Ford, 1989). Such action could be viewed as the antithesis of the problem-solving, holistic, research-based approach to care inherent in most modern philosophies of nursing and midwifery care. Such actions convey a reliance upon routines, procedures and outmoded practices that have little relevance for the contemporary critical practitioner.

The taking and recording of blood pressures at fixed and predetermined times, unrelated to the clinical status of the individual patients, could suggest a lack of clinical judgement and insight. However, the taking and recording of blood pressures are significant acts, psychologically and socially as well as clinically. For example, Menzies (1960), using a psychoanalytic approach, argued that such routines were functional in protecting individuals against anxiety.

The routinisation of procedures such as blood pressure taking contributed to the establishment of social systems that were based upon task allocation and, as such, protected the practitioner from the potential stressors of holistic nursing care. At the time that Menzies was undertaking her research, student nurses were not prepared for individualised patient care. Indeed, they were advised not to get too closely involved with patients and their problems but to focus instead upon a task-oriented approach to care. Elements of this approach are still prevalent in contemporary clinical practice as evidenced by the routine monitoring of vital observations, including the ritualisation of blood pressure measurement and recording.

Using a social action perspective, Chapman (1983) suggested that non-rational actions, eg. the routinised taking of blood pressure for no demonstrable clinical purpose, are not meaningless actions but convey meaning and concern; they demonstrate to both the patient and significant peers the caring commitment of the nurse. Such actions are learnt during professional socialisation and, like all learnt behaviours, are likely to be resistant to change and have strong symbolic significance. This can be reinforced if, for example, medical staff request rigidly timed observations that are not subsequently reviewed.

An example of the power of this learnt behaviour is a patient with diabetes who is admitted to a medical ward for routine investigation, and who might also be mildly hypertensive. Such a patient would normally have his blood pressure recorded 6-monthly by his GP, but because he is admitted to hospital it is likely to be recorded daily or more frequently even though it is unrelated to his current clinical problem.

In this situation, the effect of such routine may be disruptive and anxiety provoking for the patient. However, patients with considerable experience of hospital life often have an expectation that such routine practices are necessary and may be concerned if excluded from these unnecessary observations.

Burroughs and Hoffbrand (1990) found that, despite the absence of specific policies, 78% of nurses in their survey believed that policies did exist that required all new admissions to have their blood pressures recorded 4-hourly, and all postoperative patients to have their blood pressures recorded half-hourly. The study did not identify the time scale over which these observations were to be made.

Similarly, Kilgour and Speedie (1985) found that a significant number of patients had their postoperative blood pressure measurements continued well beyond the period that this observation was clinically stable; the reason for this continued recording was to establish routines rather than patient need.

Burroughs and Hoffbrand (1990) found that, despite the absence of specific policies, 78% of nurses in their survey believed that policies did exist that required all new admissions to have their blood pressures recorded four hourly, and all post-operative patients to have their blood pressures recorded half hourly. The study did not identify the time scale over which these observations were to be made. Similarly, Kilgour and Speedie (1985) found that a significant number of patients had their postoperative blood pressure measurements continued well beyond the period that this observation was clinically stable; the reason for this continued recording was to establish routines rather than patient need.

Burroughs and Hoffbrand (1990) found that the reasons why nurses continue with routine observations include the following: observations that have been stable for some time give nurses a sense of security; fear of missing something; and fear of medico-legal implications if such observations are not made (paradoxically, the authors argue that recording errors increase sharply with the number that have to be done, especially if the rationale for doing them is unclear).

Implications for nursing and midwifery theory and practice

During the past two decades the emphasis in nursing has evolved from routine, ritual and procedures, to individualised, problem-solving and researched-based approaches to care. This has presented considerable challenges to a profession unused to justifying the rationale for current practice.

The skilled assessment of physiological parameters, including the taking and recording of blood pressure, remains crucial to the practice of nursing, as is the justification for such observations. At one extreme it can be regarded as a common, non-problematic, nursing activity, while at the other it is an activity with suspect reliability and validity.

The ritualistic elements inherent in blood pressure measurement originate from an era of nursing where critical thought and careful reflection were not valued concepts in mainstream education. Nursing activities were based upon set procedures that could be easily applied to most nursing situations.

Once established, such rituals readily became part of the nursing culture and provided comfort and certainty to nurses in their daily work. It is not surprising that nurses are reluctant to challenge cherished and established approaches to practice, especially when the alternatives demand individualised considerations, notions of appropriate clinical decision making and professional accountability.

Conclusion

A careful and systematic look at everyday nursing actions will often reveal scope for reappraisal of practice. This appraisal will need to examine not only the rational elements of nursing actions but also the associated rituals and routines.

Key points

* Despite considerable evidence to the contrary, there is a commonly held assumption that the taking and recording of blood pressure is an unproblematic activity.
* Research indicates that nurses' knowledge, measurement and recording of blood pressure varies considerably.
* The measurement and recording of blood pressure is related to traditions and rituals that are not supported by patients' clinical needs.
* Opportunities for nurses to revise and update their knowledge and skills of blood pressure taking are sparse and need extending.
* Nurses need to use more professional judgement in deciding whether to continue or discontinue observations of blood pressure.

References

American Heart Association (1967) Recommendations for human blood pressure determination by sphygmomanometers. *Circulation* **36**: 980–8

Andersen HR, Bergsten O (1982) *Blood Pressure: Measurement and Methods.* S & W Medico Teknik, Albertslund

Boore JRP, Champion R, Furguson MC (1987) *Nursing the Physically Ill Adult.* Churchill Livingstone, Edinburgh: 613–6

Brunner LS, Suddarth DS (1990) *Lippincott Manual of Medical and Surgical Nursing.* Harper and Row, London: 356

Brunner LS, Suddarth DS (1992) *The Textbook of Adult Nursing.* Chapman and Hall, London: 316–17

Burroughs J, Hoffbrand BI (1990) A critical look at nursing observations. *Postgrad Med J* **66**: 370–2

Chapman GE (1983) Ritual and rational action in hospitals. *J Adv Nurs* **8**: 13–20

Conceicao S, Ward MK, Kerr DNS (1976) Defects in sphygmomanometers: an important source of error in blood pressure recording. *Br Med J* **i**: 886–8

Cook R (1996) Measuring and recording blood pressure. *Nurs Standard* **11**(7): 51–4

Croft PR, Cruickshank JK (1990) Blood pressure measurement in adults: large cuffs for all? *J Epidemiol Community Health* **44**: 170–3

De Swiet M, Shennan A (1996) Blood pressure management in pregnancy. *Br J Obstetrics and Gynaecology* **103**: 862–3

Draper P (1987) Nursing practice. Not a job for juniors. *Nurs Times* **83**(11 March): 58–62

Feher M, Harris-St John K, Lant A (1992) Blood pressure measurement by junior hospital doctors — a gap in medical education? *Health Trends* **24**(2): 59–61

Hill MN, Grim CM (1991) How to take a precise blood pressure. *Am J Nurs* **91**: 38–42

Hinchliff SM, Norman SE, Schober JE, eds (1993) *Nursing Practice and Health Care.* 2nd edn. Edward Arnold, London: 121–2

Jewell D (1987) Taking blood pressure. *Update* **35**: 934–41

Jolly A (1991) Taking blood pressure. *Nurs Times* **8**(15): 40–3

Kemp F, Foster C, McKinlay S (1993) Blood pressure measurement technique of clinical staff. *J Hum Hypertens* **7**: 95–102

Kilgour D, Speedie G (1985) Taking the pressure off. *Nurs Mirror* **160**(9): 39–40

Maxwell MH (1982) Error in blood pressure measurement due to incorrect cuff size in obese patients. *Lancet* **ii**: 33–6

Menzies IEP (1960) A case study in the functioning of social systems as a defence against anxiety. *Human Relations* **13**: 95–121

Petrie JC, O'Brien ET, Littler WA *et al* (1986) Recommendations on blood pressure measurement. *Br Med J* **293**: 611–5

Prichard AP, David JA (1988) *Royal Marsden Hospital: Manual of Clinical Nursing Procedures.* 2nd edn. Harper and Row, London: 259–64

Royle JA, Walsh M (1992) *Watson's Medical-Surgical Nursing and Related Physiology.* Baillière Tindall, London: 294–7

Sorensen KC, Luckmann J (1986) *Basic Nursing: A Psychophysiological Approach.* 2nd edn. WB Saunders, London: 538–46

Walsh M, Ford P (1989) *Nursing Rituals: Research and Rational Actions.* Butterworth-Heinemann, Oxford: 50–69

25

Care and management of peripherally inserted central catheters

Janice Gabriel

It is estimated that 85% of all patients admitted to hospitals in the USA in 1991 were recipients of a vascular access device (Barbone, 1995). Down-sizing of hospitals and the shift towards more outpatient and day-care procedures has meant that patients admitted to hospitals in the UK are more likely to be recipients of a vascular access device than they were ten years ago, as their conditions are more likely to be acute. This chapter will discuss how, with careful management, peripherally inserted central catheters can improve the reliability and quality of vascular access for many patients.

According to Goodwin and Carlson (1993), only vascular catheters inserted into the cephalic, median cubital or basilic veins in the antecubital fossa and which have their tips in the superior vena cava should be referred to as peripherally inserted central catheters (PICCs). Other, shorter catheters inserted by the same technique but not having their tips extend beyond the axillary vein should be described as midline peripherally inserted catheters.

Unlike other central venous catheters, a PICC line has only one or two lumens. This is because the cephalic and basilic veins are too small to accommodate a larger catheter. However, PICCs are available in a variety of sizes ranging from 2 Fr to 5 Fr. Like other central venous access devices PICCs are either open-ended or valved. The Groshong valve is a three-position valve, which is incorporated into the tip of the catheter. In the absence of a negative or positive pressure the valve remains in the closed position, thus preventing blood from the venous circulation entering the lumen or lumens. (If the patient requires more than two lumens there is no reason why two PICCs cannnot be placed, eg. a single lumen into the cephalic and a dual lumen into the basilic [Sansivero, 1997]).

Because PICCs are so fine and flexible they can easily be inserted through a smaller introducer, similar to a conventional cannula, with the minimum of trauma to the patient. Indeed, all patients in whom I have placed a PICC say that it is no more uncomfortable than having a conventional peripheral cannula inserted.

Indications

PICCs have been used in the USA since the late 1970s. Prain and Van Way (1978) advocated such devices for patients requiring infusion of hypertonic and vesicant drugs and fluids. This is because the tip of the PICC terminates in a large blood vessel, ie. the superior vena cava, thus preventing chemical irritation of the walls of smaller veins. Consequently, the incidence of chemical phlebitis is greatly diminished. Kyle and Myers (1989) reinforced the advice of Prain and Van Way (1978).

Because PICCS are placed by cannulating a peripheral vein, they are associated with markedly fewer insertion problems than other types of central venous access devices (Brown, 1989). The reason for this is that other types require more invasive surgical or percutaneous techniques for placement which can result in an increased incidence of the following:

1. Pneumothorax
2. Haemothorax
3. Air embolism
4. Venous thrombosis
5. Infection.

As highlighted above, PICCs have proved to be clinically less problematic than other central venous access devices, and their insertion procedure is relatively straightforward and comfortable for the patient. Kyle and Myers (1989) suggested that a PICC should be considered for any patient requiring vascular access for more than five days. Indeed, Barbone (1995) concluded that if a PICC is managed carefully there is no reason why it cannot remain in situ for up to 12 months.

Since PICC placements can be successfully undertaken by a suitably skilled nurse in the ward or outpatient setting, UK nurses who are currently involved in establishing short-term venous access could widen their scope of practice to include this technique (Gabriel, 1996). This would not only be cost-effective compared with the procedures required for placing tunnelled catheters and implantable injection ports, but also would allow the nurse to become involved in assessing the patient's clinical needs and lifestyle for consideration of a longer-term vascular access device. Apart from the cost savings achieved by selecting the most suitable device from the outset, there would also be an improvement in the quality and continuity of patient care.

In the clinical setting of oncology nursing I have placed a number of PICC lines in patients for no other reason than needle phobia. Each of these patients was then able to complete his/her course of treatment without having to experience any further venepunctures.

Selecting a suitable vein

If the patient has a readily accessible cephalic, basilic or median cubital vein (*Figure 25.1*), the most difficult part of the PICC placement is cannulating the vein. Once the vein has been selected, the distance from the intended insertion site to the proximal end of the clavicle should be measured; a line of this length will ensure that the tip of the PICC reaches the superior vena cava (*Figure 25.2*). The exact position of the PICC should be confirmed by a chest X-ray before using the line (Hadaway, 1989). Local hospital policy will determine whether the nurse placing the PICC can request the post-insertion X-ray. Regardless of which healthcare professional requests the X-ray, the position of the PICC should be confirmed and recorded in the patient's notes.

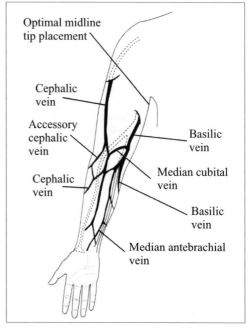

Optimal midline tip placement

Cephalic vein

Accessory cephalic vein

Cephalic vein

Basilic vein

Median cubital vein

Basilic vein

Median antebrachial vein

Figure 25.1: Venous anatomy of the arm

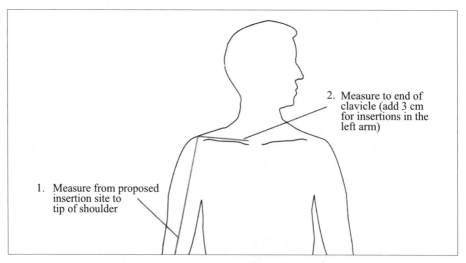

2. Measure to end of clavicle (add 3 cm for insertions in the left arm)

1. Measure from proposed insertion site to tip of shoulder

Figure 25.2: Measurement to ensure superior vena cava placement

Until recently, patients who had no accessible antecubital fossa vein were considered unsuitable candidates for a PICC. However, Andrews (1995) achieved a 99% success rate in such patients by using fluoroscopy and/or ultrasound to identify the venous anatomy of the arm and facilitate the placement of the PICC.

Today, the use of doppler ultrasound, at the patient's bedside, has assisted nurses to place PICCs in patients who were previously considered to be unsuitable, due to difficulty in identifying a suitable vein (Gabriel, 1999).

Placing the PICC

Local anaesthetic

In the USA, it is common practice to use an intradermal injection of lignocaine 1% as a local anaesthetic immediately before placing the PICC. Although this minimises the discomfort of the procedure for the patient, there is transitory discomfort from the injection. Lignocaine can also cause localised oedema, which can result in visual occlusion of the selected vein and problems for the healthcare professional inserting the PICC. To avoid subjecting the patient to the additional trauma of an intradermal injection and the possibility of oedema, a topical application of anaesthetic cream can be used. Wig and Johl (1990) proved that 'Emla' cream was highly effective in achieving painless venous cannulation in children, and 'Emla' 2ml should be applied to the skin overlying the selected vein one hour before the venepuncture is to be performed. (Other companies manufacture local anaesthetic cream and supply information relating to application times prior to undertaking venepuncture.)

Skin preparation

Goodwin and Carlson (1993) looked retrospectively at 858 PICC insertions over a period of three years and concluded that line infection is a rare occurrence. Insertion site infections are also uncommon. Goodwin and Carlson (1993) believe that such low infection rates are linked to the reduced number of bacteria on the arm compared with the chest. They also pointed out that skin temperature is lower on the arm than the chest, creating a colder climate for survival and multiplication of bacteria. Maki *et al* (1991) reported that the number of colony-forming units of bacteria on a peripheral site, eg. the arm, was approximately 10 per site, compared with 10,000 per site on the chest.

In 1991, Maki *et al* published the results of a clinical trial looking at the effectiveness of skin cleansing agents for preparing the skin before central line placement. They concluded that chlorhexidine in alcohol was the most effective. As placement of a PICC is a relatively straightforward procedure, there may be a tendency for healthcare professionals to take shortcuts. These could potentially put the patient at risk of infection. PICCs are central lines and healthcare professionals should adhere to a strict aseptic technique while placing and accessing them, to minimise the risk of infection. Adequate skin cleansing must be carried out and sterile gloves and gown should be worn during insertion of the PICC. Healthcare professionals should also wear sterile gloves when accessing the device.

Dressings

Maki (1993) carried out research to determine the most suitable dressings and dressing change intervals for PICCs. He concluded that a clear occlusive dressing was more effective in minimising the risk of infection than gauze dressings.

There can be some exudate from the venepuncture site and so it is advisable to place a small piece of sterile gauze over the area of insertion to act as a wick for the first day. This should be covered with a transparent occlusive dressing and left for 24 hours. The following day the dressing should be removed and the whole area cleaned with 0.5% chlorhexidine in alcohol. Steristrips can be applied to help stabilise the PICC, and the transparent occlusive dressing should be reapplied over the top of these. Unless there is any further exudate the dressing can be left undisturbed for seven days.

If continual access to the PICC is not required, eg. if the patient is receiving weekly cytotoxic chemotherapy, the whole of the PICC including the injection hub can be incorporated under the dressing to create a waterproof barrier for showering. The lower end of the dressing then only needs to be disturbed if access to the PICC is required for flushing or blood sampling.

Maintaining catheter patency

In 1993, Masoorli presented preliminary findings on maintaining the patency of PICCs. She suggested that if the PICC was not in continual use, it should be flushed daily with 5–10 ml of saline containing heparin, for example 10 iu/ml. In a Groshong- type PICC a weekly flush of 5–10 ml of normal saline is sufficient to maintain patency. If the PICC has two lumens, each lumen should be managed as if it were a separate catheter.

Goodwin and Carlson (1993) drew attention to the importance of the flushing technique in preventing occlusion. They recommend a rapid push/pause or pulsated flush method. This creates turbulence within the lumen of the catheter, decreasing the risk of occlusion. Goodwin and Carlson (1993) also advocate how a 'positive-pressure' flush can decrease the incidence of catheter occlusion. A 'positive-pressure' flush technique is where the catheter continues to be flushed as the syringe is removed from the vascular access device. This technique minimises the risk of blood refluxing into the lumen(s) of the catheter.

If the PICC does become occluded, then urokinase 5000 iu/ml can be instilled into the line. If difficulties are encountered when attempting to inject the urokinase, a three-way tap can be attached to the end of the catheter. Two syringes, one empty and one containing urokinase, can then be attached to the three-way tap, as shown in

Figure 25.3. A gentle rocking action between the two syringes has been found to be highly effective for injecting urokinase into the PICC. The urokinase should be left in the catheter for 10–60 minutes before being aspirated back into the syringe (Stewart, 1993).

Syringes smaller than 10 mls should not routinely be used on PICCs without consulting the device's manufacturers. This is because there is a potential for smaller size syringes to create too high a pressure when flushing the PICC which can potentially lead to rupture of the catheter (Conn, 1993).

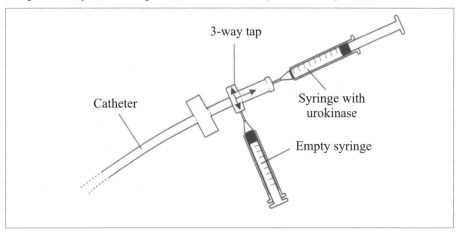

Figure 25.3: How to instil urokinase into an occluded peripherally inserted central catheter

Phlebitis

Richardson and Bruso (1993) identified three types of phlebitis (*Table 25.1*) which can occur in patients with PICC: mechanical; chemical and infective.

Mechanical

If phlebitis occurs within seven days of PICC insertion, it is likely to be due to irritation of the wall of the vein by the catheter. Richardson and Bruso (1993) advocated the application of heat in suspected cases of mechanical phlebitis. Warming the upper arm for 20 minutes three times a day usually causes this type of phlebitis to resolve within 48 hours. This is because the heat encourages the veins to dilate to accommodate the PICC. If this treatment does not work, Richardson and Bruno (1993) recommended seeking other causes for the phlebitis.

Goodwin and Carlson (1993) looked at the incidence of mechanical phlebitis in men and women and concluded that women were almost twice as likely to be affected. They reasoned that women had smaller veins, resulting in decreased blood flow around the catheter. Suturing the PICC to the patient's forearm, or using an anchoring device, and applying Steristrips can help to reduce movement of the catheter and thereby minimise the incidence of mechanical phlebitis.

Table 25.1: Management of phlebitis in patients with peripherally inserted central catheters		
Type	**Cause**	**Solution**
Mechanical phlebitis (usually occurs within seven days of PICC insertion)	Catheter too large for patient's vein. Catheter irritating the wall of the vein	Apply heat to the patient's upper arm for 20 minutes, three times per day for 48 hours
Chemical phlebitis (rare in a patient with a PICC)	Tip of PICC does not extend as far as subclavian or superior vena cava	Check where tip of PICC is terminating
Infective phlebitis (usually occurs several days after PICC inserted)	Poor aseptic technique when placing PICC Poor aseptic technique when accessing PICC Poor aseptic technique when renewing dressing	If entry site appears infected a swab should be taken for culture and sensitivity. It may be possible to treat the infection without removing the PICC. If the PICC is suspected as a source of infection, blood should be withdrawn and sent for culture and sensitivity testing (see text)
PICC = peripherally inserted central catheters		

Chemical

With a true PICC the catheter tip terminates in the superior vena cava. Consequently, Goodwin and Carlson (1993) and Richardson and Bruso (1993) argue that it is rare to see chemical phlebitis in a patient with a PICC as the drugs or fluids infused are quickly diluted by the volume of blood flowing through the superior vena cava.

Infective

Richardson and Bruso (1993) suggest that if phlebitis presents more than seven days after the PICC has been inserted, or is not resolved by the application of heat, infection should be suspected (*Table 25.1*).

Infection

Apart from inadequate skin preparation and poor aseptic technique when placing the PICC, Linares and Sitges-Serra (1985) demonstrated that the commonest cause of infected central catheters is colonisation of the injection hub by micro-organisms. This can be prevented by adequate cleaning of the hub with 0.5% chlorhexidine in alcohol before accessing it.

The development of unexplained pyrexia in a patient with a PICC in situ alone is not an indication for removing the catheter (Goodwin and Carlson, 1993). To confirm or eliminate the PICC as the cause of the infection, blood cultures should be taken from both the catheter and a peripheral vein and the microbiology results should be compared. The decision to remove an infected PICC depends on what the infection is and how ill the patient is. If the catheter is removed on the grounds that it is the suspected focus of infection, the tip should be sent for microbiological culture.

Removal

The PICC is easily removed by discarding the dressing and gently pulling on the catheter. This may be facilitated by warming the patient's arm to increase the blood flow and therefore the diameter of the vein.

Conclusion

PICCs not only offer a safer, simpler and less expensive way to achieve central venous access for many patients in the UK today, but also have the potential to decrease the trauma associated with continual site rotation in patients requiring parenteral therapy for more than five days. Nurses can now become more actively involved in improving the quality of venous access for many patients. Intermediate to long-term venous access can be achieved without the constant trauma of resiting peripheral cannulae or placing a tunnelled catheter or injection port. The arrival of PICCs is long overdue in the UK and, with careful management, PICCs will make the delivery of parenteral therapy not only more reliable but also more comfortable for many patients.

Key points

* In 1991, it was estimated that 85% of patients admitted to hospitals in the USA were recipients of a vascular access device.
* PICC lines are so fine and flexible they can easily be inserted with the minimum of trauma to the patient.
* PICCs can easily be inserted on the ward or clinic by suitably skilled nurses.
* The associated insertion problems with PICCs are markedly reduced compared with other central venous catheters.
* PICCs are a reliable, safer and less expensive alternative to pre-existing central catheters.

References

Andrews J (1995) Chronic Venous Access: The Role of Interventional Radiology. Paper presented at the 9th National Association of Vascular Access Networks (NAVAN) Conference, September, 1995, Salt Lake City, Utah

Barbone M (1995) VAD Patency. Paper presented at the 9th NAVAN Conference, September, 1995. Salt Lake City, Utah

Brown J (1989) Peripherally inserted central catheters — use in home care. *J Intravenous Nurs* **12**(2): 144–7

Conn C (1993) The importance of syringe size when using Implanted Vascular Access Devices. *J Vasc Access Network* **3**(1): 11–8

Gabriel J (1996) Peripherally inserted central catheters: expanding UK nurses' practice. *Surg Nurse* **5**(2): 71–4

Gabriel J (1999) PICCs: how doppler ultrasound can extend their use. *Nurs Times* **95**(6): 52–55

Goodwin M, Carlson I (1993) The peripherally inserted catheter: a retrospective look at 3 years of insertions. *J Intravenous Nurs* **16**(2): 92–103

Hadaway L (1989) An overview of vascular access devices inserted via the antecubital area. *J Intravenous Nurs* **13**(5): 297–305

Kyle K, Myers L (1989) Peripherally inserted central catheters — development of a hospital based program. *J Intravenous Nurs* **13**(5): 287–90

Linares J, Sitges-Serra A, Garan S (1985) Pathogenesis of catheter sepsis: a prospective study with quantitative and semi-quantitive cultures of catheter hub and segments. *J Clin Microbiol* **21**: 357–60

Maki DG (1993) Complications Associated with Intravenous Therapy. Paper presented at the 7th NAVAN Conference, September, 1993. Washington DC

Maki DG, Ringer M, Alvarado CJ (1991) Prospective randomised trial of providone iodine, alcohol and chlorhexidine for prevention of infection with central venous and arterial catheters. *Lancet* **383**: 339–43

Masoorli S (1993) Cost Containment Program for IV Nursing. Paper presented at the 7th NAVAN Conference, September 1993, Washington DC

Prain G, Van Way C (1978) The long arm Silastic catheter: a critical look at complications. *JPEN* **2**(2): 124–8

Richardson D, Bruso P (1993) Vascular access devices — management of common complications. *J Intravenous Nurs* **16**(1): 44–9

Sansivero G (1997) *Update on advanced PICC placement.* Paper presented at Board PICC meeting, Metropole Hotel, December, London

Stewart N (1993) CVC Complications. Paper presented at the 7th NAVAN Conference, September 1993, Washington DC

Wig J, Johl K (1990) Our experiences with Emla cream (for painless venous cannulation in children). *Ind J Pharmacol* **34**(2): 130–2